The Well-Woman Visit

The Well-Woman Visit

Edited by

David Chelmow, MD, FACOG
Department of Obstetrics and Gynecology, Virginia Commonwealth University School of Medicine, Richmond, VA, USA

Anita K. Blanchard, MD, FACOG
Department of Obstetrics and Gynecology, University of Chicago, Chicago, IL, USA

Lee A. Learman, MD, PhD, FACOG
Charles E. Schmidt College of Medicine, Florida Atlantic University, Boca Raton, FL, USA

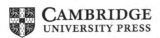
CAMBRIDGE
UNIVERSITY PRESS

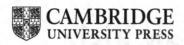

CAMBRIDGE
UNIVERSITY PRESS

Shaftesbury Road, Cambridge CB2 8EA, United Kingdom

One Liberty Plaza, 20th Floor, New York, NY 10006, USA

477 Williamstown Road, Port Melbourne, VIC 3207, Australia

314–321, 3rd Floor, Plot 3, Splendor Forum, Jasola District Centre, New Delhi – 110025, India

103 Penang Road, #05–06/07, Visioncrest Commercial, Singapore 238467

Cambridge University Press is part of Cambridge University Press & Assessment,
a department of the University of Cambridge.

We share the University's mission to contribute to society through the pursuit of
education, learning and research at the highest international levels of excellence.

www.cambridge.org
Information on this title: www.cambridge.org/9781316509982

DOI: 10.1017/9781316537459

© Cambridge University Press & Assessment 2017

First published 2017

A catalogue record for this publication is available from the British Library

Library of Congress Cataloging-in-Publication data
Names: Chelmow, David, editor. | Blanchard, Anita K., editor. | Learman, Lee A., editor.
Title: The well woman visit / edited by David Chelmow, Anita K. Blanchard, Lee A. Learman.
Description: Cambridge, United Kingdom ; New York, NY : Cambridge University Press, 2017. |
Includes bibliographical references and index.
Identifiers: LCCN 2016056414 | ISBN 9781316509982 (paperback)
Subjects: | MESH: Women's Health | Physical Examination | Gynecology – trends | Primary
Prevention – methods
Classification: LCC RC71.3 | NLM WP 141 | DDC 618.1/075–dc23
LC record available at https://lccn.loc.gov/2016056414

ISBN   978-1-316-50998-2   Paperback

....

Contents

Contributors

Melanie D. Altizer, MD
Department of Obstetrics and Gynecology, Virginia Tech Carilion School of Medicine, Roanoke, VA, USA

Janeen Arbuckle, MD, PhD
Department of Obstetrics and Gynecology, Harvard Medical School and Beth Israel Deaconess Medical Center, Boston, MA, USA

Kavita Shah Arora, MD, MBE
MetroHealth Medical Center, Case Western Reserve University, Cleveland, OH, USA

Kevin A. Ault, MD, FACOG
Department of Obstetrics and Gynecology, University of Kansas Medical Center, Kansas City, KS, USA

Amy (Meg) Autry, MD
Department of Obstetrics, Gynecology and Reproductive Sciences, University of California, San Francisco, CA, USA

Anitra Beasley, MD, MPH
Department of Obstetrics and Gynecology, Baylor College of Medicine, Houston, TX, USA

Anita K. Blanchard, MD, FACOG
Department of Obstetrics and Gynecology, University of Chicago, Chicago, IL, USA

Margaret Boozer, MD, MPH
Department of Obstetrics and Gynecology, University of Alabama at Birmingham School of Medicine, Birmingham, AL, USA

Haywood L. Brown, MD
Department of Obstetrics and Gynecology, Duke University, Durham, NC, USA

David Chelmow, MD, FACOG
Department of Obstetrics and Gynecology, Virginia Commonwealth School of Medicine, Richmond, VA, USA

Rebecca Cohen, MD, MPH
Department of Obstetrics and Gynecology, University of Colorado School of Medicine, Aurora, CO, USA

Jeanne Conry, MD, PhD
Kaiser Permanente;
Department of Obstetrics and Gynecology, University of California, Davis, CA, USA;
American College of Obstetricians and Gynecologists

Dean V. Coonrod, MD, MPH
Department of Obstetrics and Gynecology, Maricopa Integrated Health System, District Medical Group, and University of Arizona College of Medicine, Phoenix, AZ, USA

Beth Cronin, MD
Department of Obstetrics and Gynecology, Alpert Medical School of Brown University and Women & Infants Hospital, Providence, RI, USA

Julie Zemaitis DeCesare, MD
Department of Obstetrics and Gynecology, University of Florida College of Medicine Pensacola, FL, USA

Margaret L. Dow, MD
Division of Obstetrics, Mayo Clinic;
Mayo Clinic College of Medicine, Rochester, MN, USA

Marygrace Elson, MD, MME
Department of Obstetrics and Gynecology, University of Iowa Hospitals and Clinics, Iowa City, IA, USA

Maureen E. Farrell, MD
Obstetrics and Gynecology Department, Uniformed Services University of the Health Sciences, Naval Medical Center San Diego, CA, USA

Kimberly S. Gecsi, MD
Department of Reproductive Biology, Case Western Reserve University School of Medicine;

Department of Obstetrics and Gynecology, University Hospitals, MacDonald Women's Hospital, Cleveland, OH, USA

Aaron Goldberg, MD
Department of Obstetrics and Gynecology, Virginia Commonwealth University School of Medicine, Richmond, VA, USA

Vanessa H. Gregg, MD
Department of Obstetrics and Gynecology, University of Virginia School of Medicine, Charlottesville, VA, USA

David M. Haas
Department of Obstetrics and Gynecology, Indiana University School of Medicine, Indianapolis, IN, USA

Christine R. Isaacs, MD
Department of Obstetrics and Gynecology, Virginia Commonwealth University School of Medicine, Richmond, VA, USA

Michelle M. Isley, MD, MPH
Department of Obstetrics and Gynecology, The Ohio State University, Columbus, OH, USA

Moune Jabre Raughley, MD
Department of Obstetrics and Gynecology, Weill-Cornell Medicine – Qatar, Sidra Medical and Research Center, Doha, Qatar

Andrea B. Joyner, MD, FACOG, IBCLC
Department of Gynecology and Obstetrics, Emory University School of Medicine, Atlanta, GA, USA

Eduardo Lara-Torre, MD
Department of Obstetrics and Gynecology and Pediatrics, Carilion Clinic and Virginia Tech Carilion School of Medicine, Roanoke, VA, USA

Shari M. Lawson, MD, MBA, FACOG
Department of Gynecology and Obstetrics, Johns Hopkins University School of Medicine, Baltimore, MD, USA

Lee A. Learman, MD, PhD, FACOG
Department of Integrated Medical Science, Charles E. Schmidt College of Medicine, Florida Atlantic University, Boca Raton, FL, USA

Efua Leke
Department of Obstetrics and Gynecology, Baylor College of Medicine, Houston, TX, USA

Monica Mendiola, MD
Department of Obstetrics and Gynecology, Harvard Medical School and Beth Israel Deaconess Medical Center, Boston, MA, USA

Sarah Milton, MD
Department of Obstetrics and Gynecology, Virginia Commonwealth University School of Medicine, Richmond, VA, USA

Michelle H. Moniz, MD, MSc
Department of Obstetrics and Gynecology, University of Michigan, Ann Arbor, MI, USA

Tiffany A. Moore Simas, MD, MPH, MEd
Department of Obstetrics and Gynecology, University of Massachusetts Medical School, Worcester, MA, USA

Christopher M. Morosky, MD, MS, FACOG
Department of Obstetrics and Gynecology, University of Connecticut School of Medicine, Farmington, CT, USA

Erica Nelson, MD
Department of Obstetrics and Gynecology, Southern Illinois University School of Medicine, Springfield, IL, USA

Lauren E. Nelson, MD
Department of Obstetrics and Gynecology, School of Medicine and Health Sciences, The George Washington University, Washington, DC, USA

Nguyet Anh Nguyen, MD
Division of Women's Reproductive Healthcare, Department of Obstetrics & Gynecology, University of Alabama at Birmingham, Birmingham, AL, USA

Tony Ogburn, MD
Department of Obstetrics and Gynecology, University of Texas Rio Grande Valley, Harlingen, TX, USA

Sharon T. Phelan, MD
Department of Obstetrics and Gynecology, University of New Mexico School of Medicine, Albuquerque, NM, USA

Maureen G. Phipps, MD, MPH
Department of Obstetrics & Gynecology, and Professor of Epidemiology, Brown University;
Women & Infants Hospital of Rhode Island and Care New England Health System, Providence, RI, USA

Michael S. Policar, MD, MPH
University of California, San Francisco, School of Medicine, San Francisco, CA, USA

Hope Ricciotti, MD
Department of Obstetrics and Gynecology, Harvard Medical School and Beth Israel Deaconess Medical Center, Boston, MA, USA

Bryan K. Rone, MD
Department of Obstetrics and Gynecology, University of Kentucky, Lexington, KY, USA

Jonathan Schaffir, MD
Department of Obstetrics and Gynecology, The Ohio State University, Columbus, OH, USA

Sangini S. Sheth, MD, MPH
Department of Obstetrics, Gynecology and Reproductive Sciences, Yale School of Medicine, New Haven, CT, USA

Jody Stonehocker, MD
Department of Obstetrics and Gynecology, University of New Mexico, Albuquerque, NM, USA

Regan N. Theiler, MD, PhD
Department of Obstetrics and Gynecology, Dartmouth-Hitchcock Medical Center, Lebanon, NH, USA

Meghan L. Valentine, MD
Department of Obstetrics and Gynecology, School of Medicine and Health Sciences, The George Washington University, Washington, DC, USA

C. Nathan Webb, MD, MS, FACOG
Department of Obstetrics and Gynecology, Virginia Commonwealth University School of Medicine, Richmond, VA, USA

Sara Whetstone, MD
Department of Obstetrics, Gynecology and Reproductive Sciences, University of California, San Francisco, CA, USA

Brett Worly, MD
Department of Obstetrics and Gynecology, The Ohio State University Wexner College of Medicine, Columbus, OH, USA

Christopher M. Zahn, MD
American College of Obstetricians and Gynecologists, Washington, DC, USA

Introduction

Anita K. Blanchard, David Chelmow, and Lee A. Learman

Over the last decade, there have been profound changes in women's health care. Emphasis has shifted from problem-based to well-woman care. Avoiding disease through habits that maintain health has become as important as curing illness. Comprehensive prevention and risk reduction have become central to the annual visit, which used to be much more narrowly focused. For decades, women's preventive care largely centered around an "annual Pap smear" visit, where the focus was to obtain cervical cytology and perform pelvic and breast examinations. Other components of the visit were less formalized and likely varied significantly from provider to provider. The emphasis on the prior core components has drastically changed. Revised cervical screening guidelines [1,2] now allow screening intervals up to 5 years. The American College of Physicians has recommended that screening pelvic examinations not be performed [3], and both the US Preventive Services Task Force (USPSTF) [4] and American Cancer Society (ACS) [5] no longer include recommendations for screening clinical breast examinations.

Although these new recommendations are evidence informed, there is wide variability in their adoption, in part based on specialty and provider type. The composition of the visit including screening tests should rely on the shared decision-making of the health care provider and the informed patient. The Choosing Wisely initiative (www.choosingwisely.org/) advocates for conversations between practitioners and patients to choose care that is evidence based, free from harm, and truly necessary. This campaign was initiated by the American Board of Internal Medicine Foundation in partnership with other major medical societies to promote positive change. The campaign advocates reconsidering many established routine testing and screening practices based on evidence-informed decision-making. Choices are now influenced by principles of preventive care and population risk, and individualized based on personal and family history as well as signs and symptoms.

Despite these challenges, the overall value of a well-woman preventive visit is still widely accepted. This was most clearly recognized in the Affordable Care Act (ACA), which included provision for an annual well-woman examination. Although the ACA established affordability and availability of preventive care, it did not fully define the components of the well-woman visit. Evidence-based recommendations for prevention are available from many sources, covering many health areas, but there was no consensus as to which of them should be part of the Well-Woman Visit.

In 2014, the American College of Obstetrics and Gynecology (ACOG) took an important step to address this issue and convened the Well-Woman Task Force (WWTF) [6]. The Task Force was the Presidential Initiative for ACOG President Jeanne Conry, who recognized this critical need. The vision of ACOG and the Task Force organizers was much broader than just their own specialty. They recognized the need for consistency across specialties and provider types, with the focus of the well-woman visit being the woman and not the specialty or type of provider. The Task Force was convened with representatives spanning all of the major groups that provide preventive health care for women. ACOG was careful not to limit the Task Force to physicians, but ensured that advanced practice providers of all types were also included. They comprehensively identified major US guidelines. Their final report was a series of age-based recommendations, enumerating major areas for screening, counseling, and testing. Within these areas, they developed consensus recommendations for which guidelines to apply.

The Task Force report was groundbreaking. For the first time, there were comprehensive recommendations for well-woman care organized by age. Developing these recommendations also demonstrated a number of problems. Given the vast number of components of care involved and the many available recommendations for each one, guidelines were changing even while the Task Force was conducting its review. It is very clear that recommendations for well-woman care will not be static, but will continue to evolve. Good examples of this include the recent changes in breast cancer screening by the ACS [5] and USPSTF [4] and clarifications to the American Diabetes Association recommendations for postpartum screening of women with gestational diabetes [7]. In *Re-envisioning the Annual Well-Woman Visit, The Task Forward*, George Sawaya identified the additional challenge of implementation of shared, informed decision-based care [8]. *The Well-Woman Visit* was written with the specific intent of assisting with implementing exactly this type of care into the Well-Woman Visit.

The Task Force report not only presented a perfect opportunity for writing a book to assist providers in performing an evidence-based, high-value, patient-centered well-woman visit but also highlighted the challenges. In writing this book, we sought to take the Task Force recommendations and present them in book form for providers of all types. A book would allow a much more detailed presentation of the Task Force recommendations than the brief text and tables of their report. In particular, we wanted to create something very "hands on" that would help providers apply the Task Force recommendations in their practice. We were very cognizant of the volume of recommendations and that these recommendations will continuously change. We ran the risk that many would become out of date even as we edited the book. We chose to move ahead anyway. Within the Task Force recommendations are many individual guidelines and recommendations that are solid and will evolve slowly. We chose to approach the rapid evolution problem by using the book to give readers the tools to recognize excellent guidelines as they are released and facilitate integration of new recommendations and guidelines into their well-woman visit practice. To meet these two goals of outlining the current recommendations and giving providers the tools to appropriately update their practice, we organized the book in two sections.

The book begins with eight general principle chapters. These are designed to present the background for the book and the tools to understand and apply current guidelines and recognize and adopt new high-quality evidence-based guidelines. The section begins with the motivation for organizing women's preventive care as a periodic well-woman visit. Jeanne Conry and Haywood Brown, the initiator and chair of the Task Force, explain the genesis of the Task Force and how it operated. Maureen Phipps, a noted expert on preventive care and member of the USPSTF, reviews the data and theoretic framework supporting periodic health visits. The next several chapters provide tools for applying the guidelines. Lee Learman explains the principles of early diagnosis and prevention. David Haas, an expert on evidence-based medicine, describes guideline development and criteria for choosing quality guidelines. As executing many of the recommendations involves counseling and promoting behavioral change to improve health, Tony Ogburn and Michelle Moniz present useful evidence-based strategies for these important skills. One of the most significant challenges is determining how to pack all of the many potential areas of the well-woman visit into a self-contained office encounter. Chris Zahn discusses strategies for this in his chapter on practical aspects of the well-woman visit. Meg Autry and Sara Whetstone discuss considerations for special populations. Mike Policar explains how well-women care is supported by the ACA and other governmental programs, emphasizing the impact of evidence-based preventive services being available without cost sharing.

The core of the book is the actual recommendations, which are covered in Section 2. Separate chapters have been written for each component of the well-woman visit included in the Task Force report. We are deeply grateful to the authors of these chapters. We were unable to individually credit them in the introduction as we did for the background authors because of the sheer volume. This is not meant to undervalue their contributions. Many were noted experts in their chapter content. Others went out of their comfort zone to develop expertise in areas far outside of their field to write clear, complete, compact syntheses of complex areas useful to providers of many disciplines. These chapters were designed to be easy, quick references and help the provider find and apply the pertinent guidelines. They were not intended to replace the WWTF Guidelines tables, which are easily assessable online, but rather to supplement them. The chapters explain the scope of each of the problems and the rationale for screening or preventing. They have a brief summary of the guidelines reviewed by the Task Force. The heart of each chapter is a section on how to apply the guidelines. The book was meant to be very practical so people could use it as a reference in their office. In instances where the guidelines changed significantly since the Task Force convened and issued its report, authors were instructed to use their best judgement in incorporating new recommendations. This was pointed out where it occurred. To decrease the chance of the component chapters becoming rapidly obsolete, each chapter also includes a section where the author made their best predictions for factors likely to motivate upcoming changes to recommendations. While much of this needed to be handled in traditional text format, we recognized the advantages of case presentations for adult learners and have supplemented most chapters with illustrative cases.

Ideally, the Task Force recommendations should be an ongoing process instead of a one-time event. The book was written to ensure that the valuable work done by the Task Force could be disseminated and applied. We were very excited to learn that the Health Resources and Services Administration (HRSA) has funded the Women's Preventive Services Initiative, awarded to ACOG, to continue important aspects of the work of the Task Force. We look forward to the recommendations for the well-woman visit becoming a living set of centrally managed recommendations that evolve over time. Until this happens, we offer our book as a way to organize recommendations for the well-woman visit and help providers stay current with the component guidelines.

The book was written as a project of the Society of Academic Specialists in General Obstetrics and Gynecology (SASGOG). SASGOG is a new organization that was created to promote academic specialists in obstetrics and gynecology and to build careers of faculty in this specialty. Academic specialists are the largest single group of faculty of academic OB/GYN departments, but prior to SASGOG had no professional organization. Two parts of SASGOG's mission are to support career development of academic specialists and to promote health and prevent and treat disease in women and enhance the delivery of clinical care. Well-woman care has traditionally been an important role for the academic specialist. The well-woman visit book posed a superb opportunity for SASGOG to simultaneously contribute to both of these parts of our mission. Despite coming from the specialty of obstetrics and gynecology, all authors were very clear that we share our responsibility for promoting women's health care with allied health care providers and physicians in other specialties. Our book was designed to be equally useful to all providers and ensure that patients got the best, effective care, regardless of what type or specialty of provider they saw. We are deeply grateful to SASGOG and the members of the organization who met the challenge and created incredibly high-quality work. We hope that this will be the first of many useful resources written by SASGOG for providers of women's health care.

We also want to acknowledge ACOG. Their work in establishing the Task Force was visionary. They have been tremendous supporters of SASGOG, helped the organization get off the ground, and have continued to help and support us in the 4 years of our existence. We are deeply appreciative of their partnering with us on the book.

As editors, we are also deeply grateful to our families. Thanks to Fay Chelmow, Beverly Learman, and Marty Nesbitt, who tolerated each of us disappearing to our lonely editor's garrets for several months to complete the book on time.

References

1. Moyer, V.A. Screening for cervical cancer: US Preventive Services Task Force recommendation statement. US Preventive Services Task Force. *Ann Intern Med.* 2012, **156**:880–91. Available at: www .uspreventiveservicestaskforce.org/uspstf/uspscerv.htm. Retrieved May 22, 2014.

2. Saslow, D., Solomon, D., Lawson, H.W. et al. American Cancer Society, American Society for Colposcopy and Cervical Pathology, and American Society for Clinical Pathology screening guidelines for the prevention and early detection of cervical cancer. *CA Cancer J Clin.* 2012, **62**:147–72. Available at: www.asccp.org/Guidelines/Screening-Guidelines. Retrieved September 26, 2015.

3. Qaseem, A., Humphrey, L.L., Harris, R., Starkey, M., Denberg, T.D.; Clinical Guidelines Committee of the American College of Physicians. Screening pelvic examination in adult women: A clinical practice guideline from the American College of Physicians. *Ann Intern Med.* 2014, **161**:67–72.

4. Siu, A.L; US Preventive Services Task Force. Screening for breast cancer: US Preventive Services Task Force recommendation statement. *Ann Intern Med.* 2016;**164**(4):279–96.

5. Oeffinger, K.C., Fontham, E.T., Etzioni, R., et al.; American Cancer Society. Breast cancer screening for women at average risk: 2015 guideline update from the American Cancer Society. *JAMA*. 2015, **314**:1599–1614.

6. Conry, J.A. and Brown, H. Executive summary, Well-Woman Task Force, components of the Well-Woman Visit. *Obstet Gynecol*. 2015, **126**:697–701.

7. American Diabetes Association. Management of diabetes in pregnancy. *Diabetes Care*. 2016, **39**(Suppl 1):S94–8. Available at: http://care.diabetesjournals.org/content/39/Supplement_1/S94. Retrieved December 30, 2016.

8. Sawaya, G. Re-envisioning the annual Well-Woman Visit: The task forward. *Obstet Gynecol*. 2015, **126**(4): 695–6.

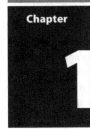

Chapter

1

The Well-Woman Task Force

Haywood L. Brown and Jeanne Conry

Learning Objectives

- Describe the motivation and rationale to convene the Well-Woman Task Force
- Define the components of well-woman's health and the background of the age-specific concerns to wellness and preventability over the life span
- Describe the collaborative organizational participation in the Well-Woman Task Force and process for the final recommendations
- Present several case scenarios relevant to the well-woman visit and the deliberations that led to the final recommendations of the Task Force

Background

The World Health Organization (WHO) defines health as "a state of complete physical, mental and social well-being and not merely the absence of disease or infirmity" [1]. To achieve this definition of health, well-woman care is critically important throughout the life span. The well-woman visit promotes health over the course of a woman's lifetime through problem detection and preventive health care. Well-woman care should consist of a history, physical examination, counseling, and screening intended to maintain well-being. The elements of well-woman's care and the intervals at which they should be performed should be individualized according to a woman's needs, characteristics, risk factors, and age. Taken together, these elements constitute the "well-woman's visit," which can be conducted as a single encounter with a provider or divided over a number of encounters.

The Well-Woman Task Force (WWTF) evolved from guidelines of the US Department of Health and Human Services (DHHS) and the Women's Preventive Services section of the Institute of Medicine (IOM) Report issued in July 2011, which recommended an annual well-woman visit. While there were clearly recommendations for having the visit, there was no good guidance for what should be done at it. The American College of Obstetrics and Gynecology (ACOG) wanted to provide a unified approach to well-woman health care, across medical specialties and providers, similar to the American Academy of Pediatrics "Bright Futures" [2]. To accomplish this, in 2013 ACOG leadership convened a broad range of organizational participants and stakeholders of the leading professional associations representing women's health care clinicians [3].

The Task Force conducted its work not only in the context of the clinical gap in defining the content of the well-woman visit but also in the context of other important societal gaps, particularly an affordability gap. Women are more likely to have lower incomes, use more health services, have higher out-of-pocket costs, and avoid needed preventive health services, and are less likely to have employer-based health coverage. Without coverage for preventive services such as age-specific cancer screening for breast and colon cancer, women are less likely to follow through on the key screening regardless of the evidence-based recommendations. Unfortunately, Americans use preventive services at half the recommended rate because of cost [4]. The work of the Task Force in defining the components of the well-woman visit is particularly important as it can set standards for what should be covered, decreasing this gap and enabling women to optimize their chance of meeting the WHO goals.

Factors Impacting Well Women's Health

There are many factors impacting women's health with significant implications for the Task Force and its recommendations. Women are living longer than in previous generations. In 2013, the life expectancy for white women was 81.2 years, black women 78.1 years, and Hispanic women 83.8 years [5]. The population size of baby boomer women aged 45–54 peaked at 22.2 million in 2010, a 34 percent increase from 1997. By 2030, it is predicted that 37.7 million women will be aged 65 and older and 30 percent of women aged 50 will live past age 80 [6]. The key areas of adult well women's health include brain, bone, breast, diet, heart, hormonal, lung, sexual, and mental.

In 2008, 107 million Americans – almost 1 out of every 2 adults aged 18 or older – had at least 1 of 6 reported chronic illnesses [6]. There are 200,000 new diagnoses of breast cancer annually. Around 7 million women are affected with depression per year. One of seven women aged 45–64 has some form of heart disease. There are 8 million women with osteoporosis. Women have twice the occurrence of multiple sclerosis and make up 90 percent of cases of rheumatoid arthritis and lupus. In all, 75 percent of the 4 million cases of Alzheimer's disease are women [7].

Women aged 55 and older are at a higher risk for coronary artery disease, and heart disease and stroke are the leading causes of death for women. Cancer is the second leading cause of death among white, black, and Native American women. Deaths from all cancers other than lung cancer have declined over the past decade. The three most common cancers among women in the United States are:

- Breast at 122.2/100,000 women, which is the most common among women of all races
- Lung at 52.1/100,000 women, which is second most common among whites, blacks, Asian/ Pacific Islanders, and American Indian/Native Americans and third among Hispanics
- Colorectal at 34.1/100,000 which is second most common among Hispanics and third among whites, blacks, Asian/Pacific Islanders, and American Indian/Alaska Natives [6].

The leading causes of cancer death among women are:

- Lung at 36.4/100,000 women, which is the most common among whites, blacks, Asian/pacific Islanders, and American Indian/Alaska Natives and second among Hispanics
- Breast at 21.3/100,000 women, which is the most common among Hispanics and second among whites, blacks, Asian/Pacific Islanders and American Indian/Alaska Natives
- Colorectal at 12.4/100,000 women, which is third most common among women of all races [8].

Leading causes of death in woman vary by age group. For example, unintentional injury is a leading cause

for women aged 18–44 and the third leading cause of death for women aged 45–64, while intentional injuries from suicide and homicide were the fourth and fifth leading causes of death for women aged 19–44 in 2010 [9]. Four causes of death increased among women between 2000 and 2010: chronic respiratory diseases, Alzheimer's disease, unintentional injury, and kidney disease. Liver disease is also now included within the top ten causes of death for women below age 65 [9].

Women are more likely than men to suffer with conditions that have activity limitations impacting quality of life and long-term health. Activity limitation occurs when an individual requires assistance from another person to perform physical tasks or requires the use of special equipment to perform routine tasks [10]. These physical activities may include walking up to ten steps, standing for two hours, carrying a 10-pound object, or engaging in social activities and recreations such as going shopping, visiting friends, or sewing. In 2007–2009, 32.8 percent of adults reported being limited in their ability to perform one or more common activities. Women are more likely than men to report having activity limitations: 37.2 compared to 28.1 percent, respectively [10]. According to a 2006 report from the National Center for Health Statistics in women aged 18 and older, in addition to back and neck problems, conditions associated with activity limitation include the following:

- Arthritis/rheumatism, which impacts activity in 27.3%, 31.2%, and 27.7% of white, black, and Hispanic women, respectively
- Chronic hypertension, which impacts activity in 9.6%, 20.1%, and 13.7% of white, black, and Hispanic women, respectively
- Diabetes, which impacts activity in 9.0%, 16.1%, and 18.4% of white, black, and Hispanic women, respectively
- Heart conditions, which impact activity in 12.8%, 13.4%, and 10.6% of white, black, and Hispanic women, respectively [11].

Activity limitations increase with age and by poverty level. In all, 43.6 percent of women aged 45–64 reported activity limitation compared to 67.9 percent of women aged 65 and older and 22.4 percent of women aged 25–44 [10]. Approximately 45 percent of women with a household income of less than 200 percent of poverty reported activity limitation compared to 34.3 percent of women with

BOX 1.1 Organizational Participants of the Well-Woman Task Force

American Academy of Family Physicians

American Academy of Pediatrics

American Academy of Physician Assistants

American College of Nurse-Midwives

American College of Obstetricians and Gynecologists

American College of Osteopathic Obstetricians and Gynecologists

American College of Physicians

Association of Reproductive Health Professionals

Association of Women's Health, Obstetric and Neonatal Nurses

National Association of Nurse Practitioners in Women's Health

National Medical Association

Planned Parenthood Federation of America

Society for Maternal-Fetal Medicine

Society of Academic Specialists in General Obstetrics and Gynecology

Society of Gynecologic Oncology

a household income of 200 percent or more of poverty [11]. Obesity is the leading chronic disease of women and impacts long-term health. It is a confounder for activity limitations, even for those who consider themselves currently in normal health. Two-thirds of all reproductive-aged women in the United States are currently overweight or obese by BMI standards [12]. Women who are overweight or obese are at increased risk for adverse health outcomes during pregnancy and comorbid conditions including cardiovascular disease, diabetes, kidney disease, and obesity-related cancers over their life course.

Why Preventive Well-Woman Care?

As noted by IOM, the Patient Protection and Affordable Care Act of 2010 (ACA) ushered in a shift from a reactive health care system to one that promotes optimal health and well-being [13]. Under the ACA, the annual well-woman visit must be included as a covered benefit with no co-payment. The visit potentially involves a wide range of clinicians who provide women's care including obstetrician-gynecologists, family physicians, internists, pediatricians, and advanced practice providers including nurse practitioners, nurse-midwives, and physician assistants. The selection of a provider for the well-woman care visit will be determined by the woman's needs and preference, access to health services, plan, and age category.

The Well-Woman Task Force

Given the many types of clinicians who provide well-woman care and the broad range of potential topics for inclusion in the visit, ACOG invited a broad range of provider types with wide-ranging clinical expertise and perspectives to be part of the Task Force. Organizational participants included the associations and organizations listed in Box 1.1. The collaboration also had ad hoc representation from several other organizations and groups dedicated to women's health care.

Each Task Force participant organization provided their organizations top three priorities for well-woman care. For example, the top three priority areas for ACOG were reproductive health management, obesity prevention, and smoking cessation. All three areas of priority were considered critical to all age levels of current and long-term women's health. These priority areas were collated and used as a starting point for inclusion of well-woman visit components.

The WWTFs objective was to develop age-specific well-woman health care guidelines with the goal of improving health outcomes and to provide specific age-appropriate guidance for an annual well-woman visit. Preventive guidelines for well-woman care are primarily based on age and reproductive potential. After careful deliberation by the Task Force, women were categorized in the following age ranges:

- Adolescents (13–18 years)
- Reproductive-aged women (19–45 years)
- Mature women (46–64 years)
- Women older than 64 years

The final recommendations for age ranges recognized that organizations typically base their recommendations on different age range categories for evidence-based screening and preventive care. The work of the group began with compilation of existing guidelines for conditions and diseases. ACOG staff compiled existing guidelines from DHHS, IOM, the US Preventive Services Task Force (USPSTF), the participating organizations on the Task Force, and other authoritative organizations not represented by the Task Force such as the Centers for Disease Control (CDC) and major subspecialty societies. Prior to the first in-person meeting, participants were provided a summary of guidelines for review, organized by topic according to the level of agreement. The level of agreement was defined as follows:

- Single source (e.g., abdominal examination)
- No agreement (e.g., mammography screening)
- Limited agreement (e.g., pelvic examination)
- General agreement (e.g., hypertension, osteoporosis)
- Sound agreement (e.g., screening for sexually transmitted infections)

The existing guidelines were then reviewed by individual workgroups, who made recommendations to the convened Task Force, who developed joint final recommendations. In developing the Task Force recommendations for the components of the well-woman visit, Task Force members focused on what should be done to optimize health for the average woman. After review of the various content areas of the well-woman visit, final recommendations relied on evidence-based guidelines derived by the IOM, USPSTF, and CDC. Where evidence-based guidelines were not applicable, evidence-informed recommendations were made based on the guidelines of medical societies and professional organizations. A minority of the recommendations were based on uniform expert agreement derived from the deliberation of the Task Force to resolve conflicting guidelines or to supplement evidence-based and evidence-informed guidelines. Recommendations were considered to be "strong" if based primarily on evidence-based or evidence-informed guidelines and "qualified" if they relied primarily on expert consensus. For example,

colorectal screening guidelines were considered evidence based and the recommendation for screening was considered "strong."

Illustrative Cases

Breast Cancer Screening

A 38-year-old woman requested a screening mammogram because her best friend was recently diagnosed with breast cancer at the time of her last screening mammogram at age 42. The woman had no family history of breast cancer.

However, evidence-based recommendations for the age to begin mammographic breast cancer screening in average risk populations remain controversial and continue to be debated. Because of the importance of this recommendation to women, clinicians, and insurers, the Task Force debated the evidence-based recommendation of the USPSTF to begin screening mammography at age 50 and the American Cancer Society to begin screening at age 40. The final WWTF recommendation for screening utilized both evidence-based and evidence-informed guidelines and based the recommendation on the uniform expert opinion that mammography screening reduces breast cancer mortality for women aged 40–69 and that data was insufficient for older women. The Task Force also recognized the concerns of the USPSTF about false-positive mammography results requiring additional imaging.

The final recommendation of the Task Force was that for women aged 40 and older, the decision to start and terminate regular screening mammography should be individualized and the patient context including assessment of breast cancer risk and comorbidities, and the patient's values regarding specific benefits and harm of screening should be taken into account. This final recommendation was categorized as "strong," as was that routine screening mammography should occur by age 50. The final recommendation on whether screening frequency should be annual or biennial was categorized as "qualified." While the source recommendations have changed since the Task Force convened, their final recommendation remains broad enough to still be useful.

Domestic Violence

A 56-year-old, long-time patient in your practice appears depressed and anxious during her annual well-

woman visit. She divorced after 30 years and started a new relationship several months ago. She has some old bruises on her forearms and wrist. When questioned, she confides her partner is "a bit rough" at times.

Low-cost screening such as for domestic or intimate partner violence is not supported by high-quality evidence, but is considered important for quality health care. In these types of cases such as domestic abuse and depression, the Task Force recommendation was phrased to be permissive as opposed to prescriptive.

One key area of concern with screening is the ability to treat or refer women with positive screens. Screening is important for the health and safety of women, but is not effective unless appropriate actions can be taken regarding identified problems. The Task Force considered the feasibility of effectively implementing the recommendations and was cognizant that there are often barriers to being able to make referrals. The Task Force felt that screening for depression and domestic/intimate partner violence needed to be elements of the well-woman visit despite these concerns, given the implications not only for the health of the woman but also for her family. The USPSTF recently updated their depression screening recommendation in line with the WWTF, calling for screening for depression to be coupled with adequate systems for diagnosis, treatment, and follow up [14].

The Pelvic Examination

A 21-year-old nulliparous woman presents for a well-woman visit. She is in a new relationship and wants to discuss contraception. She asks whether she needs a full pelvic examination. Her last examination was performed 2 years ago. She is sexually active and she and her partner use condoms.

There are no evidence-based or evidence-informed guidelines about screening pelvic examinations. Routine pelvic examinations have long been considered a key component of the annual woman visit. In July 2014, the American College of Physicians recommended against performing routine pelvic examinations [15]. Their recommendation contradicted the expert opinion-based guidelines from ACOG, which reiterated its support for the yearly pelvic examination [16]. The Task Force acknowledged that not all women require a complete external,

speculum, and bimanual pelvic examination, and took this into account in making their final recommendation. The Task Force final recommendation was that the decision whether or not to perform a screening pelvic examination should be a shared decision after a discussion between the patient and her health care provider. An inspection of the external genitalia should be offered to all women regardless of age group. The Task Force recommendation regarding the annual pelvic examination was based on expert opinion.

Other Special Considerations

Other special considerations include state and local laws and regulations, insurance coverage, cost and cost-effectiveness of preventive care, and availability of referral services. A minor's ability to consent to confidential reproductive health care without parental notification varies among states and is constantly changing through state legislation. It is a prime example of legislative decisions impacting health care decisions. The Task Force recognized that legislators and regulators could potentially impact well-woman care, especially in areas of contraception and reproductive choice.

Conclusion

Ongoing assessment of individual access to recommended screening represents an important component of ACA implementation. A full implementation of women's health-covered benefit of the ACA is not yet a reality in the United States for all women. The WWTF was convened in response to the opportunity created by the ACA and the need to define the components of the well-woman visit. The components of the well-woman visit recommended by the Task Force, as well as details of how to execute them are detailed at length later in the book. The Task Force reviewed hundreds of guidelines and recommendations in deriving their recommendations. These source guidelines continue to evolve as new evidence is obtained, and given the volume and complexity of components of the well-woman visit, recommendations will evolve over time. While for significant time the well-woman visit may have been considered to largely consist of an annual Pap smear, the WWTF clearly delineated the many other opportunities for improving health and preventing disease at a periodic well-woman visit.

Summary

1. The WWTF was convened to determine age-appropriate components of the well-woman visit and appropriate guidelines for each of these components.

2. Clinicians and women must be educated on the importance of the annual well-woman visit to achieve adherence to the WHO definition of women's health.

3. This education will ensure that a well-woman visit meets the standards of care for each Task Force recommendation and achieves satisfaction and meets the expectations for the woman and her providers.

4. The ultimate goal of the well-woman visit is age-appropriate screening and prevention based on the best available evidence.

5. The goal of counseling at the well-woman visit is to identify behaviors and situations that impact health and implement preventive strategies to achieve health and wellness over the life span.

6. The final recommendations of the WWTF will require periodic updates as more evidence-based information becomes available in specific content areas such as cancer screening.

7. Full implementation of all components of a well-woman visit and the counseling and screening requirements will not be realized for all women until the challenges for affordable care are met.

References

1. World Health Organization. Constitution of the World Health Organization. Basic Documents, 45th edition, Supplement, October 2006. Available at: www.who.int/governance/eb/who_constitution_en.pdf. Retrieved March 28, 2016.

2. Bright Futures. Available at: https://brightfutures.aap.org/Pages/default.aspx.

3. Conry, J.A. and Brown, H. Executive summary, well-woman task force, components of the well-woman visit. *Obstet Gynecol.* 2015, **126**:697–701.

4. US Department of Health and Human Services. *Affordable Care Act Rules on Expanding Access to Preventive Services for Women.* Washington, DC: US Department of Health and Human Services, 2013. Available at: www.hhs.go/healthcare/facts/factssheets/2011/08/womensprevention0801201a.html. Retrieved June 9, 2015.

5. Centers for Disease Control, National Center for Health Statistics, United States. Life expectancy at birth, by sex and race/ethnicity – United States, 2011. *Morb Mortal Wkly Rep.* September 5, 2014, **63**(35):776.

6. Heron, M.P., Hoyert, D.L., Murphy, S.L., and Jiaquan, X. Deaths: Final data for 2006. *Natl Vital Stat Rep.* 2009, **57**(14).

7. National Center for Health Statistic. *Health, United States. 2010: With Special Features on Death and Dying.* Hyattsville, MD: Library of Congress Catalog Number 76-641496, 2011.

8. US Cancer Statistics Working Group. *United States Cancer Statistics: 1999–2012 Incidence and Mortality Web-Based Report.* Atlanta, GA: US Department of Health and Human Services, Centers for Disease Control and Prevention and National Cancer Institute, 2015. Available at: www.cdc.gov/uscs.

9. US Department of Health and Human Services, Health Resources and Service Administration. *Women's Health USA 2013.* Rockville, MD: US Department of Health and Human Services, 2013.

10. US Department of Health and Human Services, Centers for Disease Control and Prevention, National Center for Health Statistics. *2009 National Health Interview Survey (NHIS) Questionnaire: Adult Health Status and Limitations.* Rockville, MD: US Department of Health and Human Services, 2011.

11. US Department of Health and Human Services, Health Resources and Services Administration. *Women's Health USA 2006.* Rockville, MD: US Department of Health and Human Services, 2006.

12. Flegal, K.M., Carroll, M.D., Ogden, C.L., and Curtin, L.R. Prevalence and trends in obesity among US adults, 1999–2008. *JAMA.* 2010, **303**:235–41.

13. Institute of Medicine. *Clinical Preventive Services for Women: Closing the Gaps.* Washington, DC: The National Academics Press, 2001.

14. Siu, A.L. Screening for depression in adults, US preventive services task force recommendation statement. *JAMA.* 2016, **315**(4):380–7.

15. Qaseem, A., Humphrey, L.L., Harris, R., Starkey, M., and Denberg, T.D. Screening pelvic examination in adult women: A clinical practice guideline from the American College of Physicians. *Ann Inter Med.* 2014, **161**:67–72.

16. ACOG. ACOG practice advisory on annual pelvic examination recommendations. Available at: www.acog.org/About-ACOG/News-Room/Practice-Advisories/ACOG-Practice-Advisory-on-Annual-Pelvic-Examination-Recommendations. Retrieved March 28, 2016.

Suggested Reading

Conry, J.A. and Brown, H. Executive summary, well-woman task force, components of the well-woman visit. *Obstet Gynecol.* 2015, **126**:697–701.

Flegal, K.M., Kit, B.K., Orpana, H., and Graubard, B.I. Association of all-cause mortality with overweight and obesity using standard body mass index categories: A systematic review and meta-analysis. *JAMA.* 2013, **309**:71–82.

Flegal, K.M., Graubard, B.I., Williamson, D.F., and Gail, M.H. Cause specific excess deaths associated with underweight, overweight, and obesity. *JAMA.* 2007, **298**: 2028–37.

US Department of Health and Human Services, Health Resources and Services Administration, Maternal and Child Health Bureau. *Women's Health USA 2013.* Rockville, MD: US Department of Health and Human Services, 2013.

Johnson, N.B., Hayes, L.D., Bown, K., Hoo, E.C., and Ethier, K.A. CDC National Health Report: Leading causes of morbidity and mortality and associated behavioral risk and protective factors – United States, 2005–2013. *Morb Mortal Wkly Rep Suppl.* October 31, 2014, **63**(04):3–27.

Chapter

2

Rationale for the Well-Woman Visit

Maureen G. Phipps

Learning Objectives

- Review existing data about the effectiveness of preventive visits
- Describe benefits of the well-woman visit including identifying health risk behaviors and conditions, discussing modifiable risk factors, promoting healthy behaviors, and prescribing interventions and counseling to improve quality of life
- Highlight the value of building the physician–patient relationship during the well-woman visit

Introduction

The purpose of the well-woman visit is to identify modifiable risk factors and address concerns that impact health and wellness. The goal of the visit is to work with the patient to understand her health-related goals and to help her understand the actions she can take to improve her long-term health and quality of life. The cost-benefit consideration for an annual physical examination is controversial and the collective components of the well-woman visit have not been robustly evaluated. Despite these concerns, there are important reasons why the well-woman visit is a critical opportunity to improve or maintain health and has the potential for a more positive effect on overall health compared with problem-focused provider visits. Although quantitatively measuring the positive impact on well-being and commitment to healthy behaviors presents challenges, much is gained when an individual woman is provided the opportunity to talk with her provider about health risk behaviors, health concerns, and personal issues impacting her overall health. By focusing on long-term health, women's health providers are able to individualize strategies for maintaining healthy behaviors, screening, and addressing modifiable conditions and risk factors to help women optimize their overall health and well-being.

Overarching Goal of the Well-Woman Visit

Through individualized discussions, the well-woman visit brings forth focused interventions and recommendations with the goal of preventing disease, optimizing health, and improving health outcomes. The specific elements of the examination are organized in the tables from the Well-Woman Task Force (WWTF) report [1] and described in detail in individual chapters. However, the overall approach to the well-woman visit centers around understanding the individual woman's health risks through screening and discussion to develop a plan that will help modify unhealthy behavior, promote healthy behavior, and implement early interventions or treatments that will benefit long-term health.

In most cases, patients with complex medical conditions benefit from having their care closely monitored and managed. It is equally important to focus on keeping individuals healthy and identifying people with modifiable health risk factors that will benefit from targeted intervention and treatment. In general, people are considered asymptomatic or healthy when they do not present for care or do not have specific complaints. Unfortunately, many women do not present for care because they do not recognize their symptoms, believe nothing can be done about their condition, or are unaware that they should seek care for their specific problem. When women present for a well-woman visit, screening can be done for unrecognized or hidden symptoms and risk factors and risk behaviors can be detected, discussed, and addressed before they become more problematic or more significant.

Promoting Health and Quality of Life

Studies evaluating the range of preventive services provided through a well-woman visit are often tangentially related studies and are further limited by only including a narrow scope of periodic health examinations or health checks. A systematic review evaluating the value of the periodic health examination showed benefit for the delivery of preventive services associated with the examination. However, it did not demonstrate long-term health benefits [2]. The systematic review was limited by heterogeneity among the included studies with poor reporting of some of the specified outcomes, variation in study design, some studies including only men, and including several studies initiated prior to 1989 when the US Preventive Services Task Force (USPSTF) guidelines were first published. Although a Cochrane systematic review by Kogsboll [3] showed that general health checks in adults did not reduce morbidity and mortality, the review had limitations similar to the earlier review by Boulware et al. [2]. The studies included had inconsistent inclusion criteria, interventions, and methodology. In addition, the included studies did not necessarily focus on preventive care or evidence-based guidelines and the topics evaluated were diverse and not consistent among the studies. Applying these findings to the well-woman visit is not appropriate because the focus of the visit is prevention of diseases and improving quality of life. Each well-woman visit is tailored to the individual patient and recommendations for intervention are based on that individual's risk factors and values. Designing a study to evaluate the impact of the multidimensional well-woman visit would be challenging. It would require measuring changes in clinical outcomes as well as quality of life based on the broad range of issues addressed at each visit and recommendations tailored to the individual's risk profile and ability to make change. Incremental improvements in quality of life are very difficult to measure, even when they may have a profound impact on an individual. Given these challenges, limited evidence is available evaluating the effect of the well-woman visit on quality of life and health outcomes.

Although data directly addressing the effectiveness of the well-woman visit is limited, there are many compelling reasons supporting the well-woman visit. The cost-effectiveness of preventive services has been debated in the literature. In response to this debate, in 2010 Maciosek et al. [4] presented an analysis showing that if proven evidence-based preventive services guidelines such as those recommended by the USPSTF are used, then the costs associated with the preventive services are neutral and health benefits are positive. Risk and problems vary by age, health status, and many other individual factors. The well-woman visit is an opportunity to gather these data for a single patient and focus on the most common problems for a woman of her age, race, and other risk factors. The conversations about risk behaviors can focus on modifiable behaviors or conditions particular to the individual patient that if addressed can improve morbidity, mortality, and quality of life. For example, women in their late teens and twenties have higher rates of death from accidents, suicide, and drug misuse compared with other age groups. For women in their late teens and twenties, an age-based assessment during the well-woman visit should focus on safety behaviors, depression symptoms, and mental health concerns as well as alcohol, tobacco, and drug use. In contrast, women in their fifties and sixties have higher rates of cardiovascular disease (CVD), lung cancer, and breast cancer, so the conversation should focus more on screening and counseling for these conditions. Useful information to help understand and prepare for counseling patients about morbidity and mortality by age and gender can be found at www.worldlifeexpectancy.com/usa-cause-of-death-by-age-and-gender. Incorporating age-specific risk assessment along with behavior-specific risk assessment is important as the recommendations for testing, behavior modification, and targeted interventions are being developed. The well-woman visit offers an opportunity not present at problem-focused provider visits to effectively do this individual assessment.

Because many of the leading causes of mortality are directly related to chronic disease, prevention, behavior modification, early detection, and intervention aimed at reducing morbidity from chronic disease are particularly important. The well-woman visit allows for extra time for detailed identification of risk behaviors, risk factors, adverse health conditions, and early disease states, which allows providers and patients to optimize interventions to improve quality of life and prevent excess morbidity and mortality. Many evidence-based screening guidelines have been developed to help prevent or improve disease states. Although different methodologies are used for their development, guidelines from different professional societies, advocacy groups, and government are available to help guide screening, counseling, health promotion, and interventions. The well-woman visit is the only structured opportunity to comprehensively apply these guidelines.

As an example, the USPSTF works to improve the health of all Americans by making evidence-based recommendations about clinical preventive services such as screening, counseling services, and preventive medications. The USPSTF develops recommendations based on rigorous review of existing peer-reviewed scientific evidence with the intention to help primary care providers and patients decide together whether a preventive service is right for that particular patient. Because the recommendations from the USPSTF apply to people who have no signs or symptoms of the specific disease or condition that the screening, counseling, or preventive medication targets, they are suited to being implemented during the well-woman visit.

Examples of recommendations from the USPSTF that can be applied at the well-woman visit include treatment of alcohol misuse, CVD assessment to guide treatment with aspirin and prevention with healthy diet and physical activity, depression screening, intimate partner violence (IPV) screening, diabetes screening, obesity screening, high blood pressure screening, tobacco use counseling, lung cancer screening for smokers with a 30-year pack history, screening for sexually transmitted infections, Hepatitis B and Hepatitis C screening, BRCA risk assessment, falls prevention, cervical cancer screening, osteoporosis screening, colon cancer screening, and breast cancer screening. (The updated list of USPSTF recommendations can be found at www.uspreventiveservicestaskforce.org.)

The well-woman visit is an essential tool for achieving the full potential of implementing prevention guidelines in all populations of women. It provides an opportunity for all women to gain access to appropriate preventive services that they might otherwise have avoided, ignored, or not had access to. Although not well understood, low health literacy is related to higher rates of morbidity and mortality. The well-woman visit with its focus on individualized counseling, screening, and intervention has the potential to mediate challenges associated with low health literacy. Developing local resource guides and collaborating across community-based health organizations will help in decreasing the barriers to care associated with low health literacy, social determinants of health, and cultural challenges. The well-woman visit provides a framework for discussing risk factors and risk behaviors, assessing appropriate testing and screening, and guiding behavioral modification

recommendations to improve health. Through promoting healthy behaviors, screening for disease, and intervening with early treatment as necessary, the provider and patient can collaborate in developing the plan for optimizing her health.

Focus on Health: The Patient–Provider Relationship

Although the medical definition of quality of life may vary, the main elements include the patient's satisfaction with her ability to engage in and enjoy the activities in her life. The definition from the Centers for Disease Control and Prevention includes: "On the individual level, this [quality of life] includes physical and mental health perceptions and their correlates – including health risks and conditions, functional status, social support, and socioeconomic status" [5]. Emphasizing a national focus on this issue, the goal of the Healthy People 2020 (HP2020) Health-Related Quality of Life and Well-Being (HRQOL) objectives is to increase the proportion of adults who self-report good or better physical health and mental health. The HP2020 objectives aim to measure improvement over time to aid health care providers and public health professionals in implementing guidance and programs to improve these measures. The well-woman visit provides an important opportunity to implement these new recommendations and programs.

Women may be unaware of the relationship between their behaviors and their health. Risk-taking behaviors including sexual risk taking, smoking, and alcohol misuse are difficult conversations that require time and focused attention. Without a well-woman visit, these behavioral issues may be ignored or pushed to the side to address acute medical issues. Medical conditions such as hypertension, high cholesterol, osteoporosis, and diabetes may not have identifiable symptoms that would prompt a woman to see her provider until she has a complication. The well-woman visit is a chance to screen for these conditions in time to prevent an adverse outcome. Cancer screening is driven by complex risk assessment that requires time to evaluate family history, risk factors, and individual values. The visit is an opportunity to help women understand that ongoing immunizations improve health by preventing disease as well as preventing the spread of disease. Evaluation and treatment for obesity and healthy lifestyle is essential to long-term health and has significant implications for morbidity, mortality, and quality of life. Screening for depression and IPV requires time for support and evaluation as well as identifying appropriate community resources for referral. In addition to screening and evaluation, understanding a woman's health goals including pregnancy planning or managing life transitions is critically important in developing individualized recommendations for optimizing her health. Without a well-woman visit, there is no other venue with adequate time to address these many important issues.

Beyond the Pelvic Examination

Although a physical examination, often including a pelvic examination, has been an expected component of a well-woman visit, it is likely among the least important components. The patient–provider conversation is essential to improving long-term health. Screening and preventive counseling discussions and interventions are essential to engaging women in health-promoting behaviors and understanding that behavior modifications can be implemented to improve long-term health, quality of life, and well-being. Screening includes a thorough family history, immunization history, social history, risk behavior assessment, goals for family planning, engagement in exercise, and overview of diet and nutrition. Effective screening helps focus conversations about behavior modification and the impact on short- and long-term health. Examples include reducing risk associated with alcohol, tobacco, and drug use, weight, cardiovascular health, diabetes, sexual risk-taking behavior, and sun exposure and skin cancer. Depending on the individual, screening for age and risk factors may lead to testing for breast cancer, colon cancer, osteoporosis, and other conditions. Screening can also lead to direct interventions for cases of depression, IPV, obesity, or updating immunizations. There is really no opportunity to do this important screening in the context of problem-focused visits, while the well-woman visit is specifically designed to do it effectively.

Although the ability to diagnose a condition early or identify risk that can be modified cannot be overstated, the benefits of the well-woman visit go beyond screening and behavior modification and disease prevention. Having a functioning relationship with a provider directly benefits the patient as well as the health care system. When a patient has an acute problem or change in health condition, having a preexisting relationship with a provider who can facilitate care is more efficient and patient centered.

Collaboration

The complex issues addressed during the well-woman visit will frequently require the provider to engage other professionals and support personnel to help implement guidelines and interventions. Providers must have experience and proficiency in discussing the significant sensitive issues that women face at all stages of their lives. Along with treating gynecologic issues, the care provider or team should be prepared to ask questions that facilitate discussion with the patient about important health issues in otherwise asymptomatic women. Building trust with patients, feeling comfortable with difficult conversations, and making patients feel at ease are essential competencies for an effective well-woman visit. These competencies relate to addressing concerns that include sexual health, sexuality, perimenopausal symptoms, menopause-specific issues, domestic violence and IPV, and mental health issues. Recognizing the importance of collaboration, the multidisciplinary provider team might include a range of women's health care providers from diverse medical backgrounds, nursing, social work, behavioral health, pharmacy, and public health. In addition to effectively addressing issues during a well-woman visit, being part of a team and knowing about community-based health resources will help facilitate the implementation of screening guidelines and interventions.

Case Scenarios

A 45-year-old woman presents without complaints for a well-woman visit and reports no concerns in her medical history or family history. Her vital signs reveal a body mass index (BMI) of 30 kg/m² with a 15-pound weight gain over the past year. Her blood pressure is 150/90. What screening, evaluation, and counseling should be recommended related to her weight and blood pressure as part of the visit?

The well-woman visit is an ideal time to address health issues that are asymptomatic and would otherwise not be detected. This patient was feeling well and would have otherwise not sought out care. The USPSTF and WWTF recommendations on screening all adults for obesity is helpful to guide the conversation about the long-term health concerns related to her weight and BMI. The recommendation includes offering or referring patients with a BMI of 30 kg/m² or higher to intensive, multicomponent behavioral interventions [1, 6]. To implement this recommendation, a clinician would need to be familiar with resources available in their community and provide information on how to access the resources. In asymptomatic patients with obesity, evaluating other risk factors is important for implementing a plan for avoiding poor health outcomes in the future. The USPSTF has separate guidance for patients presenting with a BMI consistent with obesity and confirmed elevated blood pressure or other CVD risk factors including hypertension, dyslipidemia, impaired fasting glucose, or the metabolic syndrome. The USPSTF recommends offering or referring adults who are overweight or obese and have additional CVD risk factors to intensive behavioral counseling interventions to promote a healthful diet and physical activity for CVD prevention [7].

The well-woman visit is an ideal opportunity to address serious health issues in asymptomatic women and develop strategies for behavior change and intervention. Using national or local guidelines can be very helpful in guiding discussions with patients as well as developing a plan for screening, evaluation, medical treatment, or behavioral modification. Provider knowledge about community resources is important, as is a practice's ability to access resources and provide education and support services for patients.

A 55-year-old woman presents without complaints for a well-woman visit and reports no concerns in her medical history or family history. She has gained 15 pounds over the past year and her BMI is 27 kg/m². Initially, the patient denies any problems or concerns. After further evaluation, the patient reveals that she stopped exercising over the past 9 months because she developed urinary incontinence and is embarrassed by her situation. She is stressed because exercise has always been a big part of her life and she is not sure what to do about the incontinence.

Causes for weight gain need to be explored. This patient's weight gain is related to not exercising due to her incontinence. Having the opportunity to discuss this situation with the patient before her obesity worsens and leads to other health problems is important to her future health. Managing her incontinence as well as guiding her in adopting a healthy diet will help meet this goal. This case highlights the point that without a well-woman visit to assess lifestyle and risk behaviors, many patients would be considered asymptomatic when in reality they have unrecognized or unacknowledged symptoms. Intervening early, addressing important related health issues, and supporting healthy behaviors are important to improved quality of life, long-term health, and overall wellness.

A 24-year-old woman presents without complaints for a well-woman visit and reports tobacco and alcohol use in her medical history. She has an unremarkable family history.

Based on her age and these risk behaviors, what should her assessment include?

- Screening for gonorrhea and chlamydia: The USPSTF recommends screening for chlamydia in sexually active females aged 24 or younger and in older women who are at increased risk for infection [1, 8].
- Discussing tobacco use: The USPSTF recommends that clinicians ask all adults about tobacco use, advise them to stop using tobacco, and provide behavioral interventions and US Food and Drug Administration-approved pharmacotherapy for cessation to adults who use tobacco [1, 9].
- Discuss alcohol use: The USPSTF recommends that clinicians screen adults aged 18 or older for alcohol misuse and provide persons engaged in risky or hazardous drinking with brief behavioral counseling interventions to reduce alcohol misuse [1, 10]. The USPSTF found that counseling interventions in the primary care setting can positively affect unhealthy drinking behaviors in adults engaging in risky or hazardous drinking. Positive outcomes include reducing weekly alcohol consumption and long-term adherence to recommended drinking limits.
- Screen for depression: The USPSTF recommends screening for depression in the general adult population, including pregnant and postpartum women. Screening should be implemented with adequate systems in place to ensure accurate diagnosis, effective treatment, and appropriate follow-up [1, 11].
- Screening for IPV and domestic violence: The USPSTF recommends that clinicians screen women of childbearing age for IPV, such as domestic violence, and provide or refer women who screen positive to intervention services [1, 12].
- Discuss overall safety habits including seatbelt use and helmet use: Driving safety counseling should include avoiding distracted driving and driving while under the influence of alcohol or drugs [1].

Summary

Through the well-woman visit, providers have the opportunity to engage with women to understand their health concerns, address their health goals, and help them understand what they can modify to minimize risk and enhance their health. It is also an important opportunity to reinforce positive current behaviors that will have a positive impact on their long-term health. The well-woman visit facilitates prevention and planning through understanding modifiable risk factors, prevention, and the patient's health concerns and values. Without a well-woman visit, many women will not have their unrecognized or unacknowledged symptoms, signs, or risk behaviors come to the attention of their provider in time to prevent adverse outcomes. Without a well-woman visit, the ability to identify disease at an early or asymptomatic stage is reduced and many opportunities are lost to address modifiable risk behaviors in women at risk for adverse outcomes and provide treatment or implement interventions to improve long-term health. The well-woman visit is the main opportunity to address age-related health risks and guide individualized evidence-based discussions surrounding behaviors to modify (e.g., smoking cessation) or incorporate (e.g., exercise and healthy lifestyle choices) to minimize risk and improve overall health. Challenging conversations about sexual health, unhealthy lifestyle, violence, and risk-taking behaviors are central elements of the well-woman visit that require the expertise and competency of sensitive women's health providers. The well-woman visit provides women the opportunity to work with their providers to optimize their health and address preventable morbidity and mortality in areas ranging from planning a pregnancy to planning for menopause and beyond, considering immunizations, incorporating a healthy lifestyle, and considering measures to prevent disease and applying interventions to improve health.

Resources

- National Guideline Clearinghouse. Agency for Healthcare Research and Quality. www.guideline.gov/index.aspx
- US Preventive Services Task Force Resources. www.uspreventiveservicestaskforce.org
- Causes of death by age and gender in the United States. www.worldlifeexpectancy.com/usa-cause-of-death-by-age-and-gender
- A resource for patients and providers to help guide patients toward implementing recommendations. www.Healthfinder.gov

References

1. Conry, J.A. and Brown, H. Well-Woman Task Force: Components of the well-woman visit. *Obstet Gynecol.* 2015, **126**(4):697–701.

2. Boulware, L.E., Marinopoulos, S., Phillips, K.A. et al. Systematic review: The value of the periodic health evaluation. *Ann Intern Med.* 2007, **146**:289–300.

3. Kogsboll, L.T. General health checks in adults for reducing morbidity and mortality from disease. *Cochrane systematic review and meta-analysis.* BMJ. 2012, **345**:e7191.

4. Maciosek, M.V., Coffield, A.B., Flottemesch, T.J., Edwards, N.M., and Solberg, L.I. Greater use of preventive services in US health care could save lives at little or no cost. *Health Aff (Millwood).* 2010, **29**(9):1656–60.

5. Health Related Quality of Life (HRQOL). Centers for Disease Control and Prevention. Available at: www.cdc.gov/hrqol/concept.htm. Retrieved October 4, 2016.

6. Moyer, V.A. and US Preventive Services Task Force. Screening for and management of obesity in adults: US Preventive Services Task Force recommendation statement. *Ann Intern Med.* 2012, **157**(5):373–8.

7. LeFevre, M.L. and US Preventive Services Task Force. Behavioral counseling to promote a healthful diet and physical activity for cardiovascular disease prevention in adults with cardiovascular risk factors: US Preventive Services Task Force recommendation statement. *Ann Intern Med.* 2014, **161**(8):587–93.

8. LeFevre, M.L. and US Preventive Services Task Force. Screening for chlamydia and gonorrhea: US Preventive Services Task Force recommendation statement. *Ann Intern Med.* 2014, **161**(12):902–10.

9. Siu, A.L. and US Preventive Services Task Force. Behavioral and pharmacotherapy interventions for tobacco smoking cessation in adults, including pregnant women: US Preventive Services Task Force recommendation statement. *Ann Intern Med.* 2015, **163**(8):622–34.

10. Moyer, V.A. and US Preventive Services Task Force. Screening and behavioral counseling interventions in primary care to reduce alcohol misuse: US Preventive Services Task Force recommendation statement. *Ann Intern Med.* 2013, **159**(3):210–8.

11. Siu, A.L. and US Preventive Services Task Force. Screening for depression in adults US Preventive Services Task Force recommendation statement. *JAMA.* 2016, **315**(4):380–7.

12. Moyer, V.A. and US Preventive Services Task Force. Screening for intimate partner violence and abuse of elderly and vulnerable adults: US Preventive Services Task Force recommendation statement. *Ann Intern Med.* 2013, **158**(6):478–86.

Principles of Early Diagnosis and Prevention

Lee A. Learman

Learning Objectives

- Distinguish primary, secondary, and tertiary forms of prevention
- Provide examples of population-wide and individual strategies for prevention
- Explain the criteria used in developing population-based screening programs
- Define the optimal characteristics of screening tests including sensitivity, specificity, accuracy, and likelihood ratios
- Explain the relationship between disease prevalence and the meaning of positive and negative test results
- List potential harms of screening to individuals and society

Introduction

Consistent use of appropriate screening and prevention guidelines will decrease morbidity and mortality and improve quality of life for women. Optimizing health during a woman's reproductive years benefits her and sets the stage for better pregnancy outcomes, potentially with lifelong consequences for her children. Providing preventive care at a well-woman visit could be as straightforward as implementing a set of guidelines developed by experts and based on best available evidence. However, guidelines are not static and specific recommendations change over time. Technological advances are likely to bring new screening tools to market before they appear in guidelines, and new evidence may question the effectiveness of existing methods. The aim of this chapter is to provide a foundation regarding key concepts in prevention and early diagnosis. Applying these principles will help us interpret screening results for different risk groups during the well-woman visit and decide which new screening technologies to introduce in practice.

Prevention: Choosing the Best Opportunities

Prevention begins by defining an important clinical outcome. Life or death is often cited as the best outcome because it is easily measured and obviously important. Diseases creating severe long-term morbidity are also important, particularly when they create a large burden of suffering and financial expense to the public health. Prevention efforts are classified as primary, secondary, and tertiary. Primary prevention occurs before the disease is present, even in a preclinical form. Secondary prevention permits early detection of disease, typically before it produces symptoms. Tertiary prevention aims to limit morbidity and mortality after the disease is clinically evident. The examples in Table 3.1 underscore the many opportunities for prevention at the well-woman visit.

Although screening can occur for many diseases, it would be impractical and harmful to screen all patients for all entities. Population screening decisions have huge implications for cost to the health system and health of individual patients. In 1968, the World Health Organization (WHO) established guidelines [1], also called "Wilson's Criteria," to help determine whether population-based screening is likely to be beneficial (Box 3.1). Breast and cervical cancer prevention fit these criteria well. Both diseases have a long latent stage and screening methods which are effective and acceptable to the population. The natural history of breast and cervical cancer creates multiple opportunities for the screening and treatment of precancerous lesions and early disease.

However, there are important differences between breast and cervical cancer screening guidelines. Although cervical cancer is not the most common reproductive tract cancer in women, it is cost-effective to provide population-based screening. There is general consensus on the screening population, frequency of testing, and duration of testing. Guidelines delaying

Table 3.1 Examples of Primary, Secondary, and Tertiary Prevention. The examples are strategies to prevent the onset of disease (primary), occult disease from becoming symptomatic (secondary), and progression or recurrence of symptomatic disease (tertiary). The examples are selected to illustrate prevention strategies and do not represent an exhaustive list.

Disease	Primary Prevention (Before Disease is Present)	Secondary Prevention (Early in Course of Disease)	Tertiary Prevention (Once Symptomatic to Minimize Morbidity)
Breast cancer	Multiparity Breastfeeding	Screening mammography DCIS treatment	Interventions to prevent cancer progression or recurrence
Cervical cancer	HPV vaccination Smoking cessation	Screening cytology and HPV testing HSIL treatment	Early detection of cancer progression or recurrence
Colorectal cancer	Smoking cessation Exercise High-fiber diet	Screening colonoscopy Villous adenoma excision	
Osteoporotic fractures	Smoking cessation Adequate diet and exercise	Screening bone mineral density testing Osteoporosis treatment Fall prevention	Prevention of recurrent fractures
Preterm birth	Smoking cessation Postpartum LARC Pregnancy interval spacing	Progesterone Cervical length measurement Cerclage	Corticosteroids Magnesium Neuroprotection

DCIS = ductal carcinoma in situ; HPV = human papillomavirus; HSIL = high-grade squamous intraepithelial lesion; LARC = long-acting reversible contraception

cervical cancer screening in young women until age 21 have been accepted to avoid the harms of overtreatment, including excisional and ablative cervical procedures which may impact future pregnancy. Breast cancer is the most common reproductive tract cancer in women and screening for breast cancer has been extensively investigated. Nevertheless, age of initiation of breast cancer screening and frequency of screening remain controversial. This controversy reflects the tension between the potential benefits of early cancer detection and the potential harms of overtreating benign and slow-growing lesions, particularly in 40–49-year-old women who as a cohort will undergo many diagnostic procedures to achieve a small increment in breast cancer diagnosis.

Most common cancers are not the target of screening programs. Neither ovarian nor endometrial cancer fit the WHO criteria. Ovarian cancer, with a 5-year survival of just 45.6 percent in 2015, has the highest case fatality rate of all reproductive tract malignancies [2]. Unfortunately, even in high-risk women the preclinical stage cannot be reliably detected early enough to prevent morbidity and mortality. Endometrial

cancer, with nearly 55,000 new cases in the United States in 2015, is more than twice as common as cervical or ovarian cancer; the 5-year survival rate is 82 percent [2]. Endometrial cancer is expected to become more frequent in the future as population body mass index (BMI) increases [3]. The natural history of most endometrial cancers allows for early diagnosis and successful treatment. There is no benefit to screening women who do not have abnormal uterine bleeding, as it was found in studies of asymptomatic high-risk women taking tamoxifen for breast cancer [4].

Diseases other than cancer can also be enormously burdensome for patients, costly to society, and fit the criteria for population-based screening. Prevention of hip fractures begins with nutritional and lifestyle counseling to achieve and maintain optimal bone mass (primary prevention), continues with detection of preclinical disease through screening for osteoporosis (secondary prevention), and later includes treatment of early disease (an atraumatic or "pathologic" fracture) to prevent subsequent fractures and further morbidity (tertiary prevention). Pathologic hip fracture can result in premature death and follows

19

BOX 3.1 World Health Organization Criteria for Screening Programs. The WHO criteria are used worldwide to inform governmental decisions about which diseases should be the target of publicly funded screening programs.

1. The condition should be an important health problem.
2. There should be a treatment for the condition.
3. Facilities for diagnosis and treatment should be available.
4. There should be a latent stage of the disease.
5. There should be a test or examination for the condition.
6. The test should be acceptable to the population.
7. The natural history of the disease should be adequately understood.
8. There should be an agreed policy on whom to treat.
9. The total cost of finding a case should be economically balanced in relation to medical expenditure as a whole.
10. Case-finding should be a continuous process, not just a "once–and-for-all" project.

Source: Jenabi, E. and Poorolajal J. The effect of body mass index on endometrial cancer: a meta-analysis. *Public Health*. May 27, 2015. doi: 10.1016/j.puhe.2015.04.017 [Epub ahead of print].

many years of bone loss, allowing multiple opportunities for detection and intervention. There are effective screening tests to detect osteoporosis prior to a hip fracture, and there are effective interventions to stabilize bone mass and reduce fracture risk.

Decisions about prevention strategies also depend on the existence of effective interventions. In many instances, outcomes data are scarce and extrapolation is risky. Interventions proven effective for secondary prevention are typically not tested as interventions for primary prevention, and it is usually unclear if generalization is possible. For instance, a drug effective for secondary prevention of osteoporotic fractures cannot be assumed to be effective for primary prevention. For a variety of reasons, there is no hard-and-fast rule that an intervention effective in reducing recurrence of disease also works to prevent the initial occurrence. Alendronate, a bisphosphonate, reduces hip fracture in women who have been diagnosed with low bone density or have already had a vertebral fracture (secondary prevention), but does not prevent hip fracture in women with normal bone density who have not had a vertebral fracture (primary prevention) [5]. In

contradistinction, statins are effective as primary prevention in people with hyperlipidemia but without evidence of cardiovascular disease, just as they are in people with existing cardiovascular disease [6].

Deaths in 2013 from heart disease (611,105) exceeded deaths from all cancers (584,881) in the United States [7]. Obesity, diabetes, hyperlipidemia, and chronic hypertension produce a wide range of modifiable morbidities including heart disease, stroke, renal insufficiency, and cognitive impairment. Detecting these diseases at a preclinical stage (secondary prevention) or before they create end organ damage (tertiary prevention) is effective due to highly available and relatively inexpensive screening tests and effective interventions. The well-woman visit provides opportunities for primary and secondary prevention of these chronic diseases.

Role of the Well-Woman Visit

At the well-woman visit, prevention strategies are tailored to the patient's age and risk factors and take a number of different forms. We may counsel women to promote healthy behavior and stop high-risk behavior, hoping to prevent the occurrence of obesity, cardiovascular morbidity, unplanned pregnancy, or preterm delivery. We may offer vaccinations to immunize women against infectious diseases and to promote herd immunity to facilitate eradication of specific infectious diseases. We may perform or facilitate screening for diabetes, hyperlipidemia, osteoporosis, breast cancer, and cervical cancer, as well as depression and intimate partner violence, hoping to effect early diagnosis and treatment.

The well-woman visit is a focused opportunity to provide prevention interventions. Because patients respect and value advice from their physicians, we play a critical role in motivating patients to improve their health. Behavioral counseling and motivational interviewing are important tools (covered in detail in Chapter 5), but are more effective for some diseases than for others. Motivational interviewing is a particular type of counseling in which patients are guided to confront and resolve their ambivalence to change health behavior. Motivational interviewing sessions as brief as 10 minutes may increase the likelihood of smoking cessation by 26 percent compared to brief advice or usual care; motivational interviewing by a primary care physician is more effective than when provided by a counselor [8]. Behavioral counseling combined with pharmacotherapy is more effective for smoking cessation than usual care [9]. For substance abuse, however, motivational interviewing is no more effective than usual care [10].

Cervical cancer prevention illustrates a variety of other prevention strategies that can be provided at the well-woman visit. Primary prevention starts with vaccination against high-risk human papillomavirus (HPV) subtypes but also includes advice to delay first sexual intercourse, minimize the number of sexual partners, use safe sex practices, and refrain from tobacco smoking. Secondary prevention includes detection of patients infected with high-risk HPV types or with precancerous cytologic changes and treatment of patients with high-grade squamous intraepithelial lesions (HSILs) before cancer emerges. As specialists in women's health, we realize that some strategies may have benefits extending beyond a single problem like cervical cancer prevention. Smoking cessation will also prevent a multitude of cardiovascular and pulmonary and infectious diseases. Consistent use of safe sex practices may decrease the risk of cervical pathology and infectious diseases. Effecting behavior change may require skillful counseling discussions extending over several well-woman visits.

Prevention strategies directed at individual patients are supplemented by strategies directed at populations. Some of these population-based strategies have enormous impact. Insufficient drinking water, sanitation, and hygiene were responsible for over half a million deaths from diarrheal diseases in low- and middle-income countries in 2012 [11]. In a high-resource setting like the United States, we may take for granted the availability of clean water, effective sanitation, and universal access to vaccinations. Before there was a vaccine against measles, nearly everyone in the United States became infected with the disease and hundreds died each year. In 2004, only 1 case of diphtheria was reported to the Centers for Disease Control and Prevention (CDC) compared with 15,000 deaths from diphtheria in 1921. In 2012, only 9 cases of rubella were reported to the CDC, but an epidemic less than 50 years prior infected 12.5 million Americans and resulted in 11,000 miscarriages and 2,000 infant deaths [12]. Public service announcements, media campaigns, and health insurance incentives can raise awareness about the harms of smoking, excessive alcohol consumption, drug abuse, obesity, and inactivity to motivate behavior change and create synergy with our individual efforts at the well-woman visits.

Screening Tests: Distinguishing Good from Bad

Screening tests are used to detect precursors of disease or presymptomatic "occult" disease. The ideal screening test is inexpensive, easy to administer, and causes minimal discomfort. It is also reliable (consistent across testing situations) and valid (able to distinguish disease from nondisease). The validity of a screening test relies on its accuracy, sensitivity, and specificity (Table 3.2). Evaluating the validity of a test requires a gold standard so the test results can be compared to a true positive and true negative. The gold standard can be a diagnostic laboratory test, pathologic diagnosis, or convergence of other data. Test accuracy is the percent of the total population for which the test provided true positive and true negative results. Sensitivity is defined as the proportion of patients with the disorder in whom the test result is positive. We can rely on highly sensitive tests to rule out disease because nearly all true cases are detected. We can rely on highly specific tests to rule in disease because there are so few false positives. The overall performance of a test can be depicted on a receiver operating characteristic (ROC) curve, which plots sensitivity on the y-axis (ranging from 0 to 1.00) as a function of the false positive rate on the x-axis (ranging from 0 to 1.00) (Figure 3.1). The area under the curve (AUC) reflects the trade-offs between detecting all true cases (sensitivity) and false positive cases (1 − specificity). In the example of a useless test (upper figure), there is one false positive result for each true positive result. The ROC curve is a line with slope of 1 and the AUC is 0.50 of the total graphical area. In the example of a high-performing test (lower figure), 9 true positives are identified for each false positive, yielding a very steep ROC curve with an AUC of 0.90 indicating an extremely accurate test.

Sequential testing strategies have been developed to make up for the limitations of single screening tests. Imperfect, inexpensive, and safer screening tests may be used as a first step with more definitive, expensive, and potentially harmful diagnostic testing to follow if the screening test is positive. Detection of fetal aneuploidy is a good example of the sequential approach to screening and diagnostic testing. For trisomy 21, traditional serum screening with biomarkers is 80–95 percent sensitive and 95–97 percent specific. Patients with a positive screening test are offered a diagnostic chorionic villus sampling or amniocentesis, which is

Table 3.2 Important Characteristics for Evaluating Test Validity. At the center is a 2 × 2 table depicting screening test results against a gold standard for diagnosis. The four cells comprise true positive, false positive, true negative, and false negative test results. Sensitivity, specificity, PPV, NPV, and test accuracy are defined using the information in the 2 × 2 table.

		Actual Disease Status (Based on Diagnostic Gold Standard)		Predictive Values of a Screening Test Result
		Positive	**Negative**	
Screening test result	Positive	True positive *a*	False positive *b*	PPV = True Positives / All Screened Positive = *a* / (*a* + *b*)
	Negative	False negative *c*	True negative *d*	NPV = True Negatives / All Screened Negative = *d* / (*c* + *d*)
Sensitivity, specificity, and accuracy of a screening test		Sensitivity = True Positives / All with Disease = *a* / (*a* + *c*)	Specificity = True Negatives / All without Disease = *d* / (*b* + *d*)	Test accuracy = (True Positives + True Negatives) / All Who Were Screened = (*a* + *d*) / (*a* + *b* + *c* + *d*)
		1 − Sensitivity = False Negative Rate	1 − Specificity = False Positive Rate	

PPV = positive predictive value; NPV = negative predictive value

99.99 percent sensitive and over 99 percent specific. Recent advances in technology have created a variety of noninvasive prenatal tests (NIPTs), which have greater than 99 percent sensitivity and specificity for trisomy 21, but perform less well for other aneuploidies. A recent study of 19,000 women compared cell-free DNA (cf-DNA) screening to routine screening with first-trimester nuchal translucency testing and biochemical markers. Screening results were compared against a gold standard defined by diagnostic genetic testing (amniocentesis or chorionic villus sampling) or newborn examination. Both screening modalities performed well for detection of trisomy 21, but cf-DNA was superior with an AUC of 0.999 compared with 0.958 for routine screening [13]. Despite these outstanding test characteristics, NIPT is still considered a screening test and can create false positive results particularly in a low-risk population. The American College of Obstetrics and Gynecology (ACOG) recommends that a positive cf-DNA result be followed by diagnostic chorionic villus sampling or amniocentesis to confirm the presence of trisomy 21 (particularly if it will affect pregnancy management), detect other aneuploidies, and understand the type of trisomy for recurrence risk counseling [14].

It is easier to make up for low test specificity than low sensitivity. Screening tests with low specificity produce many false positive results and are usually followed by a highly specific diagnostic or confirmatory test. For example, the most common HIV screening test is an enzyme-linked immunosorbent assay (ELISA), which is highly sensitive but less specific. A positive ELISA is followed by a highly specific "confirmatory" diagnostic test such as the Western blot or immunofluorescence test, which can be run on the same sample. Gestational diabetes is an example of sequential testing, which extends over several visits, first with a simple 1-hour glucose challenge test (screening) and then with a more complex 3-hour glucose tolerance test (diagnosis) to minimize false positive diagnoses. In contradistinction, if a screening test has imperfect sensitivity, it will fail to detect disease. The cumulative probability of detecting disease improves with each subsequent screening test and is a reasonable strategy when the disease has a long preclinical lead time. A single mammogram has a sensitivity of 77–95 percent and specificity of 94–97 percent [15]. A single Pap test has only moderate sensitivity (55 percent) but high specificity (97 percent) [16], whereas three successive Pap tests have approximately 90 percent sensitivity.

The likelihood ratio (LR) is a useful way to summarize the value of positive and negative test results. The LR (+) describes how the pretest probability is transformed when the test is abnormal. The LR (−) describes how the pretest probability is transformed when the test is normal. There are conceptual and mathematical ways to understand LRs (Table 3.3). Conceptually, LRs represent trade-offs between correct classification and erroneous classification for positive and negative test results. The LR (+) describes the test's ability to detect all people with true disease

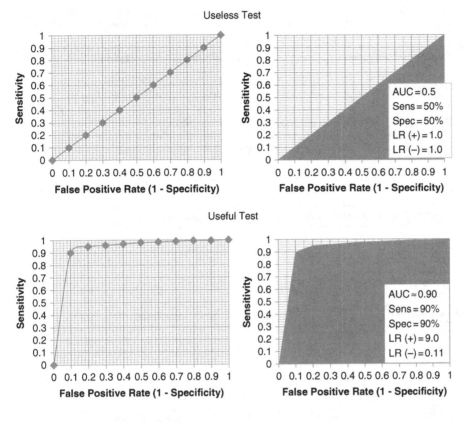

AUC: Area Under the ROC Curve (range, 0.00 to 1.00)

Sens = Sensitivity (range, 0–100%)

Spec = Specificity (range, 0–100%)

LR(+) = Positive Likelihood Ratio (range, 1.0–∞)

LR(–) = Negative Likelihood Ratio (range, 1.0–0)

Figure 3.1 Receiver Operating Characteristic (ROC) Curves. The ROC curves plot test sensitivity as a function of false positive results. The top panel depicts the performance of a useless test with low sensitivity and specificity in which each detected case of disease (sensitivity) is accompanied by a false positive result (1 – specificity); the AUC measuring accuracy for the useless test is 50 percent. The bottom panel depicts the performance of a useful test with high sensitivity and specificity with an AUC of 0.90.

relative to the price paid in false positives. The LR (–) describes the price paid in false negatives relative to the test's ability to detect all true disease-free people. The best tests have an LR (+) of 10 or more and an LR (–) of 0.1 or less.

Figure 3.2 depicts the practical impact of LRs on transforming the pretest probability (prevalence) to a hopefully more useful and precise posttest probability of disease. A useless test is depicted in the top panel as a nonrefracting lens through which the pretest probability passes unaltered. The useless test has an LR (+) and LR (–) of 1.0 meaning that the test result does nothing to change the probability of disease from

what it is in the population. Left with no additional information to inform decision-making, we are likely to pursue additional tests. The concave lens in the bottom panel represents a useful test, which refracts the probability based upon the test results and differentiates patients who are diseased and nondiseased. A positive test, while not perfect, gives us what we need to discuss treatment with the patient. A negative result, while not perfect, gives us enough information to not offer treatment and not do further testing.

The ROC curves in Figure 3.1 provide another way to understand LR. The LR (+) is the slope of the ROC curve. In the example of the useless test, the slope is 1.0

Table 3.3 Likelihood Ratios: Definition and Interpretation. The LRs summarize how well a test performs when its results are positive (LR+) or negative (LR−). The table provides conceptual and mathematical definitions of LR+ and LR−. The LRs transform the pretest probability into posttest probability that disease is present or absent.

	Conceptual Definition	Calculation/Interpretation
LR (+)	The test's ability to detect all people with disease relative to the price paid in false positives.	Sensitivity / (1 − Specificity) Range: 1−∞ HIGHER is BETTER
LR (−)	The price paid in false negatives relative to the test's ability to detect all disease-free people.	(1 − Sensitivity) / Specificity Range: 0−1 LOWER is BETTER

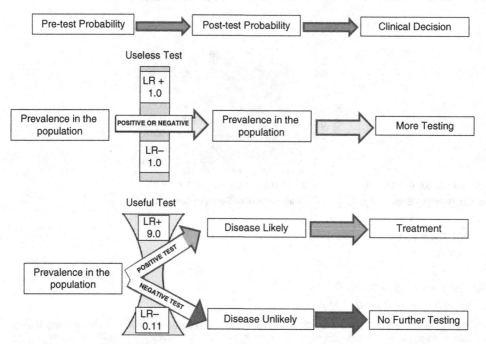

Figure 3.2 Likelihood Ratios in Action. The quality of a test is depicted as a lens which transforms a pretest probability (prevalence) into a posttest probability. The useless test (upper panel) (LR+ = 1.0 and LR− = 1.0) is depicted as a nonrefracting lens through which the pretest probability passes unaltered. The useful test (lower panel) (LR+ = 9.0 and LR− = 0.11) is depicted as a concave lens causing the pretest probability to diverge into a posttest probability high enough to warrant treatment if positive, or low enough to warrant no treatment or further testing if negative.

because each additional true positive comes with a false positive. In the example of the useful test, the slope in the initial part of the curve is 9.0, which represents the ratio of true positives to false positives. When there is a range of possible cut-points for defining a positive test, the LR changes depending on which value is being used as the cutoff. In the example in Figure 3.1, the cutoff would correspond to the value at which sensitivity is 0.9 and specificity is 0.9 (false positive = 0.1).

Interpreting Test Results: The Importance of Risk Status

The meaning of individual test results varies according to the prevalence of the disease and the patient's risk for that disease. During the well-woman visit, we will mostly screen women who have an average risk of disease. As an example, the pretest probability of cervical cancer (or HSIL) in women with an average risk should be the same as the prevalence of this disease in the population. Because Pap and HPV tests are high-quality screening tools, their results transform the pretest probability into a more informed estimate of whether the patient has HSIL or cancer, the "positive predictive value" (PPV) of the test. Negative Pap and HPV tests transform the pretest probability into a posttest probability so low that colposcopy is not indicated. This is the negative predictive value (NPV) of the test. If instead we screened women with a higher risk of HSIL and cancer than the general population, such as women with a recent history of HSIL diagnosed by colposcopy and treated with loop electrosurgical excision procedure (LEEP), the PPV of the test would be higher (more true positives to find) and the NPV of the test would be lower (fewer true negatives to find). We would be likely to perform colposcopy for a positive test, and a single negative test wouldn't completely reassure us, leading to recommendations for more frequent screening in the initial post-LEEP surveillance period. If instead we screened a low-risk population for disease, the impact on the PPV and NPV would be different. Annual screening of postmenopausal women for chlamydia would reduce the PPV of the test when compared to annual screening of women aged 25 or younger (as recommended by the CDC and ACOG). The prevalence of chlamydia infection in postmenopausal women is so low that the test is more likely to generate false positive results. For the same reason (low prevalence), the NPV would be outstanding. The pretest probability of not having chlamydia would be exceedingly high in this age group, and a negative test result would make it even higher. The principle that disease prevalence alters the PPV and NPV of test results is one of the reasons why chlamydia and cervical cancer screening recommendations are not the same in younger and older women.

Very high-risk patients do not represent the general population. In some cases, application of screening tests to this population is termed "case-finding" as opposed to screening to indicate that they are already under surveillance for the disease. The higher prevalence of disease makes a positive test more likely to be accurate than it would be an average-risk population. For example, a meta-analysis estimated the effectiveness of office-based screening for depression using questionnaires. Five randomized trials including nearly 6,000 high-risk patients showed a 27 percent increase in detection of depression (vs. no questionnaire), a statistically significant improvement. However, 7 randomized trials comprising nearly 5,500 unselected patients showed no increase in detection of depression [17]. This difference in screening effectiveness is likely due to the greater prevalence of depression in the high-risk patients, making positive screening results more likely to be true positives.

Serum CA-125 testing is not used to screen the population for ovarian cancer. However, application of this test to low- versus high-risk women with pelvic masses illustrates the relationship between disease prevalence and the predictive value of test results. CA-125 is not very useful in triaging benign from malignant masses in premenopausal women. Other tissues make CA-125, there are more physiologic ovarian cysts, and there is low prevalence of ovarian cancer in younger women with pelvic masses, all of which drive up the false positive rate. The prevalence of ovarian cancer in postmenopausal women with pelvic masses is higher and there are fewer physiologic reasons for CA-125 to be elevated. A study stratifying test performance by menopausal status found CA-125 elevation to have a PPV of 98 percent in postmenopausal women with masses (cancer prevalence of 63 percent), but only 49 percent in premenopausal women (cancer prevalence of 15 percent) [18]. The Society for Gynecologic Oncology guidelines reflect this distinction. Referral is recommended for *any* CA-125 elevation in women aged 50 or older but reserved for marked elevation (CA-125 levels >200 units/mL) in women younger than 50 years [19]. Raising the threshold value for younger women increases test specificity and decreases the number of women unnecessarily referred to a gynecologic oncologist.

The Yin and Yang: Overstated Benefits, Overdiagnosis, and Overtreatment

Doctor, should I go get a whole body CT scan? How about free carotid artery screening? Isn't it better to know if I have a ticking time bomb so I can do something to prevent it from killing me? The answer to these questions is a resounding "no" because abnormal findings on these tests are unlikely to signify an actual threat to the patient's health [20]. The goal of screening programs is to reduce mortality and morbidity while minimizing the costs and harms of screening. Early detection of some diseases and precursors can produce harms while not reducing morbidity and mortality. A well-known example of this phenomenon was the prior practice screening women less than 21 years for cervical cancer. Teenage girls have 1–2 cervical cancer cases per million girls per year [21], an extremely low risk. Despite cytologic abnormalities, particularly low-grade squamous intraepithelial lesion (LSIL), being relatively common, the high spontaneous resolution of lesions and low cancer risk makes screening this population ineffective, as evidenced by studies showing no decrease in cancer in this age group when screened [22]. Evidence on the natural history of HPV infection in this age group and the potential impact of treatment on subsequent pregnancy resulted in a US Preventive Services Task Force (USPSTF) "D" recommendation against screening for cervical cancer in women younger than 21 years because the harms outweigh the benefits [23].

There are several common biases that falsely inflate the apparent performance of some tests. Screening can appear to increase life expectancy by increasing the number of years an individual is aware they have cancer. Screening all 80-year-old women with mammography would identify women with early breast cancer who may die of other causes in the next 10 years. Screened women will live longer with a cancer diagnosis than unscreened women who present later with symptoms, creating an erroneous impression that screening improved survival (*lead time bias*). Another kind of bias occurs because indolent, slow-growing tumors can be present for many years before they are clinically detectable. The longer the time from preclinical detection to clinical findings, the greater the chance a screening program will detect the tumor. Aggressive tumors have a shorter presymptomatic window. Consequently, screening programs are more likely to detect less aggressive lesions. When this occurs, attributing longer survival to the screening program is an example of *length bias*.

Understandably, because cancer is difficult to control, we may tend to overtreat cancer precursors before there is sufficient evidence to clarify which precursors are dangerous enough to warrant treatment. Overdiagnosis refers to the detection of disease that would not have become clinically evident in a person's lifetime. Overtreatment also refers to treatment of a disease or its precursor that would not have created morbidity if left untreated. For many decades, CIN-1 lesions were treated rather than followed. More evidence then became available to understand the natural history of HPV infection and clearance, as well as the pregnancy consequences of excisional and ablative cervical procedures. Consequently, we no longer treat women with CIN-1 as it has low cancer risk and typically spontaneously clears with observation. Efforts to detect early breast cancer may also produce unintended harms, particularly for women in their forties who are more likely than older women to have false positive results and benign lesions detected, culminating in unnecessary interventions, patient anxiety, and cost.

Breast cancer prevention is faced with additional challenges. Ductal carcinoma in situ (DCIS) is a premalignant lesion, and it is estimated that 25–50 percent will progress to invasive cancer if untreated. A recent analysis of the Surveillance, Epidemiology and End Results (SEER) database from 1988 to 2011 identified that 98 percent of 57,222 DCIS cases were managed with total mastectomy, or with partial mastectomy and whole breast radiotherapy. However, the survival benefit of surgical care varied substantially according to the nuclear grade of the lesions. A 10-year breast cancer-specific survival with low-grade DCIS was 98.6 percent for the surgically treated group and 98.8 percent for the nonsurgically treated group. Surgery was associated with a small survival benefit for intermediate-grade DCIS (98.6 percent vs. 94.6 percent) and a larger benefit for high-grade DCIS (98.4 percent vs. 90.5 percent) [24]. The implications for these findings are important for all women, and particularly for women screened for breast cancer prior to age 50. The increase in breast cancer screening from 1973 to 2011 was associated with increased incidence of DCIS from 5.83 per 100,000 women to 35.54 per 100,000. Screening women younger than 50 years further increases the rate of DCIS diagnosis. The authors of the SEER study estimate that there will be over 1 million women in the United States living with DCIS by 2020. Over half of these women will have low-grade (over 150,000) or intermediate-grade (over 380,000) tumors. Until the relative effectiveness of surveillance versus aggressive treatment is established in prospective studies, detection of DCIS lesions through screening is likely to produce an enormous amount of morbidity and cost without proven benefit.

The Role of Individual Preferences in Screening Decisions

Many screening programs come with trade-offs between the benefits of early detection of diseases, which can shorten or diminish the patient's quality of life, and the harms of overtreating benign and precursor diseases that are unlikely to cause morbidity. These trade-offs are important to discuss with patients so their individual preferences can be elicited and used to inform a decision reflecting their priorities and concerns. As specialists in women's health, we play a crucial role in explaining screening recommendations and trade-offs. This duty becomes challenging when professional societies make different screening recommendations based upon the same body of evidence, as occurred with breast cancer screening. Because breast cancer is so common, most patients know an individual with the disease, and that knowledge can increase their awareness, personal anxiety, and willingness to accept the potential harms of early screening. The American Cancer Society's guideline from 2015 recommends that average-risk women aged 40–44 should have the choice to start annual breast cancer screening with mammograms if desired, that women aged 45–54 should receive annual mammography, and that women aged 55 and older should be offered to continue annual screening or switch to biennial mammography [25]. In early 2016, the USPSTF updated its position to recommend biennial mammography for women aged 50–74 (Grade B recommendation: at least moderate net benefit). Cautioning against the harms of screening including false positive results and unnecessary biopsies, the USPSTF concluded that the decision to start screening before age 50 should be made in partnership between women and their doctors (Grade C recommendation: small net benefit). The USPSTF website includes its final recommendations as well as resources to assist patients and health care providers in discussing the trade-offs of breast screening, including overdiagnosis and overtreatment [26].

Case Scenarios

1. *You are recruited by your county health department to participate in an expert panel charged to make recommendations for reducing preterm birth in your community, which is approaching 10 percent of live births, an all-time high. What strategies for prevention can you recommend, and which can be implemented at the well-woman visit?*

    Once pregnancy is underway, many opportunities for primary prevention have been missed. Although interventions for patients with a history of preterm birth can reduce the risk of recurrent preterm birth, there are many other initiatives the public health department can support. Efforts at primary prevention include community-based interventions such as public service announcements, insurance incentives, and workplace policies to minimize smoking. Removing reimbursement barriers to immediate postpartum long-acting reversible contraception (LARC) will decrease the risk of short interpregnancy interval and the burden of preterm birth from unplanned pregnancy.

    At the well-woman visit, we can reduce the risk of preterm birth by counseling about smoking cessation, healthy weight and nutrition, pregnancy spacing, and the use of effective contraception. We can coordinate care to optimize the control of chronic medical conditions that predispose to preterm birth and pregnancy loss. These community-based and individual efforts at primary prevention are just as important as interventions once a high-risk pregnancy is underway, and produce additional benefits to women's health beyond their impact on preterm birth.

2. *An 18-year-old who became sexually active presents for her first well-woman visit, accompanied by her mother. She has completed her HPV vaccination series and requests Pap and HPV testing. You explain that we don't begin cervical cancer screening until age 21. The patient's mother tells you about her own history of HSIL. In the past year, she had an ASC-H Pap result with positive HPV reflex testing followed by colposcopy and loop excision. She is worried about her daughter and has urged her to be screened now that she is sexually active. How will you explain why we don't offer Pap and HPV testing to her daughter?*

The key points in your counseling could include the following:

- Cervical cancer is an important disease to prevent. Fortunately, it takes a long time for HPV infection to create lasting changes in the cervix and for cancer to develop. This long timeline gives us multiple opportunities to find those changes early and prevent cancer.

- Early screening may cause unnecessary worry by detecting changes on the Pap smear that are temporary. Most go away as the patient's immune system clears the virus, which is why the guidelines have changed and we now delay cervical cancer screening until age 21.
- It is fantastic that your daughter completed the HPV vaccination, as it will greatly reduce her risk of becoming infected with the types of HPV which cause cervical cancer and will also reduce her risk of genital warts.

3. *A 27-year-old nulliparous woman comes to your office for a well-woman visit. Her 53-year-old godmother was recently diagnosed with ovarian cancer. She found a recent publication reporting the success of a new biomarker panel for detecting ovarian cancer in woman with a family history of the disease (defined as one first-degree relative with ovarian cancer before age 50). Despite not having a family history of ovarian or breast cancer herself, the patient requests being tested. You schedule a follow-up visit and download the publication to learn more. The biomarker panel had 90 percent sensitivity and 90 percent specificity, and the AUC was 0.90. The authors concluded, "The new biomarker panel is extremely accurate for detecting ovarian cancer with only 10 percent false positives." When the patient returns for her follow-up visit, how will you respond to her request?*

Before concluding that the test would work equally well with an individual patient, we need to compare the lifetime risk of ovarian cancer in the study population and the individual patient. We go back to the article and find that 10 percent of the patients ultimately developed ovarian cancer based on a histopathological gold standard. Because the patient has no personal or family history of ovarian cancer, her risk is closer to the general population prevalence of 1.3 percent [2] than it is to 10 percent. Altering the disease prevalence has huge impact on the PPV and NPV. Using the test in low-risk patients will create more false positives, driving downward the predictive value and LR of positive test results. In addition to acknowledging her concerns, your counseling could attempt to guide the patient's interest from detecting early ovarian cancer (secondary prevention) to making decisions which could prevent the development of ovarian cancer (primary prevention).

- The risk of developing ovarian cancer in your lifetime is the same as the risk for all women: 1 in 77 women (1.3 percent).
- There are things you can do to reduce your risk, such as using birth control pills, having multiple children, and breastfeeding your children.
- Less than 1 in 300 women carry a genetic mutation that increases their risk of ovarian cancer. Because you have no relatives with breast or ovarian cancer, you are not in a high-risk group and do not need testing for the mutation.
- Women in the biomarker study were high risk. They had a 10 percent risk of ovarian cancer, which is eight times higher than your risk. If you received the test and the result showed positive, we wouldn't be able to tell whether it is a true positive or a false positive.

The study results would be applicable to *BRCA* mutation carriers because their ovarian cancer risk (12–46 percent) is higher than the prevalence found in the study sample (10 percent). The AUC would improve as would the LR of a positive test and there would be fewer false positives. However, the patient in the scenario did not qualify for *BRCA* testing based upon her history. According to a joint recommendation by the ACOG and Society for Gynecologic Oncology, testing is warranted when there is at least a 20–25 percent chance of having an inherited predisposition to breast or ovarian cancer [27].

Summary

- The well-woman visit is a critical opportunity for primary and secondary prevention.
- Primary prevention, such as risk factor modification and vaccination, succeeds by preventing the onset of disease.
- Secondary prevention, exemplified by screening tests, aims to identify disease precursors and occult disease in time to prevent symptomatic disease.
- Population-based prevention strategies such as clean water, effective sanitation, school-based vaccinations, and universal access to preventive health care can markedly improve the health status of the population.
- Commonly used criteria for screening focus on a disease's impact on morbidity and mortality, the availability of effective diagnosis and treatment, the length of the latent stage of disease, an effective and acceptable screening test, an understanding of

the disease's natural history, and the net cost of screening (factoring in benefits and harms).

- Optimal screening tests identify most patients with disease (high sensitivity) with a minimum of false positive results (high specificity) and are at least 90 percent accurate in classifying patients as having or not having the disease.
- The ROC curve plots test sensitivity against the false positive rate (1 – specificity) and depicts test accuracy as the AUC.
- Applying results of an optimal test to individual patients transforms their pretest probability of disease into a posttest probability high enough to warrant treatment or low enough to warrant no treatment and no further testing.
- Identifying whether the patient's pretest probability is different from the population used to validate the test is important. The prevalence of disease (pretest probability) affects the predictive value of a positive or negative test. As prevalence increases, the predictive value of a positive test will increase and there will be fewer false positives. As prevalence decreases, the predictive value of a positive test will decrease and there will be more false positive results.
- False positive screening test results can lead to harmful interventions, particularly in low-risk patients. The age at first screening for cervical cancer changed to 21 years once the natural history of HPV infection and the harms of overdiagnosis were better understood. Screening cohorts of low-risk women for breast cancer is also likely to produce more harms than benefits.
- Patient preferences should be elicited to inform screening decisions in light of individual differences in how patients value the trade-offs between potential benefits and harms of screening tests.

References

1. Wilson, J.M.G. and Jungner, G. Principles and practice of screening for disease. *WHO Chronicle. Geneva: World Health Organization.* 1968, **22**(11):473. Public Health Papers, #34.

2. National Cancer Institute. Surveillance, Epidemiology, and End Results program: Cancer statistics. Available at: www.seer.cancer.gov. Retrieved August 29, 2015.

3. Jenabi, E. and Poorolajal, J. The effect of body mass index on endometrial cancer: A meta-analysis. *Public Health.* May 27, 2015. doi: 10.1016/j.puhe.2015.04.017 [Epub ahead of print].

4. American College of Obstetricians and Gynecologists. Tamoxifen and uterine cancer. Committee Opinion No. 601. *Obstet Gynecol.* 2014, **123**:1394–7.

5. Wells, G.A., Cranney, A., Peterson, J. et al. Alendronate for the primary and secondary prevention of osteoporotic fractures in postmenopausal women. *Cochrane Database Syst Rev.* 2008, (**1**):CD001155. doi: 10.1002/14651858.CD001155.pub2.

6. Taylor, F., Huffman, M.D., Macedo, A.F. et al. Statins for the primary prevention of cardiovascular disease. *Cochrane Database Syst Rev.* 2013, (**1**):CD004816. doi: 10.1002/14651858.CD004816.pub5.

7. Centers for Disease Control and Prevention. Leading causes of death. Available at: www.cdc.gov/nchs/fastats/leading-causes-of-death.htm. Retrieved August 29, 2015.

8. Lindson-Hawley, N., Thompson, T.P., and Begh, R. Motivational interviewing for smoking cessation. *Cochrane Database Syst Rev.* 2015, (**3**):CD006936. doi: 10.1002/14651858.CD006936.pub3.

9. Stead, L.F. and Lancaster, T. Combined pharmacotherapy and behavioural interventions for smoking cessation. *Cochrane Database Syst Rev.* 2012, (**10**):CD008286. doi: 10.1002/14651858.CD008286.pub2.

10. Smedslund, G., Berg, R.C., Hammerstrøm, K.T. et al. Motivational interviewing for substance abuse. *Cochrane Database Syst Rev.* 2011, (**5**):CD008063. doi: 10.1002/14651858.CD008063.pub2.

11. World Health Organization. Preventing diarrhoea through better water, sanitation and hygiene: exposures and impacts in low- and middle-income countries. 2014. Available at: www.who.int/water_sanitation_health/gbd_poor_water/en/. Retrieved August 25, 2015.

12. Centers for Disease Control and Prevention. What would happen if we stopped vaccinations? 2014. Available at: www.cdc.gov/vaccines/vac-gen/whatifstop.htm. Retrieved August 25, 2015.

13. Norton, M.E., Jacobsson, B., Swamy, G.K. et al. Cell-free DNA analysis for noninvasive examination of trisomy. *N Engl J Med.* 2015, **372**(17):1589–97.

14. American College of Obstetricians and Gynecologists. Cell-free DNA screening for fetal aneuploidy. Committee Opinion No. 640. *Obstet Gynecol.* 2015, **126**:e31–7.

15. Humphrey, L.L., Helfand, M., Chan, B.K., and Woolf, S.H. Breast cancer screening: A summary of the evidence for the US Preventive Services Task Force. *Ann Intern Med.* 2002, **137**:347–60.

16. Mayrand, M.H., Duarte-Franco, E., Rodrigues, I. et al.; Canadian Cervical Cancer Screening Trial Study Group. Human papillomavirus DNA versus

papanicolaou screening tests for cervical cancer. *N Engl J Med*. 2007, **357**(16):1579–88.

17. Gilbody, S., Sheldon, T., and House, A. Screening and case-finding instruments for depression: A meta-analysis. *CMAJ*. 2008, **178**(8):997–1003.

18. Malkasian, G.D. Jr., Knapp, R.C., Lavin, P.T. et al. Preoperative evaluation of serum CA 125 levels in premenopausal and postmenopausal patients with pelvic masses: Discrimination of benign from malignant disease. *Am J Obstet Gynecol*. 1988, **159**(2):341–6.

19. Im, S.S., Gordon, A.N., Buttin, B.M. et al. Validation of referral guidelines for women with pelvic masses. *Obstet Gynecol*. 2005, **105**(1):35–41.

20. US Preventive Services Task Force. Carotid artery stenosis: Screening. July 2014. Available at: www.uspreventiveservicestaskforce.org/Page/Document/UpdateSummaryFinal/carotid-artery-stenosis-screening. Retrieved August 29, 2015.

21. American College of Obstetricians and Gynecologists. Screening for cervical cancer. Practice Bulletin No. 131. *Obstet Gynecol*. 2012, **120**:1222–38.

22. Sasieni, P., Castanon, A., and Cuzick, J. Effectiveness of cervical screening with age: Population based case–control study of prospectively recorded data [published erratum appears in BMJ 2009;339: b3115]. *BMJ*. 2009, **339**:b2968.

23. US Preventive Services Task Force Recommendation. Cervical cancer: Screening. March 2012. Available at: www.uspreventiveservicestaskforce.org/Page/Document/UpdateSummaryFinal/cervical-cancer-screening. Retrieved September 26, 2015.

24. Sagara, Y., Mallory, M.A., Wong, S. et al. Survival benefit of breast surgery for low-grade ductal carcinoma in situ: A population-based cohort study. *JAMA Surg*. 2015, **150**(8):739–45.

25. American Cancer Society. Breast cancer prevention and early detection. Available at: www.cancer.org/cancer/breastcancer/moreinformation/breastcancerearlydetection/breast-cancer-early-detection-acs-recs. Retrieved May 10, 2016.

26. US Preventive Services Task Force. Breast cancer screening: Final recommendation statement. www.uspreventiveservicestaskforce.org/Page/Document/UpdateSummaryFinal/breast-cancer-screening1?ds=1&s=Breast cancer. Retrieved March 7, 2017.

27. American College of Obstetricians and Gynecologists. Hereditary breast and ovarian cancer syndrome. Practice Bulletin No. 103. *Obstet Gynecol*. 2009, **113**:957–66.

Suggested Reading

Bhandari, M. and Guyatt, G.H. How to appraise a diagnostic test. *World J Surg*. 2005, **29**(5):561–6.

Cox, B. and Sneyd, M.J. Bias in breast cancer research in the screening era. *Breast*. 2013, **22**(6):1041–5.

Goetzinger, K.R. and Odibo, A.O. Statistical analysis and interpretation of prenatal diagnostic imaging studies, Part 1: Evaluating the efficiency of screening and diagnostic tests. *J Ultrasound Med*. 2011, **30**(8):1121–7.

Grimes, D.A. and Schulz, K.F. Refining clinical diagnosis with likelihood ratios. *Lancet*. 2005, **365**(9469):1500–5.

Iams, J.D., Romero, R., Culhane, J.F., and Goldenberg, R.L. Primary, secondary, and tertiary interventions to reduce the morbidity and mortality of preterm birth. *Lancet*. 2008, **371**(9607):164–75.

Chapter

4

Guidelines
Deciding What Belongs in the Well-Woman Visit

David M. Haas

Learning Objectives

- Understand how guidelines and their recommendations are used in clinical care and policy development
- Explain the sources of guideline recommendations and how they relate to the focus of the organization developing the guideline
- Understand the process of guideline development, including the initial question, data retrieval and synthesis, and the final publication
- Describe the different systems used in evaluating the quality of evidence utilized in guideline development (e.g., GRADE and USPTF)
- Locate guidelines on different topics in women's health care
- Develop tools to decide which guidelines to follow and how to implement them in clinical practice through examples

Introduction

How should we practice? What should inform our clinical decisions and recommendations for patients? Typically, providers make clinical decisions and form recommendations based on a complicated and informal synthesis of their training, habits based on clinical experience, prevailing evidence for care, special patient considerations, and local patterns. Of these, evidence of effectiveness should be a major driver. The goal of women's health providers is to optimize the health of women [1], so remaining informed of new evidence for screening, treatment, and prevention is critical. Most relevant primary evidence appears in medical journals. With over 5,600 medical journals included in Index Medicus alone, keeping up with the flow of new information in a narrow area is difficult and essentially impossible for an individual provider across an entire specialty. Keeping up with the evidence for well-woman care is especially challenging given the broad range of specialties encompassed.

Guidelines are an extremely important strategy for helping provide evidence-based, effective, quality care. They are developed to contain recommendations about health interventions and behaviors and can come from clinical, public health, or policy perspectives [2, 3]. The federal government through the US Preventive Services Task Force (USPSTF) and many major professional societies actively develop and maintain guidelines for important clinical problems. Guidelines are recommendations intended to assist providers and recipients of health care and other stakeholders to make informed decisions [2]. Practice guidelines attempt to synthesize the most relevant, highest-quality evidence to inform decisions. The quality of recommendations varies with the quality and strength of the supporting evidence [4]. Guidelines may be evidence based, evidence informed, or consensus based. Guidelines from different organizations may be derived from different perspectives or methodologies, and result in conflicting recommendations. Guidelines also need periodic updating as new evidence becomes available. Guidelines are not meant to be rigid rules that replace clinical judgment and patient autonomy. However, as guidelines often consider cost of care, health systems and insurers are increasingly looking at guideline compliance. As greater use of preventive services could save lives at little or no cost [5], compliance with guidelines is being used as a quality of care measure and could be used to guide reimbursement.

This chapter will discuss the sources of guideline recommendations, highlight the processes that various organizations use to develop guidelines, and discuss tools used to evaluate the levels of evidence and strength of recommendations. It will also provide suggestions for assessing the quality of guidelines and selecting the most appropriate from among multiple conflicting ones.

Sources of Guideline Recommendations

Guidelines are generally developed by organizations or groups that have an interest in the subject. These can be specialty societies such as the American College of Physicians or the Royal College in the United Kingdom, international organizations such as the World Health Organization (WHO), the Institute of Medicine (IOM), or governmental agencies such as the Centers for Disease Control and Prevention (CDC) or the Agency for Healthcare Research and Quality (part of the US Department of Health and Human Services). All of these organizations have a vested interest in aiding providers and consumers of health care with recommendations to optimize health.

Some organizations focus mainly on optimizing health outcomes while others also take into consideration the impact of cost of care [1, 4]. Whether or not cost considerations are taken into account in guideline recommendations is important. In the United States, it has been shown that patients may only receive about half of their recommended preventive primary care interventions [6]. Patients often receive care that is not needed or could be harmful to them [7]. For instance, years after removing recommendations for cervical cancer screening for adolescents, half of young women under the age of 21 were still receiving Pap tests [8]. As cost is often a factor in these decisions, the health system and costs surrounding health care guideline recommendations are important. Some organizations from regions of universal health coverage or that represent large health care payers may have a perspective more focused on cost of care. Other organizations may be more focused on efficacy and quality-adjusted life years as measures. Thus, the perspectives of the recommending organization may affect their recommendations even when working from the same body of evidence.

In the United States, the USPSTF is often considered the leading independent panel of experts in prevention and primary care. Their recommendations are based on rigorous, impartial assessments of the scientific evidence for the effectiveness of a broad range of clinical preventive services, including screening, counseling, and preventive medications [9]. They have provided many recommendations regarding women's health and were a principal source of guidelines assessed by the Well-Woman Task Force (WWTF) [1]. The USPSTF makes an annual report to the US Congress and their recommendations are the basis for many health care and insurance policies [9]. Under the Affordable Care Act, all preventive services recommended by the USPSTF (A or B rating) must be covered by group or individual health insurance without cost sharing. Highlighting their importance, the USPSTF recommendations are central to many decisions determining insurance coverage of tests and procedures.

Processes for Guideline Development

Effective guideline development requires formal, well-described, and transparent processes. Although organizations such as the WHO, CDC, USPSTF, American Cancer Society (ACS), and others have small variations, their guideline development processes follow similar steps (Figure 4.1).

Initially, it is determined that a guideline is needed to help synthesize evidence or incorporate new evidence into a clinical practice or public health area. Specific key questions of clinical relevance, such as "Is human papillomavirus (HPV) testing better than a Pap test for routine screening for cervical cancer?", are first selected. The specific questions are often determined by a needs assessment [2]. Developing a question for a guideline generally is modeled in a PICO (Population, Intervention, Comparison, Outcome) format. In the example above, the question might be restated as, "For women at average risk for cervical cancer who are undergoing screening, is HPV testing alone superior to Pap test alone (or co-testing) to prevent cervical cancer."

An appropriate group must be selected to be responsible for developing the guideline. Broad stakeholders and groups representing a wide array of organizations and relevant perspectives can be important during the implementation of guideline recommendations. This allows for consensus during the development, facilitating uniform distribution and, more importantly, widespread implementation across groups. Guidelines often need to speak to multiple audiences [2]. Involvement of stakeholders from many groups, including consumers, facilitates better constructed and useful guidelines. Broad stakeholder involvement in guideline development is a best practice. For instance, the ACS appoints a group of 12 members to develop guidelines. The group includes a patient advocate and health care professionals in both clinical and population health [10].

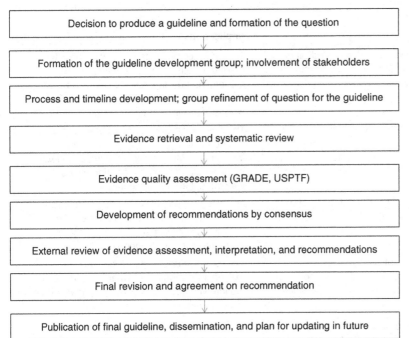

Figure 4.1 Processes for guideline development.

Once the key questions are determined, a coordinated and systematic review of all available evidence related to the question is performed. An explicit and reproducible method of exhaustively searching for primary studies on the topic and selection based on predetermined eligibility criteria is performed [2, 10, 11]. The studies are then critically appraised for quality. Typically, several group members will independently evaluate the evidence from the search, then compare findings and resolve any differences by consensus or with other members mediating. When the evidence includes data from more than a few trials and there appears to be consistency in interventions and outcomes, the findings can often be quantitatively synthesized in a meta-analysis. If a meta-analysis is not feasible, the results can be synthesized with a qualitative narrative synthesis [2, 11]. Narrative summaries typically use summary tables to display differences between important study characteristics and outcomes across studies for each key question [11].

After synthesizing and assessing the evidence in various working groups, draft recommendations for care are developed and approved by consensus of the entire guideline development group. Most organizations will then distribute these draft guidelines for external review and public comment. After external review, final revisions will be approved and the practice guideline published and disseminated widely for implementation. Plans for updating the guideline are often specified [2].

Levels of Evidence and Strength of Recommendations

During the guideline development process, the group writing the guideline evaluates the evidence for the specific intervention. Different systems have been developed to evaluate the quality of the evidence and make summary statements regarding the strength of recommendations. For instance, a recommendation based on several large randomized controlled trials all showing similar benefit to an intervention should be stronger than a recommendation based entirely on expert opinion without supportive evidence. While this example is straightforward, most bodies of data are less clear, with combinations of observational and randomized controlled studies, which may not all show consistent effects. These systems are useful for describing the degree of support for individual recommendations in a consistent and useful way. They allow the

Table 4.1 GRADE Ratings of the Certainty of Evidence

Ratings	Definitions	Implications
High	This research provides a very good indication of the likely effect. The likelihood that the effect will be substantially different is low.	This evidence provides a very good basis for making a decision about whether to implement the intervention. Impact evaluation and monitoring of the impact are unlikely to be needed if it is implemented.
Moderate	This research provides a good indication of the likely effect. The likelihood that the effect will be substantially different is moderate.	This evidence provides a good basis for making a decision about whether to implement the intervention. Monitoring of the impact is likely to be needed and impact evaluation may be warranted if it is implemented.
Low	This research provides some indication of the likely effect. However, the likelihood that it will be substantially different is high.	This evidence provides some basis for making a decision about whether to implement the intervention. Impact evaluation is likely to be warranted if it is implemented.
Very low	This research does not provide a reliable indication of the likely effect. The likelihood that the effect will be substantially different is very high.	This evidence does not provide a good basis for making a decision about whether to implement the intervention. Impact evaluation is very likely to be warranted if it is implemented.

Source: GRADE Working Group. Grading quality of evidence and strength of recommendations. BMJ. 2004, 328(7454):1490.

ability to prioritize interventions, allowing focus on the most effective methods with the best evidence for more significant problems.

The level of scientific evidence can be summarized in several ways. The individual studies obtained in the systematic search are usually evaluated and characterized based on tools such as the Cochrane Handbook methodology [12]. To assess the quality of a body of evidence and then to develop and report recommendations, WHO and many other major guideline developers use the Grading of Recommendations, Assessment, Development, and Evaluation (GRADE) approach [13]. The GRADE is a systematic and explicit approach to making judgments for evaluating evidence and recommendations (Table 4.1). It was proposed to be a single system to overcome the shortcomings of other grading systems while including their strengths. It is used as the principal system to summarize evidence and health technology assessments by a long list of international groups, including WHO, the Cochrane Collaboration, the American College of Physicians, BMJ Clinical Evidence, and the CDC's Advisory Committee on Immunization Practices. A full list can be found at www.gradeworkinggroup.org/society/index.htm.

In the United States, the strength of a recommendation from the USPSTF is most commonly reported based on a letter grade system (A, B, C, D, or I) (Table 4.2) [14]. In general, Task Force grades of "A" or "B" will recommend the evaluated service, "C" suggests to only provide the service for selected patients in certain circumstances, and a "D" grade suggests discouraging the use of the service. An "I" or "Insufficient" grade is given when there is insufficient evidence to assess the balance of benefits and harms or the evidence is lacking or of poor quality [14]. In addition, any recommendation letter grades are paired with an evaluation of the level of certainty regarding that recommendation based upon the evaluation of the evidence summary [14]. In general, a high level of certainty is assigned to recommendations based on consistent, well-designed and -conducted studies that are representative of the populations and outcomes in the guideline. Low level of certainty is derived from evidence that is insufficient to assess the impact of the intervention on health outcomes due to limited studies or inconsistent findings. Moderate level of certainty is assigned when there are well-conducted studies but the confidence in the estimate is constrained by several factors (Table 4.2).

Table 4.2 US Preventive Services Task Force (USPSTF) Grade Definitions and Level of Certainty Regarding Level of Evidence

Grade	Definition	Suggestions for Practice
A	The USPSTF recommends the service. There is high certainty that the net benefit is substantial.	Offer or provide this service.
B	The USPSTF recommends the service. There is high certainty that the net benefit is moderate or there is moderate certainty that the net benefit is moderate to substantial.	Offer or provide this service.
C	The USPSTF recommends selectively offering or providing this service to individual patients based on professional judgment and patient preferences. There is at least moderate certainty that the net benefit is small.	Offer or provide this service for selected patients depending on individual circumstances.
D	The USPSTF recommends against the service. There is moderate or high certainty that the service has no net benefit or that the harms outweigh the benefits.	Discourage the use of this service.
I	The USPSTF concludes that the current evidence is insufficient to assess the balance of benefits and harms of the service. Evidence is lacking, of poor quality, or conflicting, and the balance of benefits and harms cannot be determined.	Read the clinical considerations section of USPSTF Recommendation Statement. If the service is offered, patients should understand the uncertainty about the balance of benefits and harms.

Level of Certainty*	Description
High	The available evidence usually includes consistent results from well-designed, well-conducted studies in representative primary care populations. These studies assess the effects of the preventive service on health outcomes. This conclusion is therefore unlikely to be strongly affected by the results of future studies.
Moderate	The available evidence is sufficient to determine the effects of the preventive service on health outcomes, but confidence in the estimate is constrained by such factors as: • The number, size, or quality of individual studies. • Inconsistency of findings across individual studies. • Limited generalizability of findings to routine primary care practice. • Lack of coherence in the chain of evidence. As more information becomes available, the magnitude or direction of the observed effect could change, and this change may be large enough to alter the conclusion.
Low	The available evidence is insufficient to assess effects on health outcomes. Evidence is insufficient because of: • The limited number or size of studies. • Important flaws in study design or methods. • Inconsistency of findings across individual studies. • Gaps in the chain of evidence. • Findings not generalizable to routine primary care practice. • Lack of information on important health outcomes. More information may allow estimation of effects on health outcomes.

Source: USPSTF website: www.uspreventiveservicestaskforce.org/Page/Name/grade-definitions (accessed January 7, 2016)
* The USPSTF defines certainty as "likelihood that the USPSTF assessment of the net benefit of a preventive service is correct." The net benefit is defined as benefit minus harm of the preventive service as implemented in a general, primary care population. The USPSTF assigns a certainty level based on the nature of the overall evidence available to assess the net benefit of a preventive service.

Where to Find Guidelines

There are several resources where busy clinicians can quickly locate guidelines to assist in patient care decisions. The component chapters of this book list guidelines for specific aspects of well-woman care recommended by the WWTF from the "Components of the Well-Woman Visit" section of their report [1]. Useful websites for finding guidelines are listed in Box 4.1. These sources are useful for finding guidelines for topics not covered by the WWTF, and ones updated since the completion of their report. Going straight to a specialty society website will usually allow a provider to see that organization's guidelines on a topic. In addition, there are several national guideline clearinghouses such as the AHRQ's National Guideline Clearinghouse (www.guide line.gov), which collects guidelines from multiple organizations on a single topic. This site houses over 3,100 published guidelines categorized by Medical Subject Headings.

Deciding Which Guideline to Follow

With so many different organizations producing practice recommendations and guidelines, how is a provider or policy maker to decide which one to follow? The IOM produced a report providing guidance for identifying guidelines to trust [15]. Ideally, each organization's guidelines will have evaluated the evidence similarly and the guidelines will be largely congruent in their recommendations. The process of guideline review and achieving a consensus when guidelines are conflicted was a key focus of the WWTF. During selection of the well-woman visit guidelines, the American College of Obstetrics and Gynecology (ACOG) involved representatives from a very broad range of organizations to ensure a broad range of perspectives [1]. In addition to the Society of Academic Specialists in General Obstetrics and Gynecology, these 14 organizations included representatives from the American Academy of Pediatrics, the American Academy of Family Physicians, the National Association of Nurse Practitioners in Women's Health, the National Medical Association, and several others (see Table 4.1). This broad representation helps make the well-woman visit summary recommendations a true synthesis and consensus of guidelines that is helpful for clinicians. Absent this type of consensus, it is left to individual providers, insurers, and patients to review guidelines and choose the one that they are most comfortable with.

Determining guidelines to follow can be relatively easy when different organizations have similar recommendations, as is the case with cervical cancer screening. In other cases, such as mammography recommendations, where the recommendations differ somewhat widely, this can be more difficult. In general, it is appropriate to select a major organization's guidelines if they meet the IOM criteria [15] and are constructed from the same perspective as the provider's needs.

Cervical Cancer Screening Recommendations

Over the last two decades, there have been significant advances in understanding cervical cancer precursors and the consequent introduction of HPV testing. These types of advances highlight the need to continually update guidelines, a process that is built into the plans for most guideline development [2, 11].

The recommendations for cervical cancer screening have undergone a tremendous evolution over this time. Currently, the USPSTF, ACS, and ACOG all recommend beginning cervical cancer screening at age 21 with Pap test screening every 3 years until age 30. For women aged 30–65, ACS recommends co-testing with HPV testing and Pap every 5 years. The USPSTF recommends either Pap testing every 3 years or co-testing every 5 years over this age interval. These recommendations are largely in concert, making it relatively easy to select from among them. The WHO has slightly different recommendations but has a global health perspective, whereas the other organizations listed focus on the high-resource setting of the United States.

Mammography Recommendations

One of the most controversial examples of guideline differences in women's health is in the area of screening mammography for average-risk women. In 2009, the USPSTF updated their guidelines for screening for breast cancer in average-risk women [16]. Their new recommendation was for biennial screening mammography for women aged 50–75. They recommended against routine screening for women aged between 40 and 49, citing minimal reduction in mortality and higher rates of interventions for false positive results [16, 17]. This recommendation for women aged 40–49 was later clarified that "the decision to start regular biennial screening mammography before the age of 50 years should be an individual one." The USPSTF's recently updated guidelines on mammography recommend biennial mammography from 50 to 74 and individualized decisions (C recommendation) for women aged 40–49 [18]. These recommendations were met with a strong reaction from special interest groups, other organizations, and providers, as many did not agree with the evidence-based recommendations [19–22]. Some isolated decreases in mammography in the 40–49-year-old group occurred [23], but in general the US public and providers did not follow the guideline [20].

Table 4.3 highlights the different recommendations from different organizations. These differences may stem in part from the different perspectives of the organizations. For instance, the American College of Radiology recommends annual screening mammography starting at "age 40 for general populations" [24]. As they represent radiologists performing mammography, this may have influenced these recommendations. In the United Kingdom, where there is universal health coverage and population cost-effectiveness is a large consideration, the

Table 4.3 Mammography Guideline Recommendations* for Average-Risk Women from Selected Organizations

Organization	Age (years)	Guideline Recommendation
American College of Obstetricians and Gynecologists	40 and older	• Annual mammography
US Preventive Services Task Force	40–49 50–74	• Individualized decision but not routinely recommended • Mammography every 2 years
American College of Radiology	40 and older	• Annual mammography
American Cancer Society	40–44 45–54 55 and older	• Should have the choice about starting mammography • Annual mammography • Mammography every 2 years
National Health Service, UK	40–49 50–70	• Mammography not recommended • Mammography every 3 years
World Health Organization	40–49 50–69	• Screening mammography only if the program is conducted in the context of rigorous research and monitoring and evaluation • Mammography every 2 years

* As of February 1, 2016 [27, 28].

National Health Service (NHS) recommends mammography every 3 years for women aged between 50 and 70. While in England women as young as 47 years may be invited to be screened, in general average-risk women in their forties are not invited for screening mammography [25]. The WHO recommendations reflect their global perspective that includes low-resource settings [26]. Different recommendations by different organizations are arrived at based on the perspectives or key outcomes or costs they are looking at. Some recommendations come from the perspective of maximizing finding every case of breast cancer. Others may be from the perspective of maximizing quality of life and minimizing false positive results. Key differences between USPSTF and other US recommendations derive from differing interpretations of potential harms of screening including additional biopsies and follow-up testing not leading to cancer diagnoses and the risks over overdiagnosis.

When there are wide differences in recommendations, as there are for mammography, it is difficult for patients, providers, and policy makers to determine their best choice. Differences in recommendations may be based on scientific, public health, cost, weighting of benefits or harms, or other influences. An individual women's health care provider must choose a guideline to follow for the individual patient in his or her office. Their choice of guidelines can be driven by local practice, insurance provider mandate, or quality-improvement initiatives. In the absence of these drivers, it is left up to the individual provider to choose the guidelines he or she believes are the best for his or her patients. Guideline recommendations should be chosen that best fit the population being cared for by the provider or other stakeholder. Until a global (or at least regional) consensus that harmonizes the guidelines for screening mammography is reached, providers must nonetheless choose. Major societies recognize the problems conflicting guidelines cause and the need to harmonize them. The ACOG sponsored a meeting of major guideline making groups in January 2016 to achieve common ground on mammography recommendations. Luckily, for most other areas of well-woman care, there is more harmony in guideline recommendations. The process of the WWTF in comparing guidelines and utilizing experts to find consensus is a great model for finding harmony when guidelines conflict.

Utilizing Guidelines in Practice

There are tools to help individuals or groups determine how to use guidelines and apply findings of systematic reviews of evidence to patient care [29, 30]. When presented with a clinical scenario, finding a guideline on the topic can be accomplished by searching one of the sites in Box 4.1. Typically, the guideline document will outline its recommendations and the strength of the recommendation. The clinician is then able to decide if the guideline applies to their patient and can utilize the guideline and strength of recommendation to engage in a discussion with the patient in a shared decision-making model of care.

Developing guidelines and practice recommendations does not automatically translate into practice change or consistent care. Implementation science is now gathering momentum to hasten the use of evidence-based guidelines into clinical practice and policy. As an example, the NIH has convened an annual conference series on the science of dissemination and implementation in health (diconference.academyhealth.org/home). In this way, agencies are attempting to help maximize the usefulness of guideline development to truly impact public health by getting these recommendations to clinicians, the public, and policy makers.

Illustrative Case

A 49-year-old generally healthy woman presents for her well-woman visit. You consult the components of the Well-Woman Visit Guidance and note that she does not need cervical cancer screening since she had a negative Pap and HPV test last year. Additionally, she is not due for colorectal cancer screening until age 50, so you counsel her that you will be recommending it in 1 year. As it is flu season, the CDC guidelines state she should get an influenza vaccine and a Td booster if she has not had one in the last ten years. You are aware of the controversy in mammography screening guidelines, and in conjunction with other providers at your multispecialty practice, have chosen to follow the ACS screening guidelines and recommend a mammogram to her. She enquires about stroke prevention. You note that the WWTF has adopted the USPSTF recommendations and go to the USPSTF website for the source guideline document. Per the USPSTF recommendations, it is not recommended that she use aspirin for stroke prevention until age 55 (Grade A recommendation). These are just a few of the health recommendations that are easy to access during her visit. The CDC has an online tool where a patient can enter their gender and age and get a list of preventive health recommendations (www.cdc.gov/prevention). Thus, very quickly, these guidelines coalesce into the well-woman visit procedures that are aimed at optimizing your patient's health.

Summary

Guidelines are developed by stakeholders to make recommendations about health interventions. While always underscoring the importance of individual patient care, guidelines generally are robust and informed to also optimize public health. Development of useful guidelines is a rigorous and defined process. Effective guideline producing groups carefully evaluate the level of evidence and declare the strength of their recommendations using tools such as GRADE and the USPSTF letter grade system. In the end, clinicians, the public, and policy makers incorporate guideline recommendations into their daily decisions about health care. Through this process, we can assess and combine the components of the well-woman visit to be the most effective encounter to promote health for women.

References

1. Conry, J.A., and Brown, H. Well-Woman Task Force: Components of the well-woman visit. *Obstet Gynecol.* 2015, **126**(4):697–701.

2. World Health Organization. *WHO Handbook for Guideline Development.* Geneva, Switzerland: World Health Organization, 2012.

3. Institute of Medicine. Committee to advise the public health service on clinical practice guidelines. In Field, M.J. and Lohr, K.N. *Clinical Practice Guidelines: Directions for a New Program.* Washington, DC: National Academy Press, 1990.

4. Brouwers, M.C., Kho, M.E., Browman, G.P. et al. AGREE II: Advancing guideline development, reporting and evaluation in health care. *CMAJ: Canadian Medical Association Journal.* 2010, **182**(18):E839–E42.

5. Maciosek, M.V., Coffield, A.B., Flottemesch, T.J., Edwards, N.M., and Solberg, L.I. Greater use of preventive services in US health care could save lives at little or no cost. *Health Aff.* 2010, **29**(9):1656–60.

6. McGlynn, E.A., Asch, S.M., Adams, J. et al. The quality of health care delivered to adults in the United States. *N Engl J Med.* 2003, **348**(26):2635–45.

7. Schuster, M.A., McGlynn, E.A., and Brook, R.H. How good is the quality of health care in the United States? *Milbank Q.* 2005, **83**:843–95.

8. Hirth, J.M., Tan, A., Wilkinson, G.S., and Berenson, A.B. Compliance with cervical cancer screening and human papillomavirus testing guidelines among insured young women. *Am J Obstet Gynecol.* 2013, **209**(3):200. e1–e7.

9. US Preventive Services Task Force. About the USPSTF. 2016. Available at: www.uspreventiveservicestaskforce .org/Page/Name/about-the-uspstf. Retrieved February 16, 2016.

10. Brawley, O., Byers, T., Chen, A. et al. New American cancer society process for creating trustworthy cancer screening guidelines. *JAMA.* 2011, **306**(22):2495–9.

11. US Preventive Services Task Force. *US Preventive Services Task Force Procedure Manual.* Rockville, MD: USPSTF Program Office, 2015.

12. Higgins, J.P. and Green, S., editors. *Cochrane Handbook for Systematic Reviews of Interventions 5.1.0.* 2009. Chapter 8: Available at: www.cochrane-hand book.org. Retrieved March 2011.

13. GRADE Working Group. Grading quality of evidence and strength of recommendations. *BMJ.* 2004, **328**(7454):1490.

14. US Preventive Services Task Force. Grade Definitions. 2014. Available at: www.uspreventiveservicestaskforce .org/Page/Name/grade-definitions. Retrieved January 7, 2016.

15. Institute of Medicine. *Clinical Practice Guidelines We Can Trust.* Washington, DC: National Academy Press, 2011.

16. US Preventive Services Task Force. Screening for breast cancer: US Preventive Services Task Force recommendation statement. *Ann Intern Med.* 2009, **151**(10):716–26.

17. Mandelblatt, J.S., Cronin, K.A., Bailey, S. et al. Effects of mammography screening under different screening schedules: Model estimates of potential benefits and harms. *Ann Intern Med.* 2009, **151**(10):738–47.

18. US Preventive Services Task Force. Final recommendation statement: Breast cancer: Screening. February 2016. Available at:www.uspreventiveservices taskforce.org/Page/Document/RecommendationState mentFinal/breast-cancer-screening1. Retrieved February 16, 2016.

19. Allen, J.D., Bluethmann, S.M., Sheets, M. et al. Women's responses to changes in U.S. Preventive Task Force's mammography screening guidelines: Results of focus groups with ethnically diverse women. *BMC Public Health.* 2013, **13**:1169.

20. Corbelli, J., Borrero, S., Bonnema, R. et al. Physician adherence to US Preventive Services Task Force mammography guidelines. *Womens Health Issues.* 2014, **24**(3):e313–9.

21. Hendrick, R.E. and Helvie, M.A. United States Preventive Services Task Force screening mammography recommendations: Science ignored. *AJR Am J Roentgenol.* 2011, **196**(2):W112–6.

22. Squiers, L.B., Holden, D.J., Dolina, S.E. et al. The public's response to the US Preventive Services Task Force's 2009 recommendations on mammography screening. *Am J Prevent Med.* 2011, **40**(5):497–504.

23. Wharam, J.F., Landon, B., Zhang, F. et al. Mammography rates 3 years after the 2009 US Preventive Services Task Force guidelines changes. *J Clin Oncol.* 2015, **33**(9):1067–74.

24. American College of Radiology. ACR appropriateness criteria: Breast cancer screening. 2012. Available at: www.acr.org/~/media/ACR/Documents/AppCriteria/Diagnostic/BreastCancerScreening.pdf. Retrieved January 7, 2016.

25. National Health Service. Breast screening: Programme overview. 2015. Available at: www.gov .uk/guidance/breast-screening-programme-over view. Retrieved January 7, 2016.

26. World Health Organization. *WHO Position Paper on Mammography Screening.* Geneva, Switzerland: World Health Organization, 2014.

27. The American Cancer Society. American Cancer Society recommendations for early breast cancer detection in women without breast symptoms. Available at: www.cancer.org/cancer/breastcancer/mor einformation/breastcancerearlydetection/breast-can cer-early-detection-acs-recs. Retrieved January 7, 2016.

28. Breast cancer screening. Practice Bulletin No. 122. *Obstet Gynecol.* 2011, **118**:372–82.

29. Murad, M., Montori, V.M., Ioannidis, J.A. et al. How to read a systematic review and meta-analysis and apply the results to patient care: Users' guides to the medical literature. *JAMA.* 2014, **312**(2):171–9.

30. Agency for Healthcare Research and Quality. *Implementing US Preventive Services Task Force (USPSTF) Recommendations into Health Professions Education.* Rockville, MD: Agency for Healthcare Research and Quality, 2010. Available at: www.ahrq.gov/cpi/centers/ockt/kt/tools/impuspstf/impuspstf1.html. Retrieved October 2014.

Chapter 5

Promoting Lifestyle Modification and Behavior Change in the Context of Shared Decision-Making

Michelle H. Moniz and Tony Ogburn

Learning Objectives

- Define the key health promotion activities in women's health
- Describe the role of the provider in promoting lifestyle modification and behavior change at the well-woman exam
- Discuss the various theories of health promotion and behavior change
- Understand the value of shared decision-making and motivational interviewing for promoting lifestyle modification and behavior change
- List practical tips to promote lifestyle modification and behavior change
- Describe emerging strategies to promote and sustain lifestyle modification and behavior change

Introduction

Guidelines and recommendations for health promotion and lifestyle modification are readily available to guide the provider during the well-woman visit. Frequently, the greater challenge is how to effectively partner with patients to implement beneficial lifestyle changes such as increasing physical activity or quitting smoking.

Effective patient–provider communication and patient-centered care are essential to health promotion. A variety of approaches and tools are available to the provider to optimize communication with patients, effectively promote healthy behaviors, and improve their patients' health outcomes.

The aim of this chapter is to review the common theories regarding health behavior change and provide the clinician with an understanding of practical approaches and tools to utilize in their practice and to assist their patients in achieving their health goals.

The Role of the Provider in Health Promotion and Lifestyle Modification

The World Health Organization defines health promotion as the process of enabling people to increase control over and to improve their health [1]. Health promotion encompasses a broad scope of individual, social, and environmental interventions that improve individual, community, and population health outcomes. Key health promotion activities for women's health include reproductive life planning; safe sexual decision-making and prevention of sexually transmitted infections; immunization; healthy weight maintenance, physical activity, and nutritional intake; mental health promotion; substance use management; reducing gun violence risk; and promoting motor vehicular safety. Lifestyle modification refers to the behavior changes recommended to prevent chronic conditions such as cardiovascular disease, diabetes, and obesity, which are among the leading causes of mortality in the United States and worldwide. Behavior modifications for these conditions include improving dietary patterns, increasing physical activity, reducing tobacco use, and reducing excessive alcohol consumption. The well-woman visit provides a critical opportunity to engage in conversations about health promotion and lifestyle modification and provide patients with evidence-based interventions to improve their health. Effective patient–provider communication is critical for health promotion (Figure 5.1). The key goals of patient–provider communication are to foster a strong therapeutic relationship, promote accurate information exchange, validate and respond to emotions, help patients manage uncertainty and make health decisions, and encourage self-management [2]. Successful communication can increase patient engagement and satisfaction, produce health behavior changes, and ultimately improve health outcomes [3, 4].

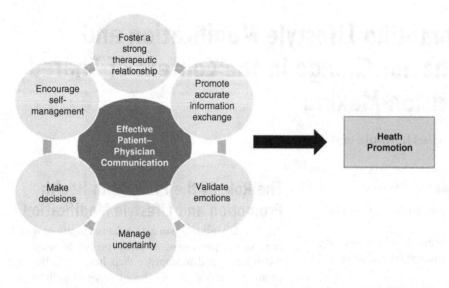

Figure 5.1 Effective Patient–Provider Communication as Critical for Health Promotion. Effective patient–provider communication involves a number of skills in action (light gray boxes). Effective communication can lead to health promotion.

Theories of Behavior Change: An Overview of Modern Theories to Guide Clinical Intervention

Health behavior change is the most promising means of reducing the burden of preventable disease affecting women. Health behavior change theories help articulate the processes and key factors that shape behavior and the potential levers that can be used to promote behavior change [2, 5]. Theories exist to guide health promotion at the individual level (e.g., Health Belief Model, Integrated Behavioral Model), the interpersonal level (e.g., Social Cognitive Theory), the community level (e.g., Health Communication Theory), the organizational level (e.g., Theoretical Domains Framework), and across individual, environmental, and policy levels (e.g., Social Ecological Model).

Behavior change theories propose specific strategies that can be used by clinicians to promote effective patient–clinician communication. For example, the Health Belief Model posits that an individual's perceived susceptibility to and severity of a disease, as well as the perceived benefits outweighing the costs of an intervention are critical factors influencing health behaviors. For example, when promoting vaccination during pregnancy, the Health Belief Model suggests emphasizing pregnant women's increased risk of

severe influenza and the benefits of maternal vaccination for both mother and child in avoiding the disease (Figure 5.2a). Similarly, the Integrated Behavioral Model highlights the importance of knowledge and skills to perform a health behavior, perceived social norms, intention to perform the behavior, and environmental constraints. This theory suggests that clinicians conducting contraceptive counseling should seek to provide accurate contraceptive knowledge, assess normative beliefs about childbearing and contraception, characterize a woman's immediate and long-term childbearing intentions, and remove environmental barriers that threaten access to a woman's preferred contraceptive method (Figure 5.2b). Central to both models is the importance of addressing the patient's beliefs and perceptions about the behavior change, providing factual information about the disease and impact of the behavior change, and addressing real and perceived barriers to the behavior change.

Shared Decision-Making as One Tool for Patient-Centered Promotion of Behavior Change

The Institute of Medicine's landmark report *Crossing the Quality Chasm* defined patient-centered care as "care that is respectful of and responsive to individual

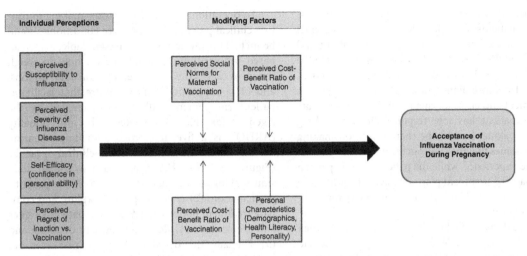

Figure 5.2a Modified Health Belief Model as a Theoretical Framework for Acceptance of Vaccination during Pregnancy. This depicts the Health Belief Model as a conceptual framework that describes factors that affect patient's willingness to accept vaccines during pregnancy. Individual perceptions are depicted in gray boxes. Factors that modify these perceptions and their relationship with vaccine acceptance are depicted in white boxes.

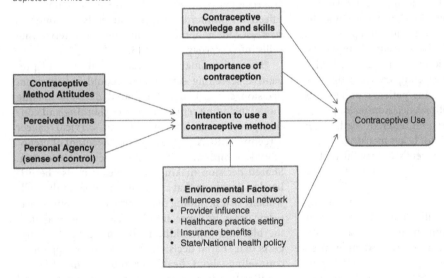

Figure 5.2b Integrative Behavioral Model as a Theoretical Framework for Contraceptive Behaviors. This depicts the Integrative Behavioral Model as a conceptual framework that describes factors affecting contraceptive utilization. Contraceptive use is influenced by factors such as contraceptive knowledge and skills, perceived importance of contraception, intention to use a method, and environmental factors (gray boxes). An individual's intention to use a method may also be influenced by attitudes toward the method, perceived contraceptive norms, and sense of personal agency (white boxes), as well as environmental factors (e.g., insurance coverage and out-of-pocket cost for a given method).

patient preferences, needs and values" and that ensures "that patient values guide all clinical decisions" [6]. Shared decision-making is a tool for achieving patient-centered communication and care [7]. Shared decision-making refers to a collaborative process in which the clinician and patient share information with the goal of developing a management plan that aligns with the patient's goals, values, and preferences. The clinician provides an evidence-based description of the risks and benefits of appropriate options, and the patient expresses values and personal information that might make one treatment option more desirable than the other(s) [3]. The hallmark of shared decision-making is bidirectional flow of information – often accompanied by deliberation and negotiation – between patients and providers. This bidirectional information exchange is followed by the patient and clinician jointly selecting a management plan. Unlike paternalistic or informed decision-making models, shared decision-making aims to optimize patient engagement and empowerment, but does not mandate that the patient has sole responsibility for making a decision alone. Rather, the shared decision-making model assumes that the clinician brings medical knowledge and experience, while the patient is the expert on the impact the treatment plan will have on her life, and that the expertise of both parties is necessary for effective patient care [8].

Shared decision-making is particularly useful when two or more reasonable treatment options exist and differ in their immediate and long-term implications for a patient. In these situations, patient engagement in decision-making is critical to determining the management approach that best aligns with her personal preferences and values. Shared decision-making may be particularly useful in decision-making in reproductive health since often the available options are medically equivocal (i.e., no one option is clearly more effective than the other) or involve complex trade-offs for patients. In such instances, the patient's preferences and values are key to optimal decision-making. For example, optimal counseling on different methods of contraception or treatments for heavy menstrual bleeding must incorporate the patient's individual preferences and values in the development of the best management plan for her.

It is worth noting that shared decision-making may not be appropriate in all situations; nor does it preclude provider recommendation of a clearly beneficial medical intervention. For example, provider recommendation is a powerful predictor of a woman's decision to receive indicated vaccinations during pregnancy [9]. Clinicians should clearly and unequivocally recommend medical interventions with clear evidence of benefit, such as indicated vaccines, tobacco cessation, and seat belt use. Patients' willingness to accept these medical recommendations, however, can vary. Shared decision-making, along with other evidence-based approaches discussed subsequently, can provide a framework to explore patient perceptions about available options, assist patients in making health decisions, and promote behavior changes that can optimize health.

To operationalize shared decision-making in routine clinical practice, at least three conditions should be met: (1) ready access to understandable, evidence-based information; (2) guidance on how to weigh the pros and cons of different available options; and (3) a supportive clinical culture that facilitates patient engagement [10]. SHARE, created by the Agency for Healthcare Research and Quality (ARHQ), is a five-step process for implementing shared decision-making within clinical practice (Figure 5.3). The SHARE approach to shared decision-making involves five steps: (1) *S*eek the patient's participation; (2) *H*elp the patient explore and compare treatment options; (3) *A*ssess the patient's values and preferences; (4) *R*each a treatment decision; and (5) *E*valuate the decision. Multiple resources are available on the ARHQ website to assist clinicians in implementing the SHARE framework in their practice [11]. The American College of Obstetrics and Gynecology (ACOG) Committee Opinion on Effective Communication recommends and outlines strategies for adopting patient-centered interviewing skills into everyday practice [3].

The well-woman visit includes an array of preventive screening services that could benefit from decision support and the shared decision-making model including reproductive life planning and contraceptive counseling, breast and cervical cancer screening, BRCA testing, and management of menopausal symptoms and osteoporosis prevention. Shared decision-making principles can also be utilized to problems that commonly present at the well-woman visit including management of incontinence, pelvic organ prolapse, infertility, and abnormal uterine bleeding [8]. Additionally, emerging data suggests that shared decision-making can be applied to counseling about health promotion and lifestyle modification in areas such as tobacco cessation and weight control [12].

Practical Tips for Promoting and Sustaining Engagement in Health Behavior Change

A variety of evidence-based tools and approaches are available to clinicians pursuing health promotion and lifestyle modification counseling at the well-woman visit.

Decision Support – Operationalizing Shared Decision-Making: One of the most widely studied

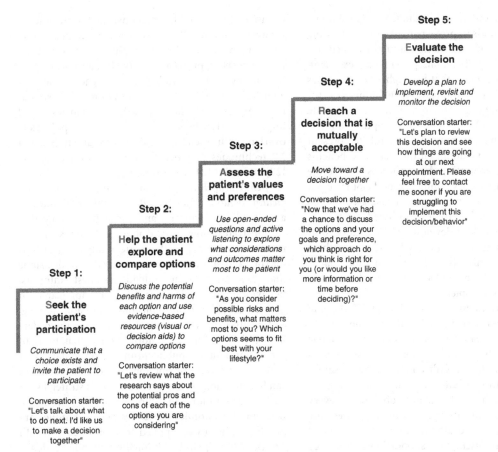

Step 1:

Seek the patient's participation

Communicate that a choice exists and invite the patient to participate

Conversation starter: "Let's talk about what to do next. I'd like us to make a decision together"

Step 2:

Help the patient explore and compare options

Discuss the potential benefits and harms of each option and use evidence-based resources (visual or decision aids) to compare options

Conversation starter: "Let's review what the research says about the potential pros and cons of each of the options you are considering"

Step 3:

Assess the patient's values and preferences

Use open-ended questions and active listening to explore what considerations and outcomes matter most to the patient

Conversation starter: "As you consider possible risks and benefits, what matters most to you? Which options seems to fit best with your lifestyle?"

Step 4:

Reach a decision that is mutually acceptable

Move toward a decision together

Conversation starter: "Now that we've had a chance to discuss the options and your goals and preference, which approach do you think is right for you (or would you like more information or time before deciding)?"

Step 5:

Evaluate the decision

Develop a plan to implement, revisit and monitor the decision

Conversation starter: "Let's plan to review this decision and see how things are going at our next appointment. Please feel free to contact me sooner if you are struggling to implement this decision/behavior"

Figure 5.3 The SHARE Approach for Shared Decision-Making. The figure depicts a five-step process for shared decision-making that includes exploring and comparing the benefits, harms, and risks of each option through meaningful dialogue about the patient's preferences, values, and priorities. Adapted from the Agency for Healthcare Research and Quality's "The SHARE Approach – Essential Steps of Shared Decision Making: Quick Reference Guide." Available at: www.ahrq.gov/professionals/education/curriculum-tools/shareddecisionmaking/tools/tool-1/index.html. Retrieved April 19, 2016).

tools is the decision aid – an intervention that can assist patients in understanding available treatment options and possible outcomes. Decision aids often incorporate exercises that help patients clarify and articulate their values and preferences. Usually designed to supplement counseling, decision aids can provide background information about treatment options, tailored estimates of potential benefits and harms, an explicit values clarification exercise, and guidance in decision-making, sometimes with a personalized recommendation for an individual patient. A recent Cochrane review suggests that the shared decision-making process can improve the quality of patient–provider communication, increase patient knowledge and decrease decisional conflict, promote patient engagement, and reduce

overtreatment [3]. In this review, 31 of 155 studies (29 percent) specifically evaluated tools related to reproductive health screening and treatment decisions [8, 13]. Currently available evidence does not allow for conclusive comment about the effect of decision aids on health outcomes, adherence to treatment, or cost of care. However, decision aids have consistently been shown to offer important benefits to patients, including improved knowledge and satisfaction and reduced decisional conflict.

Evidence-Based Risk Communication: Clinicians frequently communicate risk estimates to patients, often under circumstances where emotions and clinical complexity requires complicated information exchange. Also, some patients have limited literacy, which can be an additional barrier to effective communication and understanding. Multiple empirically tested methods improve patients' understanding of risk and benefit information and their decision-making [14]. Fagerlin et al. provide an excellent, brief, practical overview that highlights key strategies for effective risk communication, including tips for using plain language, pictographs, and absolute (instead of relative) risks. For contraceptive counseling, for example, it may be helpful to present a summary table including all the risks and benefits of each option, presenting data in terms of absolute risk (i.e., "the risk of developing a blood clot is 10 per 10,000 women years among women using combined contraceptives," rather than "combined contraceptives double the risk of developing blood clots compared to nonpregnant women who don't use these methods"), and only discussing information that is most critical to the patient's decision-making (even at the expense of completeness).

Assessing Readiness to Change – The 5 A's and Motivational Interviewing (MI): It is important to assess a woman's readiness and motivation to change behavior. One brief intervention with substantial research support for its utility in smoking cessation is the 5 A's method. Clinicians using this brief, goal-directed approach (1) **Ask** about tobacco use every time; (2) **Advise** the patient to quit; (3) **Assess** the patient's willingness to attempt cessation; (4) **Assist** the patient's quit attempt by supporting self-efficacy and developing a plan to deal with challenges; and (5) **Arrange** follow-up contact. This approach may be used to assess readiness and motivation in other areas.

Motivational interviewing (MI) is another approach for catalyzing behavior change [15]. MI focuses on eliciting and strengthening an individual's personal, intrinsic motivation for change. Key clinical activities within MI involve eliciting change talk ("What would you like to see different about your current situation?"), exploring ambivalence ("So on the one hand it sounds like . . . And, yet, on the other hand . . . "), reflective listening ("It sounds like you're not ready to quit smoking at this time"), rolling with resistance ("Naturally, the choice is up to you, and you may decide not to make any changes in your diet at this time"), and supporting self-efficacy to change ("It seems like you've put a lot of thought into these goals and have a good plan of action"). While shared decision-making is helpful when more than one reasonable option exists, MI is particularly useful for the patient with ambivalence to medically indicated

behavior change. MI has demonstrated some efficacy for a variety of health promotion activities, including smoking cessation [16], managing substance abuse [17], increasing physical activity [18], and promoting weight loss [19]. Studies also suggest that MI approaches may increase the duration of breastfeeding, prevent alcohol-exposed pregnancies, and improve lifestyle behaviors in women with polycystic ovarian syndrome [15]. Clinicians seeking training in MI techniques may benefit from a variety of online [20] and print [21] resources.

Behavioral Economics for Decision-Making and Health Behavior Change: Behavioral economics is a subfield of economics and social psychology that demonstrates how predictable, sometimes flawed mental shortcuts (i.e., heuristics) impact decision-making and sometimes promote irrational decisions that are not in an individual's best interests. Behavioral economics strategies are applicable to patient–provider communication, decision-making, and health behavior change. For example, the ordering and framing of information, elicitation of a commitment or public promise, presentation of only key, tailored information, and use of incentives can be efficacious behavioral economics strategies for health promotion in clinical settings [22–25]. Behavioral economics principles and techniques are just beginning to be applied to reproductive health practice [26, 27], and additional research is needed.

Adaptive Interventions: While much of this chapter has focused on tools for *initiating* health behavior change, novel approaches are emerging to support patients in long-term *adherence* to health-promoting behaviors [28]. A variety of adaptive interventions are under investigation to promote sustained engagement in smoking cessation, avoidance of alcohol abuse, physical activity, substance cessation, and other behaviors [29]. Adaptive interventions augment the efforts of clinicians during clinical encounters by providing the right support at the right time in the right location as an individual attempts to maintain a health behavior change.

Case Scenarios

1. *Mary, a nulliparous 23-year-old graduate student, comes to your office for a well-woman visit and requests contraception. She has been sexually active intermittently for several years and has been using condoms to prevent pregnancy and sexually*

transmitted infections. She is now in a relationship and wants a more effective method of contraception that is "easy to use." She has never used any other method of contraception. A friend suggested an intrauterine device (IUD), although her older sister told her she couldn't use one since she had never been pregnant.

Contraceptive counseling and implementation of an effective method is a critical component of preventive health for reproductive-aged women. For many years, the most common reversible method recommended and utilized in the United States was oral contraceptive pills. Recently, there has been a renewed interest in long-acting reversible contraceptives (LARCs; IUDs and the subdermal implant) that provide ease of use with high typical use effectiveness. Many patients may not be aware of these methods, or like Mary, have inaccurate information about them.

The **SHARE** approach is one effective way to assist patients in decision-making about contraception. First, *S*eek her participation in the process. A helpful first step is to discuss her reproductive life plan – does she want children, if so when, how many, etc. Excellent tools for patients and providers are available online from the Centers for Disease Control and Prevention [29]. Mary clarifies that she wants children but would like to at least wait until she has completed her graduate studies in 3–5 years. Next, *H*elp her to explore the options available to her including benefits and risks. A variety of evidence-based decision aids are available including "Your Birth Control Choices" from the Reproductive Health Access project, and Effectiveness of Family Planning Methods from the Centers for Disease Control and Prevention [30, 31]. Next it is important to *A*ssess her preferences and values – e.g. is she concerned about side effects such as amenorrhea with a levonorgestrel IUD, or about being able to remember to take a pill each day. It is essential that the provider respect the patient's preferences and values in the process. In this case, Mary expressed great reluctance to having a foreign body in her uterus. Now it is time to *R*each a decision. Many patients will be ready to move forward immediately with selection of a method, while others may need time to consider the options. If her decision is to take more time, additional decision aids may be helpful for the patient to utilize. In this case, Mary decided upon an implant, and it was placed that day. Finally, *E*valuate the decision and see how it is working for the patient. Routine follow-up visits for placement of an implant are not required, but patients should be provided information about typical expectations and instructions in how to contact the provider if issues arise. Mary contacted your office 5 weeks later and was concerned about persistent light intermittent spotting. She was reassured that this was common and instructed to make an appointment for follow-up if it increased or persisted beyond 3 months. She agreed with this plan.

2. *Maria, a 24-year-old G1P1, comes to your office for a well-woman visit. She gave birth to her first child 2 years ago and is planning to become pregnant over the next several months. She did not breastfeed her first child, because she had to go back to work after only 4 weeks. She did not feel she could breastfeed once she went back to work and assumed that breastfeeding for only 4 weeks would not be beneficial. Maria shares that she would like to breastfeed her next child.*

Breastfeeding counseling and support is an area in which MI can often be utilized effectively to catalyze behavior change. The first step is to engage the patient in a discussion about the behavior to be changed or modified and explore their motivation for change, their concerns or ambivalence to change, and to establish a trusting, respectful dialogue about the topic. An introductory statement about the general benefits of breastfeeding and then asking about the patient's thoughts on breastfeeding is a good approach. Maria expresses a desire to breastfeed but has concerns about the short-term benefits and the feasibility for her doing so once she returns to work.

The next step is to focus the conversation on her concerns and areas of ambivalence. This should be done in a manner that affirms her concerns and provides information that may help her explore, clarify, and resolve her ambivalence. For example, it may be helpful to acknowledge that breastfeeding after returning to work is a major challenge for many of your patients and there are many strategies she might utilize to enable her to continue. Also discussing the benefits to breastfeeding, even for a short interval, may solidify her intrinsic motivation to initiate breastfeeding. In this case, she was provided follow-up reading material on the benefits of breastfeeding from ACOG, information about breastfeeding classes offered by the hospital lactation consultants, and reassurance that the decision was hers to make.

Next, the patient's ongoing motivation for change should be assessed and supported. At Maria's next visit, she is establishing prenatal care and is planning to attend the breastfeeding class you recommended. She later reports that she found the class very helpful and connected with several women with similar issues. She plans to initiate breastfeed exclusively and continue to breastfeed when she returns to work, either pumping and storing breast milk or supplementing with formula. You affirm her decision and then offer assistance with action steps for success.

When you see her for a 6-week postpartum visit, she has returned to work and is successfully pumping, so her infant is receiving only breast milk. She is optimistic that she will be able to continue for the foreseeable future.

3. *Laura, a 48-year-old G2P2, comes to your office for a well-woman visit. She has gained 10 pounds since her last visit 2 years ago. She weighs 232 pounds with a body mass index (BMI) of approximately 37. Her BMI places her in the category of Obesity – Class II. She also has hypertension. She was diagnosed with hypertension 6 months ago by her Family Medicine provider and is well controlled on a single agent. Other than her weight, the remainder of her examination and recommended screening tests for her age are normal.*

Obesity is a common problem and with an increasing prevalence throughout the United States. All patients should be screened for obesity and once identified, should be offered intervention. One approach is to utilize the 5 A's in the obese patient.

a. **Ask** permission to discuss the patient's weight – e.g. with Laura, "I see you have gained 10 pounds since your visit 2 years ago. Would you be open to talking about your weight?" She is relieved when you asked about her weight as her other physician had given her a low-calorie diet, and she has had no success with it.

b. **Assess** the patient's motivation and willingness to lose weight, what concerns she has, and her barriers to success. Laura shares that she is very interested in losing weight but has failed many times in the past. She has tried several "fad diets" and typically loses a small amount of weight but always regains it within a few months. She is quite concerned about her blood pressure as her mother had a stroke that she thinks was caused by hypertension. She says the biggest barrier to

success is her and her husband's "love of eating out" – it's their time together.

c. **Advise** the patient about the health risk of obesity in general as well as specifically for her given her diagnosis of hypertension. Share with her the health benefits of weight loss and that often comorbid conditions can be mitigated or reversed with weight loss. Advise her to lose weight and discuss the importance of developing a plan for loss that is realistic and acceptable for her. Finally, review the treatment options with the patient. Laura reports she has tried multiple diets, a medication prescribed by her primary care physician, and exercise. She has never received longitudinal counseling. She would be interested in learning more about bariatric surgery as an option.

d. **Assist** the patient with developing a plan, addressing barriers, and building her confidence that she can succeed. Laura decides she would like to see a nutritionist for longitudinal counseling and incorporate walking into her daily routine. She and her husband live in a neighborhood that is quite "walkable," and they can spend time together on a daily walk after work instead of eating out.

e. **Arrange** follow-up with appropriate referrals for the patient and regular follow-up to reinforce the plan, evaluate success, and make modifications to the plan if needed. Laura was referred to a nutritionist who saw her for regular counseling. She started walking 4–5 times per week but after 3 months has lost only 4 pounds. She is frustrated and discouraged. After reassessment she is referred to a bariatric surgeon for possible surgical management.

Suggestions for Additional Reading

1. ACOG Committee Opinion No. 587: Effective patient–physician communication. *Obstet Gynecol.* 2014, 123(2 Pt 1):389–93.

2. Glanz, K. et al. (2008). *Health Behavior and Health Education: Theory, Research, and Practice.* San Francisco, CA: Jossey-Bass.

3. Department of Health & Human Services, National Institutes of Health, and National Cancer Institute. Theory at a Glance: A Guide for Health Promotion Practice. NIH Publication No. 05-3896. Available at: www

.sbccimplementationkits.org/demandrmnch/wp-content/uploads/2014/02/Theory-at-a-Glance-A-Guide-For-Health-Promotion-Practice.pdf.

4. Tucker Edmonds, B. Shared decision-making and decision support: Their role in obstetrics and gynecology. *Curr Opin Obstet Gynecol.* 2014, 26(6):523–30.

Summary

1. Health promotion encompasses a broad scope of individual, social, and environmental interventions that improve individual, community, and population health outcomes.

2. Clinicians play a pivotal role in women's health promotion by engaging women in such activities as reproductive life planning; safe sexual decision-making and prevention of sexually transmitted infections; healthy weight maintenance, physical activity, and nutritional intake; mental health promotion; substance use management; reducing gun violence risk; and promoting motor vehicular safety.

3. Effective patient–provider communication is critical for health promotion.

4. Health behavior change theories articulate the processes and key factors that shape behavior and offer strategies to promote behavior change and effective patient–clinician communication.

5. Shared decision-making is one tool for achieving patient-centered communication and care. Shared decision-making refers to a collaborative process in which both providers and patients share information, with the goal of together developing a management plan that aligns with the patient's goals, values, and preferences.

6. The SHARE approach to shared decision-making involves five steps: (1) Seek the patient's participation; (2) Help the patient explore and compare treatment options; (3) Assess the patient's values and preferences; (4) Reach a treatment decision; and (5) Evaluate the decision.

7. Decision aids, evidence-based risk communication strategies, the 5 A's approach, MI, and behavioral economics techniques may be useful tools for clinicians encouraging health-promoting behaviors and lifestyle modification at the well-woman exam.

References

1. Damschroder, L.J., Lutes, L.D., Goodrich, D.E., Gillon, L., and Lowery, J.C. A small-change approach delivered via telephone promotes weight loss in veterans: Results from the ASPIRE-VA pilot study. *Patient Educ Couns.* 2010, 79(2):262–6.

2. Glanz, K. et al. *Health Behavior and Health Education: Theory, Research, and Practice*, 4th edition. 2008. San Francisco, CA: Jossey-Bass. xxxiii, p. 552.

3. American College of Obstetricians and Gynecologists. ACOG Committee Opinion No. 587. Effective patient–physician communication. *Obstet Gynecol.* 2014, 123(2 Pt 1):389–93.

4. de Haes, H. Dilemmas in patient centeredness and shared decision making: A case for vulnerability. *Patient Educ Couns.* 2006, 62(3):291–8.

5. Damschroder, L.J. et al. Fostering implementation of health services research findings into practice: A consolidated framework for advancing implementation science. *Implement Sci.* 2009, 4:50.

6. Institute of Medicine (US) Committee on Quality of Health Care in America. *Crossing the Quality Chasm: A New Health System for the 21st Century*. Washington, DC: National Academy Press, 2001. xx, p. 337.

7. Barry, M.J. and Edgman-Levitan, S. Shared decision making – pinnacle of patient-centered care. *N Engl J Med.* 2012, 366(9):780–1.

8. Tucker Edmonds, B. Shared decision-making and decision support: Their role in obstetrics and gynecology. *Curr Opin Obstet Gynecol.* 2014, 26(6):523–30.

9. Shavell, V.I. et al. Influenza immunization in pregnancy: Overcoming patient and health care provider barriers. *Am J Obstet Gynecol.* 2012, 207 (Suppl 3):S67–74.

10. Ogburn, T. Shared decision making and informed consent for hysterectomy. *Clin Obstet Gynecol.* 2014, 57(1):3–13.

11. Au, B. et al. The longitudinal associations between C-reactive protein and depressive symptoms: Evidence from the English Longitudinal Study of Ageing (ELSA). *Int J Geriatr Psychiatry.* 2015, 30(9):976–84.

12. Hamera, E. et al. Descriptive study of shared decision making about lifestyle modifications with individuals who have psychiatric disabilities. *J Am Psychiatr Nurses Assoc.* 2010, 16(5):280–7.

13. Stacey, D. et al. Decision aids for people facing health treatment or screening decisions. *Cochrane Database Syst Rev.* 2014, (1):CD001431.

14. Fagerlin, A., Zikmund-Fisher, B.J., and Ubel, P.A. Helping patients decide: Ten steps to better risk communication. *J Natl Cancer Inst.* 2011, 103(19): 1436–43.

15. American College of Obstetricians and Gynecologists. ACOG Committee Opinion No. 423. Motivational interviewing: a tool for behavioral change. *Obstet Gynecol.* 2009, **113**(1):243–6.

16. Lindson-Hawley, N., Thompson, T.P., and Begh, R. Motivational interviewing for smoking cessation. *Cochrane Database Syst Rev.* 2015, (**3**):CD006936.

17. Smedslund, G. et al. Motivational interviewing for substance abuse. *Cochrane Database Syst Rev.* 2011, (5):CD008063.

18. O'Halloran, P.D. et al. Motivational interviewing to increase physical activity in people with chronic health conditions: A systematic review and meta-analysis. *Clin Rehabil.* 2014, **28**(12):1159–71.

19. Barnes, R.D. and Ivezaj, V. A systematic review of motivational interviewing for weight loss among adults in primary care. *Obes Rev.* 2015, **16**(4):304–18.

20. Motivational Interviewing. *Videos and Other Materials.* Available at: http://motivationalinterview .net/training/videos.html. Retrieved December 24, 2015.

21. Rollnick, S., Miller, W.R., and Butler, C. *Motivational Interviewing in Health Care: Helping Patients Change Behavior.* New York, NY: Guilford Press, 2008.

22. Shafir, E., editor. *The Behavioral Foundations of Public Policy.* Princeton, NJ: Princeton University Press, 2013.

23. Haff, N. et al. The role of behavioral economic incentive design and demographic characteristics in financial incentive-based approaches to changing health behaviors: A meta-analysis. *Am J Health Promot.* 2015, **29**(5):314–23.

24. Cahill, K., Hartmann-Boyce, J., and Perera, R. Incentives for smoking cessation. *Cochrane Database Syst Rev.* 2015, (**5**):CD004307.

25. Mitchell, M.S. et al. Financial incentives for exercise adherence in adults: Systematic review and meta-analysis. *Am J Prev Med.* 2013, **45**(5):658–67.

26. Center for Effective Global Action. A Review of Behavioral Economics in Reproductive Health. Available at: www.beri-research.org/wp-content/uplo ads/2015/01/BERI-White-Paper_version_1.20.15.pdf. Retrieved December 24, 2015.

27. Stevens, J. and Berlan, E.D. Applying principles from behavioral economics to promote long-acting reversible contraceptive (LARC) methods. *Perspect Sex Reprod Health.* 2014, **46**(3):165–70.

28. Klasnja, P. et al. Microrandomized trials: An experimental design for developing just-in-time adaptive interventions. *Health Psychol.* 2015, **34** (Suppl):1220–8.

29. ClinicalTrials.gov. Search for "adaptive interventions." Available at: https://clinicaltrials.gov/ct2/results?ter m=adaptive+intervention&Search=Search. Retrieved April 20, 2016.

30. Your Birth Control Choices Fact Sheet. Available at: www.reproductiveaccess.org/resource/birth-control- choices-fact-sheet/ Retrieved December 29, 2016.

31. Effectiveness of Family Planning Methods. Available at: www.cdc.gov/reproductivehealth/contraception/un intendedpregnancy/pdf/family-planning-methods-20 14.pdf. Retrieved December 30, 2016.

Practical Aspects of the Well-Woman Visit

Christopher M. Zahn

Learning Objectives

- Describe the challenges facing providers in addressing preventive and primary care during a well-woman visit, including barriers to optimizing preventive services during clinic visits and addressing preventive care in patients with multimorbidities
- Describe the effective use of multiple visits to address preventive care issues over time
- Describe potential tools to aid in prioritization of patient and provider agendas in addressing preventive and "problem" care issues
- Summarize the use of patient-centered medical homes in enhancing efficiency and optimization of preventive care services, and describe techniques to potentially enhance efficiency in the outpatient clinic

Introduction

Medicine has been defined as both an "art" and a "science." In most situations, the reference to both "art" and "science" applies to the care of the patient, involving the application of knowledge, skills, and experience in evaluation and treatment. Medicine also involves the practical aspects of providing health care, such as patient flow, organizing outpatient visits, workflow, prioritizing the health care issues specific to the individual patient, documentation, communication with the patients and fellow health care providers, and the business aspects. Arguably, in contrast to the care of the patient for which a good amount of "science" is available, the practical aspects are much more of an "art" than a "science." In this chapter, we will address several of the practical aspects related to the care provided in a well-woman visit.

Background and Challenges

Before considering the practical aspects related to the care of women, one must consider the components of the well-woman visit. The annual examination, or health assessment, is considered a "fundamental part" of the care of women [1]. It is described that this visit is valuable to promote prevention, to identify risk factors for disease and specific medical problems, and to establish the patient–clinician relationship [1]. Also included is counseling patients about maintaining a healthy lifestyle and reducing potential risks. This visit typically involves screening, evaluation, counseling, and discussion of immunizations [1]. This visit should also include assessment of family history, obstetric history, social history, review of medications, and a physical examination. Specific history should also be obtained related to patient safety in her surroundings, sexual function, general mental health, family planning as applicable, and bowel/bladder function. These activities can be summarized as obtaining history and relevant facts, performing a physical examination, and counseling related to management of conditions, prevention strategies, and risk reduction. It should be apparent that all of these activities amount to "a lot to do"! As a result, the provision of preventive care is challenging.

While primary and preventive care is emphasized in graduate medical education and comprises a significant proportion of the care provided by obstetrician-gynecologists, most of the published literature about providing well-woman care comes from primary care specialty journals from both the United States and the United Kingdom.

Volume of Work – Tasks to be Accomplished

Several studies have evaluated the time necessary to provide primary and preventive care. Time is one of the most significant challenges to the provision of preventive care due to the sheer volume of issues to be addressed during a well-woman visit. The standard components of the well-woman visit are poorly defined. In a study of patients in a Family Practice clinic, an average of 25 services defined by the US

Preventive Services Task Force (USPSTF) was recommended for each patient visit [2]. Another study reported a range from 12 to 74 total required tasks [3]. In a study of the development of a primary care physician task list to evaluate clinic visit workflow, the task list included 12 major tasks and 189 subtasks [4]. It is also worth noting that the number of recommended preventive services will increase as new screening tests are developed and the potential value of prevention related to chronic disease is identified [5]. This is particularly true for those conditions which may be affected by addressing modifiable risk factors [6]. These studies further highlight the time-consuming aspect of primary and preventive care.

Implementation of Preventive Care

Although preventive care services have been promulgated as an effective way to reduce the impact of chronic disease, the implementation and delivery of preventive services is far less than optimal [7–9]. In an older study of family practices in Michigan, completion of all age-appropriate screening tests for men and women over age 50 was 5 percent and 3 percent, respectively [10]. Other studies have demonstrated inadequate counseling or screening for items such as smoking cessation and obesity, mammography, cervical cancer screening, fecal occult blood testing, or colon cancer screening [5, 11, 12]. The most recent data from the Centers for Disease Control and Prevention (CDC) Behavioral Risk Factor Surveillance System (BRFSS) demonstrate the following statistics for the United States [13]:

- Only 67.3 percent of patients over age 50 have completed colorectal cancer screening (2012).
- Only 76.4 percent of adults have had cholesterol screening within the last 5 years and 20.1 percent of adults have never been checked (2013).
- Only 62.8 percent of patients over age 65 have received the influenza vaccine (2013).
- Only 77 percent of women over age 50 have had mammography (2012).
- Only 78 percent of women over age 18 have undergone cervical cytology screening within the last 3 years (2012).

Poor adherence to preventive service guidelines is a worldwide problem. In Australia, screening rates for breast and cervical cancer are only 56 percent and 61 percent, respectively [14]. It is therefore obvious that even with efforts at promoting preventive care, both the United States and other countries still fall short even for those "highly publicized" preventive measures.

Barriers

Suboptimal provision of preventive care has been attributed to a number of factors; numerous studies have analyzed barriers to the provision of preventive care. Many of these studies specifically looked at physician practices, but it is likely that the same issues are present in all practices, regardless of provider type. Some of the more common barriers cited include lack of time during the encounter, problems with insurance reimbursement, lack of patient compliance with recommendations and provider expertise in counseling [15–20]. Varying or inconsistent clinical guidelines, and poor implementation of guidelines into health care systems, may also be a barrier [21]. Indeed, time seems to be the most consistent and problematic barrier, even if time allotted to office visits has increased [22–25]. Furthermore, high-volume physicians may perform fewer preventive services, again likely due to time constraints [5, 26].

Additionally, complicating the problem is the setting in which the preventive services are provided. One study evaluated the time spent on discussing preventive care during chronic care visits [27]. More than half of the physician's time was spent obtaining history; only 20 percent of the time was spent on health education [11, 27]. Very little time (<3 percent) was spent on counseling for topics such as nutrition, exercise, or smoking. In another study in which acute and chronic care visits were used to provide preventive care, preventive services were only offered in approximately one-third of visits, increasing the length of these visits by nearly 3 minutes [28]. In addition to the time needed to address clinical services, time spent in setting up referrals and time spent in the billing and coding process may also be barriers [21]. Last, but certainly not least, is the effect of the electronic health record (EHR). Although the implementation and use of EHR in well-woman visits is not the focus of this chapter, it is nonetheless a critical component in the provision of clinical services. Although data are mixed on the effect of EHR implementation on provider time, a systematic review demonstrated that time inefficiencies exist relative to the use of an EHR, particularly for physicians [29].

Time

Further highlighting the time issue is the actual time spent on preventive services. In a study using a model to evaluate the time needed to address preventive services in a representative adult primary care patient panel of 2,500 patients with an age and gender distribution similar to the US population, it was estimated that 4.4 hours of a physician's daily working time would be needed for the provision of preventive services sanctioned by the USPSTF [5]. When children, pregnant patients, and high-risk groups were added, the requirement increased to 7.4 hours per day. Interestingly, only slightly more than 2 hours were used to address USPSTF "A" recommendations; an additional 5.2 hours were used to address "B" recommendations. Another study analyzed the amount of time spent on particular preventive services [11]. In this study, the preventive topics addressed and the time spent on them varied as to whether the visit was for chronic or preventive care. For example, during chronic care visits, more time was spent on items such as cholesterol screening, cervical cytology, mammography, exercise counseling, and blood pressure, whereas during preventive care visits, less time was spent on cervical cytology and tobacco cessation counseling. Additionally, time spent on individual "A"- and "B"-rated services varied; some exceeded the time recommended to address specific topics, whereas others involved less than the recommended time. Time spent on several "I"-recommended services was considered relatively high, although that may not be surprising given that counseling for "I" recommendations may be more involved for a patient to decide whether to pursue an "I"-rated recommendation.

Multimorbidity and Preventive Care during "Problem" Visits

Related to the concept of preventive care during chronic visits is the concept of multimorbidity. Multimorbidity is defined as the existence of two or more medical or psychiatric conditions which may or may not interact with each other individually [30, 31]. This is analogous to patients having multiple chronic conditions. It is estimated that approximately 25 percent of American patients meet these criteria [30]. Multimorbidity is associated with clinical challenges, not only because of the number of conditions present, but because of the potential interaction between the conditions themselves, or the treatments of these conditions [32]. For example, a treatment strategy for one condition may actually worsen the manifestations of another condition. This issue is further complicated by the fact that many clinical guidelines are disease- or condition-specific, and do not account for the presence

of additional morbidities that may impact the recommended intervention or that may be impacted by the particular intervention being considered [32–34].

These concerns, relative to multimorbidity, unquestionably affect the provision of preventive care and increase time per visit. Importantly, patients also describe their own challenges with multimorbidity. In a UK study evaluating "hassles" experienced by patients with multimorbidity, several were identified, including lack of information about conditions and treatment options, poor communication between clinicians involved in specific condition-related care, poor access to specialist care, and logistical issues [35]. Interestingly, one of the variables associated with an increased perception of "hassles" included younger age [35]. A US study identified similar "hassles" in patients with multimorbidity; lack of information was clearly identified as a major contributor [36].

Clinical Workflow

Compounding the issue of preventive care, potential barriers, and efficiency is the concept of clinical workflow. It has been suggested that the ineffectiveness of some tools designed to aid in the primary care delivery process may be due to a lack of knowledge about the specific workflow processes in a primary and preventive care setting [3]. It might be theorized that there is a "standard" workflow in a primary care or preventive setting, and that by identifying the standard or common workflow patterns, tools or guidelines might be developed and implemented to facilitate the provider–patient interaction. However, that is not the case. A recent study analyzed, in detail, primary care workflow patterns [3]. Workflow patterns in primary care provider clinics varied significantly, even for individual physicians and even for patients with similar problems. Studies show that there was no single or common workflow pattern identified; the workflow patterns were unpredictable. In fact, workflow was described as a "dance" between the physician and the patient, based on the interaction between the patient's and physician's agendas [3]. The lack of efficiency initially predicted to be associated with EHRs may be due to a false assumption that physician workflow patterns are standardized and consistent., EHRs do not facilitate workflow patterns that are unpredictable [3, 37, 38].

Provider Well-Being

While the focus of the preceding paragraphs has been the patient and patient–provider interaction, one cannot exclude the provider's own attributes relative to primary and preventive care. While many of the studies specifically looked at physicians, all types of providers are subject to similar pressures, and the findings likely generalize to all provider types. Primary care physicians have a high risk of "burnout," and may be deeply dissatisfied [39–42]. Reasons given for dissatisfaction include spending significant amounts of time performing functions outside of their training, time pressures, increased administrative and regulatory demands, fragmentation of care, and work–life balance challenges [42–44]. Many of these concerns are not unique to primary care physicians; indeed obstetrician-gynecologists face similar challenges [45–48]. In identifying potential solutions, it is critical that the provider's well-being also be addressed.

Possible Solutions

The previous section highlights the challenges associated with the provision of primary and preventive care. It is not feasible to expect a clinician to deliver all recommended preventive services to a panel of patients in one visit [5]. Indeed, the American College of Obstetrics and Gynecology (ACOG) Well-Woman Task Force, in the Executive Summary addressing the components of the well-woman visit, concluded that not all of the recommended components "must be performed" at the same visit or by the same provider [49]. Further highlighting the inability to perform each task in a particular visit is the "Bright Futures" guidelines addressing care for infants, children, and adolescents [50]. The Bright Futures guidelines specifically describe that no health care professional has the time to do every possible recommended intervention for a particular age-related visit [50]. So the question is . . . How do we do it? The answer lies in the use of multiple visits, prioritization, coordinated systems of care, and optimizing efficiency.

Multiple Visits

Additional visits are often required to accomplish all the activities related to preventive care. Determining the number, duration, and scheduling of each visit can be challenging. The "art" of medicine allows solutions that are individualized. Prioritization should aid in the decision of how to plan for subsequent visits, both in the time needed and the topics to be addressed. Coordination of care may also aid in setting the

timing and need for additional visits, particularly by incorporating additional health care providers.

An interesting concept related to the interpretation of "visits" and "encounters" is offered in the Bright Futures guidelines. In these guidelines, many health care professionals view a visit as a single encounter, which is also encouraged by payers and the view supported by educators [50]. These visits are "counted" as one visit, but in contrast to a "sick" visit, in which a specific condition is addressed with a desired focused outcome, a preventive care visit is associated with multiple potential outcomes, which may lead to many separate interventions within the one encounter. Based on this view, one might consider the concept of viewing one "visit" as a series of "multiple encounters" [50]. Furthermore, these "encounters" may have different goals, including disease detection, disease prevention, health promotion, and anticipatory guidance [50]. Each of these goals utilize different approaches, content, tone, and interventions; does it therefore make sense to combine them all into a single "encounter" or "visit"? Furthermore, consider the potentially vast amount of information that may be communicated relative to each of these goals and the potential for patients to be overwhelmed. According to Bright Futures, inherent incongruence between the goals of preventive visits will lead to incongruent practice and related frustrations [50]. Perhaps if providers, and payers, viewed the use of multiple "encounters" instead of multiple "visits" to achieve all of the goals related to preventive care, the distribution of care across multiple effectively timed and coordinated encounters would be more readily acceptable.

While the use of multiple visits may provide one potential solution, one must also consider the patient's perspective. Certainly, additional visits may be inconvenient for patients to attend, especially those with multimorbidity [32]. Furthermore, depending on the patient's health insurance, multiple visits may not be financially practical or feasible.

Prioritization

Unquestionably, with the inability to achieve all preventive care goals in one visit, and the likely need for multiple visits, a provider must be able to prioritize the patient's problems and goals, in order to provide effective and subsequent coordinated care. While prioritizing might on the surface seem relatively "easy," it in fact is not. This may be particularly true in prioritizing medical problems and preventive care goals in patients with multimorbidity, or for those patients seen for a problem-oriented visit in which an attempt at addressing prevention is made. This may be further challenging in the current focus on patient-centered care, because the patient's agenda may not necessarily be the same as the provider's perspective, and thus the skills needed to effectively prioritize to meet both agendas is particularly important [32]. In fact, in a study of several outpatient primary care clinics, the patient's and physician's priorities aligned only 69 percent of the time·[51]. For those situations in which priorities were not aligned, patients focused on symptomatic concerns, while physicians focused more on asymptomatic but potentially dangerous conditions or difficult-to-manage chronic conditions [51]. Nonetheless, some sort of prioritization is essential.

The Bright Futures guidelines offer good practical information related to prioritization; although the information is geared toward infants, children, and adolescents, the principles can be applied to other patient populations. Bright Futures describes activities that are considered "must dos," those that providers "need to do," and those that providers "want to do" [50]. Additionally, families have an agenda that needs to be incorporated. In order to effect the most optimal time management, it is suggested that the providers clarify the goals of the visit, identify family needs, prioritize *shared* goals for the visit (shared with the family), and consider other methods to address issues that may not be covered in a particular visit [50, 52]. In addition, Bright Futures offers a model, using a "strength-based" approach, for setting priorities [50]. In this outline, the first priorities, regardless of the visit, are the parent's concerns. Bright Futures then offers five additional topics to address at each visit, which vary depending on the age of the patient [50]. These topics are "prioritized" according to health supervision and anticipatory guidance. A similar "prioritization guide" does not exist for women's health care; indeed it would be beneficial for a guide to be developed.

There is additional guidance to aid providers in prioritization. Certainly, prioritization will depend on patient factors, including age, behavioral and risk factors, and gender, among other considerations. It is also suggested to individualize screening and prevention interventions in order to maximize the value of a particular consideration, taking into account the potential benefits, costs, and harms [53, 54]. The USPSTF preventive services guidelines may aid in prioritization via the use of the grading recommendations, in which case "A" and "B" recommendations may be prioritized over "C" recommendations. The American Academy of Family Physicians (AAFP) also provides an "Agenda-Setting Algorithm" to aid providers in setting an agenda for a particular visit and to help prioritize the goals of the visit in order to identify what will be achieved in the current visit (Figure 6.1) [55]. The Agency for Healthcare Research and Quality (AHRQ) provides a useful electronic tool, the Electronic Preventive Services Selector (ePSS) to identify patient-specific preventive services, based on the USPSTF guidelines [56]. This tool is available on a number of electronic formats. This tool allows a provider to enter certain characteristics, including age, risk factors such as tobacco use, and gender, and generates a list of recommendations to consider for a particular patient, which can be prioritized according to the USPSTF grade. Another potential tool is a scoring system, incorporating a 10-point scale, for prioritizing preventive services [57, 58]. In the previously cited study addressing the time required to provide preventive services, these authors calculated that according to the scoring system, if those services considered to be the highest priority (score of 7 through 10) were provided, 1 hour per day would be required, as opposed to the 2.2 hours per day to provide the USPSTF "A"-graded services in their study [5].

Related to multimorbidity, one study of primary care from the United Kingdom described an "additive-sequential" model to accommodate care for patients with multiple problems [32]. In this model, clinicians made a list of the patient's problems and their associated complexity, identifying priorities among the patient's and clinician's agendas. These problems were then managed sequentially until time was ended, with remaining problems deferred until future visits [32]. While this model seemingly aids in management of complex patients, it was not clearly defined how the patients' conditions were prioritized. It was noted, however, that continuity of care provided more effective use of the "additive-sequential" model, since the patient returned to the same provider to address subsequent problems [32].

Patient-Centered Homes and Other Alternatives

One solution suggested to provide a venue to coordinate care, prioritization, and flexibility, is the

AGENDA-SETTING ALGORITHM

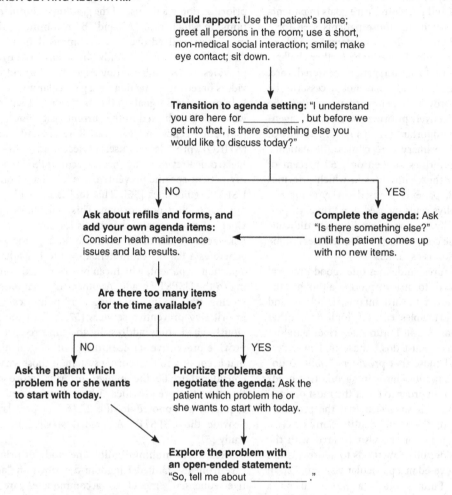

Build rapport: Use the patient's name; greet all persons in the room; use a short, non-medical social interaction; smile; make eye contact; sit down.

Transition to agenda setting: "I understand you are here for _____ , but before we get into that, is there something else you would like to discuss today?"

NO

YES

Ask about refills and forms, and add your own agenda items: Consider heath maintenance issues and lab results.

Complete the agenda: Ask "Is there something else?" until the patient comes up with no new items.

Are there too many items for the time available?

NO

YES

Ask the patient which problem he or she wants to start with today.

Prioritize problems and negotiate the agenda: Ask the patient which problem he or she wants to start with today.

Explore the problem with an open-ended statement: "So, tell me about _____ ."

This tool was developed by Egnew TR, Tacoma Family Medicine, Tacoma, Wash. Copyright © 2012 Thomas R. Egnew. Physicians may photocopy or adapt for use in their own practices; all other rights reserved. http://www.aafp.org/fpm/2014/0700/p25.html.

Family Practice Management®

Figure 6.1 Agenda-Setting Algorithm That Could be Used to Facilitate Prioritization of Goals during a Particular Clinical Visit Agenda, Reprinted with permission from The Art of Medicine: Seven Skills That Promote Mastery, 2014, Vol 21(4), Family Practice Management, Copyright © 2014, American Academy of Family Physicians. All Rights Reserved.

patient-centered medical home. These "homes" are one way of organizing care that emphasizes coordination and communication [49, 59]. The advantage of the patient-centered medical home is described as providing a platform for prioritizing, personalizing, delivering care, and referring patients for needed services [60]. Aspects related to the patient-centered medical home, including concepts, incentives, recognition, and accreditation programs, are also available on the AAFP website [61]. The patient-centered

medical home has been associated with improvements in patient satisfaction, provider work environment, and quality of care; cost savings are also a reported benefit [62]. Related to the care of patients with complex health conditions, the American Medical Association (AMA) provides a module to deliver "intensive primary care" [63]. While the specifics of this model may be outside of the realm of an obstetrician-gynecologist, it nonetheless describes the creation of a team-based approach to provide health care. In the previously addressed study considering provider satisfaction, those practices recognized as patient-centered homes were identified as "high-performing" and associated with physician work–life satisfaction [42]. These "high-performing" homes implemented a number of solutions to common problems in primary and preventive care, including proactive planned care, utilization of previsit planning and previsit laboratory tests, shared clinical care among a team, sharing of clerical tasks including "scribing" and nonphysician order entry, improvements in communication, and enhancements in team function through colocation, team meetings, and workflow mapping [42].

Related to women-centered medical homes, ACOG supports the concept of developing medical homes related to women's health care [49, 59, 64]. In addition, ACOG has developed a toolkit to help women's health practices assess whether they would be interested in developing a medical home [65]. However, in contrast to publications regarding the implementation and benefits of a patient-centered home in primary care practice, little has been published relative to the development and study of a woman-centered medical home especially related to primary and preventive care for women. The use of a patient-centered home by internists to provide comprehensive preconception care may be one example of how a woman-centered home could be modeled and implemented [66]. Interestingly, a bill was introduced in Congress in 2009 to direct the Secretary of Health and Human Services to establish a 3-year women's medical home demonstration project; however, this bill was not enacted [67].

Other alternatives that have been suggested include those that go beyond the traditional face-to-face encounter. These alternatives include group visits, use of health educators, incorporating other health care providers in the care of a patient, using a team-based approach (maybe not necessarily as part of a "home" model), and extending methods of patient education [5, 68, 69]. The concept of "group" care specific to obstetrics and gynecology has been demonstrated through group prenatal care, which has been shown to be positively viewed by women and associated with no adverse effects [70].

Interestingly, not all data on team-based approaches demonstrate effectiveness, although this may be limited to studying a particular population. In a systematic review analyzing various interventions to manage patients with multimorbidity, organizational interventions such as case management to coordinate care through multidisciplinary teams was not as effective as patient-oriented interventions focused on functional difficulties [71].

Enhancing Efficiency

In addition to team-based care or incorporation of the patient-centered home, additional tools and interventions have been described to potentially enhance efficiency in the provision of primary and preventive care. The Bright Futures guidelines provide some solutions to enhance clinical and organizational processes related to the provision of care for infants, children, and adolescents [50]. Again, although tailored to care of these groups of patients, it is possible that some of the strategies may be applicable to the care of adults.

The AAFP also provide resources designed to improve efficiency in the provision of primary and preventive care, including a number of modules [72]. Some of these modules include tools and resources addressing office efficiency, such as tools to identify common inefficiencies and strategies for creating a more efficient practice. There are also tools and guidance relative to patient efficiency, including tips to improve practice efficiency and patient satisfaction, and a module on team-based care in improving efficiency. Similar to the consideration of the Bright Futures guidelines, although these modules are geared toward family medicine practitioners, there are likely useful aspects that could be applied to the provision of well-woman and preventive care. Additionally, the AHRQ also provides a number of resources under the heading "Improving Primary Care Practice" that address the ability of primary care and preventive practices to be involved in quality improvement activities [73].

Other potential methods to improve efficiency and enhance uptake of preventive services include optimizing office systems, such as using decision aids or training medical assistants to discuss preventive services *before* a visit in order to improve provider efficiency and help patients make informed decisions [74].

Although the issue of provider time efficiency associated with EHR implementation was previously addressed, computer-based information-gathering systems and the EHR have been promulgated as having a role in trying to improve overall clinical environment efficiency. For example, a study evaluating the acceptability of a waiting room touch-screen computer system to collect patient health behavior information was found to be positively received by patients, and general practitioners noted that this system was not disruptive of practice [9]. This system was both feasible and acceptable, and one of the implications for practice was that this system may aid in the prioritization process [9]. In a review of the role of "e-health" in optimizing preventive care, this electronic system was noted to be beneficial in facilitating collection of patient-reported data on health and lifestyle behaviors and improving clinical management through the provision of tailored feedback, educational materials, and reminders [6]. Collection of patient self-reported data was found to be accurate as well, thus self-reported data was considered feasible, especially if standardized questions were asked. Reported advantages of incorporating an electronic system included more comprehensive collection of information, point-of-care feedback, more effective transfer of data, allowing providers the ability to identify those issues considered more concerning and thus assisting with prioritization, and promoting patient-centered care [6]. In summary, electronic systems and the EHR have some potential to improve care and efficiency, but there are issues to overcome in order to reach these systems' true potential.

Another technology that may have a role in enhancing efficiency in the preventive care setting is telehealth and telemedicine. There are a number of studies and reports that have evaluated the role of telehealth and smart technology in a variety of settings or specific disease conditions, including mental health, intensive care, management of chronic obstructive pulmonary disease, emergency medicine, wound care, dermatology, radiology, and ophthalmology [75–80]. The application of telemedicine in more general primary and preventive care is not as robust, however. A systematic review published in 2010 did not identify any studies in which telemedicine could serve as a "replacement" for general practice visits [81]. An updated systematic review is in process to evaluate subsequent data regarding the use of telemedicine in general practice care [80]. Certainly as technology advances, it is theoretically possible that telehealth could improve the efficiency of providing primary and preventive care.

Coding, Billing, and Reimbursement

General Considerations

A detailed and comprehensive description of issues related to billing, coding, and reimbursement is beyond the scope of this chapter; there are a number of resources, including coding courses offered by ACOG [82], to aid in coding and related documentation. These resources often provide specific examples to highlight coding and billing issues and considerations. However, several points are important to highlight.

Preventive medicine services, which are a type of evaluation and management (E/M) service, do not require a chief complaint. There are generally two types: counseling for risk factor reduction and behavioral change intervention (codes 99401–99412) and preventive medicine E/M services (codes 99381–99387 and 99391–99397). It is important to note that counseling related to risk factor reduction or behavioral change must be provided at a separate encounter from the preventive medicine service; this consideration may be important when setting priorities and planning for multiple visits. It is also important to highlight that although it must be separately coded from the preventive E/M, behavioral change interventions for behaviors such as tobacco use, obesity, and substance abuse are a billable service.

Additionally, it is significant to highlight the distinction between the comprehensive history and examination obtained during preventive services compared to other E/M services. The comprehensive history for preventive services should first be appropriate for the patient's age, gender, and identified risk factors and should include a comprehensive review of systems and assessment of risk factors, family history, and social history. The examination should be multisystem, with the extent based on the patient's age, gender, and risk factors. The history and examination do **not** have to meet the criteria for a comprehensive history or examination as defined by the Centers for Medicare and Medicaid Services (CMS) E/M documentation guidelines.

Coverage

Coverage of preventive services is certainly a complex environment, although the Affordable Care Act (ACA) does provide some consistency related to coverage of at least some preventive services. The ACA requires private health plans to cover several evidence-based preventive services, including mammography, colonoscopy, and childhood immunizations, currently without cost sharing. Medicare also covers certain screening services that are often performed during a preventive care visit. Of note, Medicare does **not** cover the comprehensive preventive medicine codes 999387 or 99397.

Importantly, related to the issue of addressing specific problems and preventive services, for non-Medicare payers, the CPT* (current procedural terminology) rules state that if problems are identified during a preventive visit, that an appropriate office outpatient code (99201–99215) should be reported in addition to the preventive medicine code if an abnormality is encountered or a preexisting problem is addressed during the preventive E/M encounter. The problem must be significant enough to require additional activities to perform the key components of the problem-oriented E/M service. In this case, the Modifier 25 may be used to identify a significant and separate E/M service.

Medicare polices related to preventive coverage are certainly complex and are beyond the scope of this chapter. Resources addressing Medicare-related issues may be found in a number of areas, including ACOG and the CMS [83].

Summary

1. Providers of preventive care face numerous challenges, including the sheer volume of tasks to be addressed and accomplished, gathering comprehensive information regarding the patient's health status, and counseling to address management, prevention strategies, and risk reduction.

2. Barriers to optimizing preventive care include lack of time, lack of patient compliance, billing and reimbursement issues, and varying guidelines; time is the more commonly cited barrier.

3. Multimorbidity adds to the complexity of patient visits and adds to the difficulty in the provision of preventive care when also having to address several chronic conditions.

4. Multiple visits, when planned effectively and closely aligned with prioritization, enhance efficiency of the office visit and coverage of multiple health care issues.

5. Prioritization aids in addressing patient and provider agendas, especially when not aligned, and

includes tools such as the ePSS and tools suggested by organizations such as the AAFP, American Academy of Pediatrics (AAP), and the AHRQ.

6. Patient-centered medical homes may enhance efficiency and adherence to preventive care by organizing care that emphasizes coordination and communication.

7. Techniques that may improve efficiency in the outpatient clinic include tolls to recognize inefficiencies, use of organizational modules such as those provided by the AAFP and AHRQ, effective use of EHRs, and telemedicine/telehealth.

References

1. American College of Obstetricians and Gynecologists. Well-woman visit. Committee Opinion Number 534. *Obstet Gynecol.* 2012, **120**:420–4.

2. Meddler, J.D., Kahn, N.B. Jr., and Susman, J.L. Risk factors and recommendations for 230 primary care adult patients, based on US Preventive Services Task Force guidelines. *Am J Prev Med.* 1992, **8**:150–3.

3. Holman, G.T., Beasley, J.W., Karsh, B.T. et al. The myth of standardized workflow in primary care. *J Am Med Inform Assoc.* 2015, September 2. doi: 10.1093/jamia/ocv107.

4. Wetterneck, T.B., Lapin, J.A., Krueger, D.J. et al. Development of a primary care physician task list to evaluate clinic visit workflow. *BMJ Qual Saf.* 2012, **21**:47–53.

5. Yarnall, K.S.H., Pollak, K.I., Østbye, T., Krause, K.M., and Michener, J.L. Primary care: Is there enough time for prevention? *Am J Public Health.* 2003, **93**:635–41.

6. Carey, M., Noble, N., Mansfield, E. et al. The role of ehealth in optimizing preventive care in the primary care setting. *J Med Internet Res.* 2015, **17**:e126.

7. McGlynn, E.A., Asch, S.M., Adams, J. et al. The quality of health care delivered to adults in the United States. *N Engl J Med.* 2003, **348**:2635–45.

8. Anderson, L.M. and May, D.S. Has the use of cervical, breast, and colorectal cancer screening increased in the Unites States? *Am J Public Health.* 1995, **85**:840–2.

9. Paul, C.L., Carey, M., Yoong, S.L. et al. Access to chronic disease care in general practice: The acceptability of implementing systematic waiting-room screening using computer-based patient-reported risk status. *Br J Gen Pract.* 2013, **63**:e620–6.

10. Ruffin, M.T., Gorenflo, D.W., and Woodman, B. Predictors of screening for breast, cervical, colorectal, and prostatic cancer among community-based primary care practices. *J Am Board Fam Pract.* 2000, **13**:1–10.

11. Pollak, K.I., Krause, K.M., Yarnall, K.S.H. et al. Estimated time spent on preventive services by primary care physicians. *BMC Health Serv Res.* 2008, **8**:245.

12. Sonntag, U., Henkel, J., Renneberg, B. et al. Counseling overweight patients: Analysis of preventive encounters in primary care. *Int J Qual Health Care.* 2010, **22**:486–92.

13. Centers for Disease Control and Prevention. Behavioral Risk Factor Surveillance System. Available at: www.cdc.gov/brfss. Retrieved December 22, 2015.

14. Cancer Council Australia. National Cancer Prevention Policy, 2007–2009. Cancer Council Australia, 2011. Available at: www.cancer.org/au/content/pdf/Cancer ControlPolicy/NationalCancerPreventionPolicy/NCP P07-09breastcacner.pdf.

15. Burack, R.C. Barriers to clinical preventive medicine. *Prim Care.* 1989, **16**:245–50.

16. Kottke, T.E., Brekke, M.L., and Solberg, L.I. Making "time" for preventive services. *Mayo Clin Proc.* 1993, **68**:785–91.

17. McPhee, S.J., Richard, S.J., and Solkowitz, S.N. Performance of cancer screening in a university general internal medicine practice: Comparison with the 1980 American Cancer Society Guidelines. *J Gen Intern Med.* 1986, **1**:275–81.

18. Spitz, M.R., Chamberlain, R.M., Sider, J.G., and Fueger, J.J. Cancer prevention practices among Texas primary care physicians. *J Cancer Educ.* 1992, **7**:55–60.

19. Wender, R.C. Cancer screening and prevention in primary care. Obstacles for physicians. *Cancer.* 1993, **72**(Suppl 3):1093–9.

20. Passey, M., Fanaian, M., Lyle, D., and Harris, M.F. Assessment and management of lifestyle risk factors in rural and urban general practices in Australia. *Aust J Prim Health.* 2010, **16**:81–6.

21. Ayres, C.G. and Griffith, H.M. Perceived barriers to and facilitators of the implementation of priority clinical preventive service guidelines. *Am J Manag Care.* 2007, **13**:150–5.

22. Campion, E.W. A symptom of discontent. *N Engl J Med.* 2001, **344**:223–5.

23. Collins, K.S., Schoen, C., and Sandman, D.R. *The Commonwealth Fund Survey of Physician Experiences with Managed Care.* New York, NY: The Commonwealth Fund, 1997.

24. Hadley, J., Mitchell, J.M., Sulmasy, D.P., and Bloche, M.G. Perceived financial incentives, HMO market penetration, and physicians' practice styles and satisfaction. *Health Surv Res.* 1999, **34**:307–21.

25. Dennis, S., Williams, A., Taggart, J. et al. Which providers can bridge the health literacy gap in lifestyle risk factor modification education: A systematic review and narrative synthesis. *BMC Fam Pract*, 2012, **13**:44.

26. Zyzanski, S.J., Stange, K.C., Langa, D., and Flocke, S.A. Trade-offs in high-volume primary care practice. *J Fam Pract.* 1998, **46**:397–402.

27. Yawn, B., Goodwin, M.A., Zyzanski, S.J., and Stange, K.C. Time use during acute and chronic illness visits to a family physician. *Fam Pract.* 2003, **20**:474–7.

28. Stange, K.C., Flocke, S.A., and Goodwin, M.A. Opportunistic preventive services delivery. Are time limitations and patient satisfaction barriers? *J Fam Pract.* 1998, **46**:419–24.

29. Poissant, L., Pereira, J., Tamblyn, R., and Kawasumi, Y. The impact of electronic health records on time efficiency of physicians and nurses: A systematic review. *J Am Med Inform Assoc.* 2005, **112**:505–16.

30. Mercer, S.W., Smith, S.M., Wyke, S., O'Dowd, T., and Watt, G.C. Multimorbidity in primary care: Developing the research agendas. *Fam Pract.* 2009, **26**:79–80.

31. Uijen, A.A. and van de Lisdonk, E.H. Multimorbidity in primary care: Prevalence and trend over the past 20 years. *Eur J Gen Pract.* 2008, **14**(Suppl 1):28–32.

32. Bower, P., Macdonald, W., Harkness, E. et al. Multimorbidity, service organization and clinical decision making in primary care: A qualitative study. *Fam Pract.* 2011, **28**:579–87.

33. Tinetti, M.E., Bogardus, S.T. Jr., and Agostini, J.V. Potential pitfalls of disease-specific guidelines for patients with multiple conditions. *N Engl J Med.* 2004, **351**:2870–4.

34. Safford, M.M., Allison, J.J., and Kiefe, C.I. Patient complexity: More than comorbidity, the vector model of complexity. *J Gen Intern Med.* 2007, **22**(Suppl 3):382–90.

35. Adeniji, C., Kenning, C., Coventry, P.A., and Bower, P. What are the core predictors of "hassles" among patients with multimorbidity in primary care? A cross-sectional study. *BMC Health Serv Res.* 2015, **15**:255.

36. Parchman, M.L., Noël, P.H., and Lee, S. Primary care attributes, health care system hassles, and chronic illness. *Med Care.* 2005, **43**:1123–9.

37. Harrison, M.I., Koppel, R., and Bar-Lev, S. Unintended consequences of information technologies in health care – An interactive sociotechnical analysis. *J Am Med Inform Assoc.* 2007, **14**:542–9.

38. Avitzur, O. In practice: The worst features of EHRs and how to fix them. *Neurol Today.* 2012, **12**:22–7.

39. Shanafelt, T.D., Boone, S., Tan, L. et al. Burnout and satisfaction with work-life balance among US physicians relative to the general US population. *Arch Intern Med.* 2012, **172**:1377–85.

40. Dyrbye, L.N. and Shanafelt, T.D. Physician burnout: A potential threat to successful health care reform. *JAMA*. 2011, **305**:2009–10.

41. Okie, S. Innovation in primary care – Staying one step ahead of burnout. *N Engl J Med*. 2008, **359**:2305–9.

42. Sinsky, C.A., Willard-Grace, R., Schutzbank, A.M. et al. In search of joy in practice; a report of 23 high-functioning primary care practices. *Ann Fam Med*. 2013, **11**:272–8.

43. Altschuler, J., Margolius, D., Bodenheimer, T., and Grumbach, K. Estimating a reasonable patient panel size for primary care physicians with team-based task delegation. *Ann Fam Med*. 2012, **10**:396–400.

44. Grumbach, K., and Bodenheimer, T. A primary care home for Americans; putting the house in order. *JAMA*. 2002, **288**:889–93.

45. Rayburn, W.F. *The Obstetrician-Gynecologists Workforce in the United States. Facts, Figures, and Implications – 2011*. Washington, DC: American College of Obstetricians and Gynecologists, 2011.

46. Weinstein, L. and Wolfe, H.M. The downward spiral of physician satisfaction: An attempt to avert a crisis within the medical profession. *Obstet Gynecol*. 2007, **109**:1181–3.

47. Bettes, B.A., Chalas, E., Coleman, V.H., and Schulkin, J. Heavier workload, less personal control: Impact of delivery on obstetrician/gynecologists' career satisfaction. *Am J Obstet Gynecol*. 2004, **190**:851–7.

48. Keeton, K., Fenner, D.E., Johnson, T.R., and Hayward, R.A. Predictors of physician career satisfaction, work–life balance, and burnout. *Obstet Gynecol*, 2007, **109**:949–55.

49. Conry, J.A. and Brown, H. Executive Summary: Well-Woman Task Force. Components of the well-woman visit. *Obstet Gynecol*. 2015, **126**:697–701.

50. Hagan, J.F., Shaw, J.S., and Duncan, P.M., editors. *Bright Futures: Guidelines for Health Supervision of Infants, Children, and Adolescents*, 3rd edition. Elk Grove Village, IL: American Academy of Pediatrics, 2008. pp. 203–19.

51. Tomsik, P.E., Witt, A.M., Raddock, M.L. et al. How well do physician and patient visit priorities align? *J Fam Pract*. 2014, **63**:e8–e13.

52. Green, M. and Palfrey, J.S., editors. *Bright Futures: Guidelines for Health Supervision of Infants, Children, and Adolescents*, 2nd edition. Arlington, VA: National Center for Education in Maternal and Child Health, 2002.

53. Saini, S.D., van Hees, F., and Vijan, S. Smarter screening for cancer: Possibilities and challenges of personalization. *JAMA*. 2014, **312**:2211–2.

54. Harris, R.P., Wilt, T.J., and Qaseem, A.; High Value Care Task Force of the American College of Physicians. A value framework for cancer screening: Advice for high-value care from the American College of Physicians. *Ann Intern Med*. 2015, **162**:712–7.

55. Egnew, T.R; American Academy of Family Physicians. Agenda-Setting Algorithm. Available at: www.aafp.org/fpm/2014/0700/fpm20140700p25-rt1.pdf. Retrieved December 22, 2015.

56. Agency for Healthcare Research and Quality. Electronic Preventive Services Selector (ePSS). Available at: epss.ahrq.gov/PDA/index.jsp. Retrieved December 22, 2015.

57. Maciosek, M.V., Coffield, A.B., McGinnis, J.M. et al. Methods for priority setting among clinical preventive services. *Am J Prev Med*. 2001, **21**:10–9.

58. Maciosek, M.V., Coffield, A.B., Edwards, N.M. et al. Priorities among effective clinical preventive services: Results of a systematic review and analysis. *Am J Prev Med*, 2006, **31**:52–61.

59. Sawaya, G.F. Re-envisioning the annual well-woman visit (editorial). *Obstet Gynecol*. 2015, **126**:695–6.

60. Stange, K.C. and Woolf, S.H. Policy options in support of high-value preventive care. A prevention policy paper commissioned by the Partnership for Prevention. Partnership for Prevention, 2008. Available at: www.prevent.org/data/files/initiatives/policyoptionssupporthighvaluepreventivecare.pdf. Retrieved December 22, 2015.

61. American Academy of Family Physicians. The patient-centered medical home (PCMH). Available at: www.aafp.org/practice-management/transformation/pcmh.html. Retrieved December 22, 2015.

62. Reid, R.J., Coleman, K., Johnson, E.A. et al. The Group Health medical home at year two: Cost savings, higher patient satisfaction, and less burnout for providers. *Health Aff (Millwood)*. 2010, **29**:835–43.

63. American Medical Association. Steps Forward: Building an intensive primary care practice (online module). Available at: www.stepsforward.org/modules/intensive-primary-care. Retrieved December 22, 2015.

64. American College of Obstetricians and Gynecologists. Medical home answers to some questions. Available at: www.acog.org/About-ACOG/ACOG-Departments/Practice-Management-and-Managed-Care/Medical-Home–Answers-to-Some-Questions. Retrieved December 22, 2015.

65. American College of Obstetricians and Gynecologists. ACOG medical home toolkit. Available at: www.acog.org/About-ACOG/ACOG-Departments/Practice-Management-and-Managed-Care/ACOG-Medical-Home-Toolkit. Retrieved December 22, 2015.

66. Files, J.A., David, P.S., and Frey, K.A. The patient-centered medical home and preconception

care: An opportunity for internists. *J Gen Intern Med.* 2008, **23**:1518–20.

67. United States Congress. United States Senate Bill S. 1303 (111th): Women's Medical Home Demonstration Act. Available at: www.govtrack.us/congress/bills/111/s1301. Retrieved December 22, 2015.

68. Moore, G. and Showstack, J. Primary care medicine in crisis: Toward reconstruction and renewal. *Ann Intern Med.* 2003, **138**:244–7.

69. Whitcomb, M.E. and Cohen, J.J. The future of primary care medicine. *N Engl J Med.* 2004, **351**:710–2.

70. Catling, C.J., Medley, N., Foureur, M. et al. Group versus conventional antenatal care for women. *Cochrane Database Syst Rev.* 2015, (**2**): CD007622.

71. Smith, S.M., Soubhi, H., Fortin, M., Hudon, C., and O'Dowd, T. Managing patients with multimorbidity: Systematic review of interventions in primary care and community settings. *BMJ.* 2012, **345**:e5205.

72. American Academy of Family Physicians. Family Practice Management: Practice Efficiency. Available at: www.aafp.org/fpm/topicModules/viewTopicModule.htm?topicModuleid=44. Retrieved December 22, 2015.

73. Agency for Healthcare Research and Quality. Improving primacy care practice. Available at: www.ahrq.gov/professionals/prevention-chronic-care/improve.html. Retrieved December 22, 2015.

74. Ghorob, A. and Brodenheimer, T. Sharing the care to improve access to primary care. *N Engl J Med.* 2012, **366**:1955–7.

75. Salmoiraghi, A. and Hussain, S. A systematic review of the use of telepsychiatry in acute settings. *J Psychiatr Pract.* 2015, **21**:389–93.

76. Pedone, C. and Lelli, D. Systematic review of telemonitoring in COPD: An update. *Pneumonol Alergol Pol.* 2015, **83**:476–84.

77. Bashshur, R.L., Shannon, G.W., Tejasvi, T., Kvedar, J.C., and Gates, M. The empirical foundations of teledermatology: A review of the research evidence. *Telemed J E Health.* 2015, **21**:953–79.

78. Wilson, L.S. and Maeder, A.J. Recent directions in telemedicine: Review of trends in research and practice. *Healthc Inform Res.* 2015, **21**:213–22.

79. Bossen, A.L., Kim, H., Williams, K.N., Steinhoff, A.E., and Strieker, M. Emerging roles for telemedicine and smart technologies in dementia care. *Smart Homecare Technol Telehealth.* 2015, **3**:49–57.

80. Downes, M.J., Mervin, M.C., Byrnes, J.M., and Scuffham, P.A. Telemedicine for general practice: A systematic review protocol. *Syst Rev.* 2015, **4**:134.

81. Ekeland, A.G., Bowes, A. and Flottorp, S. Effectiveness of telemedicine: A systematic review of reviews. *Int J Med Inform.* 2010, **79**:736–71.

82. Coding resources. The American College of Obstetricians and Gynecologists. Available at: www.acog.org/About-ACOG/ACOG-Departments/Coding. Retrieved December 22, 2015.

83. Centers for Medicare and Medicaid Services. Preventive services. Available at: www.cms.gov/Outreach-and-Education/Medicare-Learning-Network-MLN/MLNProducts/PreventiveServices.html. Retrieved February 5, 2016.

Considerations for Medically Underserved Populations

Amy (Meg) Autry and Sara Whetstone

Learning Objectives

- Identify unique well-woman care needs in selected special populations of women including lesbian, gay, bisexual, and transgender (LGBT) individuals, disabled women, and vulnerable marginalized women who are homeless or incarcerated
- Provide guidelines for care in the context of general women's health recommendations
- Highlight culturally sensitive issues and provide resources for unbiased health care
- Explore unique health risks and provide approaches to care for these populations of women

Introduction

In this chapter, we are charged with identifying special populations of women who have unique needs with regard to the well-woman visit. Typically, these women have been treated poorly by the medical community or the health care system in general so they have frequently delayed or avoided initiating health care, particularly preventive services. We have chosen the broad categories of lesbian, gay, bisexual, and transgender (LGBT) individuals, obese and disabled women, vulnerable or marginalized populations including incarcerated and homeless women; but acknowledge that there are additional unique populations that we do not address due to space constraints. We do not address issues related to well-woman care for women of racial and ethnic minorities; these special considerations are highlighted in the component chapters addressing specific health care issues. Nonetheless, it is important to recognize the well-documented disparities in health and health care experienced by women of color. In general, racial and ethnic minorities experience a lower quality of health services and are less likely to receive even routine medical procedures than are white

Americans. Providers must recognize that racial and ethnic disparities in health care occur in the context of broader historic and contemporary social and economic inequality. We hope that women's health providers strive to care for diverse populations, to provide excellent, evidence-based care to all women, and to recognize the discrimination and reproductive coercion that minority women have experienced. Most of the women in these categories should receive the standard care recommended in the well-woman visit, but providers must be aware of unique risks as well as special accommodations for these populations and provide nonbiased culturally appropriate sensitive patient-centered care.

Reproductive Health Care for LGBT Patients and Patients with Disorders of Sexual Development

Prior to the discussion of reproductive health care for LGBT patients as well as patients with disorders of sexual development (DSD), it is imperative that reproductive health providers understand and adopt appropriate and acceptable terminology for this population that has been traditionally marginalized particularly by the health care system. LGBT and DSD designations are oversimplifications. These categories are not well delineated and can be fluid over an individual's lifetime. It is critical to differentiate between sex (i.e., the biological and physiologic characteristics that define phenotypic males and females) and gender (i.e., the socially constructed roles, behaviors, activities and attributes considered appropriate for men and women). Further delineation in the differences between sexual identity, attraction, and behavior are often grouped together under sexual orientation but they may not be concordant.

Sexual Orientation refers to whom one is physically, romantically, or emotionally attracted to. Lesbian women are attracted to and are usually sexually involved with other women; however, 30 percent of self-identified lesbian women are also sexually active with men. Ninety percent of lesbians have had sexual relationships with men in their past. Bisexual women are attracted to and are usually sexually involved with both men and women either sequentially or concurrently. There are also other notable but less often discussed orientations including asexuality, pansexuality, and polysexuality.

Gender Identity refers to one's basic sense of being male, female, or another gender.

Gender Expression refers to characteristics in appearance, personality, and behavior culturally defined as masculine or feminine.

Cisgender refers to a person whose self-identity conforms to the female or male sex they were assigned at birth.

Gender Nonconforming refers to people who do not follow other people's ideas or stereotypes about how they should look or act based on the female or male sex they were assigned at birth.

Transgender individuals are those whose gender identity differs from their assigned sex at birth. Transgender is an umbrella term that can mean (1) someone whose gender identity or expression does not fit dominant social constructs of sex and gender, (2) a gender outside of the man/woman/binary (i.e., gender nonconforming), (3) having no gender or multiple genders, or (4) someone who is transitioning from one gender to another. Gender transition may include change in gender identity or expression (i.e., social transition), administration of gender-affirming hormones (i.e., medical transition), or surgeries (i.e., surgical transition).

Those who are transitioning from a female sex assigned at birth and identify as men are referred to as transgender men. Those assigned male sex at birth who identify as women are referred to as transgender women. In medical literature often these individuals will be referred to as female to male (FTM) and male to female (MTF), respectively, but these are terms not necessarily used by individuals themselves.

Transsexual refers to an individual who seeks hormonal and (often, but not always) surgical treatment to modify the body so they may live full-time as a member of the sex category opposite to their birth assignment. This term is falling out of favor.

Transvestite or cross-dresser refers to someone who enjoys dressing in the clothing of a gender that is not consistent with their sex assigned at birth, but whose gender identity is still consistent with their sex assigned at birth (i.e., a man who wears female clothing periodically). This is increasingly considered a derogatory term.

Transgender individuals may have any sexual orientation and be heterosexual, homosexual, or have any number of sexual orientations before and after transition.

In general, 1 in 100 people are born with some atypical feature in their sex chromosomes, gonadal development, or anatomical sex. Although this group of individuals was classified previously under the stigmatizing term "hermaphroditism," now the most commonly used medical terminology is DSD, although there is still some concern with the use of the word "disorder" and some prefer alternative terminology such as intersex, variations of sex anatomy, and difference in sex development. Clinician's reluctance to abandon the term disorder stems from the fact that while most DSD persons do not have serious health consequences, there are health risks that are associated with some. Others worry that physicians will continue to focus on unnecessary and frequently harmful procedures such as cosmetic genital "normalization" surgeries. Like LGBT, DSD is an umbrella term and does not confer any statements about one's gender identity or sexual orientation.

Sexual orientation and gender identity are distinct from a person's sex, sexual history, or sexual practices. Health care providers must respect patients' self-identities, use their preferred terminology, and ask open-ended questions in a nonjudgmental fashion.

The Genderbread person is an easy pictorial representation of the concepts of gender identity and expression (Figure 7.1).

History of Medicine and the LGBT Community

The medical community and individuals in the LGBT and DSD communities have a storied past that has led to mistrust of the health care system in general and has contributed to health disparities in this population. Although this has improved recently, historically the health care system and individual practitioners have "pathologized" homosexuality and devalued minority sexual orientations and gender identities. Homosexuality was included in the *Diagnostic and Statistical Manual of Mental Disorders* until 1973, and it was only recently in 2012, that the American Psychiatric Association removed Gender Identity

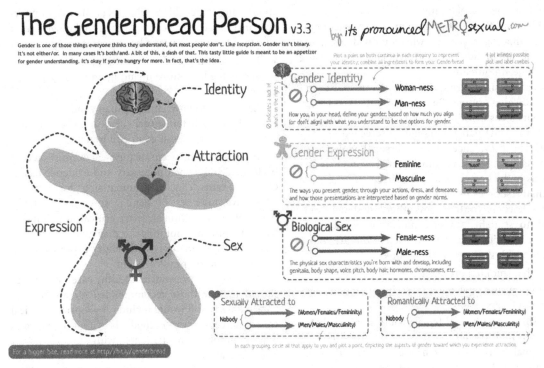

Figure 7.1 The Genderbread Person

Disorder from the Diagnostic and Statistical Manual of Mental Disorders (DSM-5), replacing it with Gender Dysphoria and shifting the focus of pathology away from any individual who is gender nonconfirming to the experience of living in a society which stigmatizes gender nonconformity.

In 2013, the United Nations called for an end to "reparative therapies" as well as unnecessary medical approaches that harm children born with DSD. To this day, efforts to "treat" homosexuality persist. Violence based on sexual orientation and gender identity was only federally categorized as a hate crime beginning in 2009 with the passage of the Matthew Shepard Act. Sterilization has, until recently, been considered a necessary legal and medical component of transition-related processes. In many countries, sterilization of trans people continues to be a prerequisite of gender identity recognition. In the United States, 14 states require proof of sexual reassignment surgery, court order, or amended birth certificate to change driver's licenses.

Individuals who are LGBT, gender nonconforming, or born with DSD often experience inadequate or inappropriate medical care ranging from unconscious bias to overtly discriminatory acts. In all, 9 percent of LGB and 52 percent of transgender individuals report being refused medical services because of their sexual orientation or gender identity. These interactions cause patients to delay seeking care or to avoid care altogether and translate into disparities in access and quality of care. Lack of provider knowledge and comfort in providing care results in absent or suboptimal risk factor assessment and medical management that is not grounded in the current best evidence and can lead to preventable harms.

LGBT individuals are twice as likely as the non-LGBT population to lack health insurance and plans often do not include provisions for same-sex partners or medical care for gender-affirming therapies. With the Affordable Care Act, the uninsured rates of LGBT adults have dropped from 24.2 to 17.6 percent. Transgender individuals are more likely than cisgender individuals to be uninsured and to postpone medical care. Transgender individuals of color are even more likely to report denial of care.

Preventive Health Care: LGBT individuals experience high rates of physical and emotional trauma throughout their lifetime. Trauma victims may present as disengaged, unfriendly, and defensive. Providers and their staff in turn may then react negatively, initiating a pattern where individuals avoid care and adopt additional risky behaviors causing adverse health outcomes.

Most resources group health risks in LGBT and DSD individuals by age. Being cognizant of risks helps providers focus their history and screening efforts. All LGBT and DSD patients should be screened for violence. The prevalence of interpersonal violence in relationships of lesbian and bisexual women is the same as in the heterosexual population, but there are minimal resources in the community for them.

Adolescents/youth (unless otherwise stated, compared to straight gender-conforming population): Gender identity and sexual orientation are more fluid in youth than other age groups.

- Higher smoking prevalence
- More misuse of alcohol, prescription opioids, and tranquilizers
- Lesbian and bisexual female youth more likely to report multiple sex partners and unprotected vaginal intercourse, and have a higher incidence of unintended pregnancies as well as chlamydia infections
- More eating disordered behaviors
- Less engagement in physical activity or team sports
- Increased depression, anxiety, and suicide attempts
- Increased violence from harassment
- Increased homelessness

Adults (unless otherwise stated, compared to straight gender-conforming population). Of Note: These data do not apply to transgender adults as there is too little data.

- Increased obesity
- Increased asthma
- Increased risk of cardiovascular disease
- Increased smoking prevalence
- Increased risk of becoming disabled and at an earlier age
- Transgender women (MTF) are at elevated risk for HIV/AIDS and other sexually transmitted infections (STIs)
- Increased incidence of depression and suicide attempts

Late adult/elders (unless otherwise stated, compared to straight gender-conforming population). Of Note: There is a significant dearth of knowledge about transgender elders, which is particularly important in this group because of lack of knowledge of effects of long-term use of hormonal therapy

- Increased stigma, discrimination, and violence across the life course including in nursing home settings
- Less likely to have children than gender-conforming heterosexual elders and are less likely to receive care from adult children

A complete and accurate physical exam should be performed only when necessary and evidence based. Genital exams can be traumatizing for patients who have histories of genital surgeries or DSD. Appropriate speculum sizes are critical. It is imperative that clinicians not judge or display inappropriate reactions when anatomy and gender expressions are not congruent on physical exam.

In general, preventive health care screenings should include those recommended for an individual's natal sex and would include appropriate cervical cancer screening for individuals with a cervix and mammography for patients with breast tissue. Mammography may also be appropriate for individuals taking either estrogen or testosterone. Chest reconstruction or "top surgery" for transgender men often does NOT remove all breast tissue and it is unclear at what age or level of estrogen exposure transgender women should start having mammograms. It is also important to note that patients who have had a vaginectomy still have a prostate and that vaginoplasty can be associated with discharge.

Appropriate immunizations should be recommended based on age, exposure, and risk factors. All patients should have received the Hepatitis B vaccination series. If a patient is at high risk for HIV infection, prophylactic medication should be discussed and possibly prescribed. Emerging literature suggests lesbians may be less likely to be immunized for human papillomavirus (HPV) when in fact HPV can be transmitted woman to woman with resultant cervical dysplasia/cancer.

Family planning, including options for parenting, and contraception should be discussed with all individuals regardless of sexual orientation, gender identity, or history of DSD. Extensive studies of children of lesbian parents have shown that the outcomes of the children through young adulthood are equivalent to those children who have heterosexual parents. Some lesbian couples select IVF in order to share the biology of the pregnancy: one partner donates the egg and the other partner carries the pregnancy.

Transgender men and their physicians must consider when to stop testosterone prior to attempting conception and when to restart postpartum. There is increased risk of gender dysphoria associated with pregnancy and delivery in transgender men. Preservation of gametes prior to surgical transitioning is available in many reproductive centers and should be discussed prior to initiation of gender-affirming hormones as the long-term fertility impact of hormonal therapy is unclear.

STI prevention should be addressed with everyone, regardless of stated sexual orientation.

LGBT and DSD patients may be at more risk for endometrial, breast, and ovarian cancer because of certain risk factors including nulliparity, delayed childbearing, alcohol consumption, obesity and anovulation, smoking, and decreased likelihood of using oral contraception.

Special Considerations for Transgender Patients and Individuals with DSD

It is likely that most women's health providers will have an inadequate knowledge base to adequately address the health needs of transgender patients and patients with DSD. Referral to practitioners who specialize in transgender or DSD care is appropriate. Self-education and national care hotlines, such as the ones listed below, are available when referral is not possible.

www.lgbthealtheducation.org/training/learning-modules/

Project Health – Transline – http://project-health.org/transline/

The Association of American Medical College's (AAMC) Advisory Committee on Sexual Orientation, Gender Identity, and Sex Development recommends that medical students graduate with the following competencies for transgender and DSD care:

- Describe the special health care needs and available options for quality care for transgender patients and for patients born with DSD (e.g., specialist counseling, pubertal suppression, elective and nonelective hormone therapies, elective and nonelective surgeries, etc.).

- Understand that medical consensus calls for referral to specialist DSD teams when a newborn, infant, child, or adolescent is identified as possibly having DSD.

- Recognize the lack of evidence to support many genital "normalizing" surgeries, including "repair" of minor benign hypospadias, clitoroplasty to reduce clitoral size in girls born with large clitorises, etc.

- Analyze the history of clinical practice regarding people born with DSD and its effect on this population. For example, historically boys born with a micropenis were sex changed into girls as babies in order to make them appear more sexually typical of their gender assignment and then withholding this medical history from the patients when they got older. Today, consensus on DSD calls for full disclosure to patients with DSD medical histories and a more patient-centered, evidence-based approach to outcomes.

- Understand surgical and hormonal options available for transitioning individuals, including pubertal suppression (in youth) and/or cross-sex treatment; know when to refer to a specialist in pediatric, adolescent, or adult gender care.

- Be aware of the lack of consensus about how health care professionals should support a prepubertal gender variant child and his or her family as they face various challenges (e.g., identifying as a new gender at school) and be aware of the lack of data on benefits and risks of gender transition, and specific circumstances when gender transition may or may not be indicated.

- Recognize there is little evidence to prevent physicians from supporting and affirming a child's current gender identity and/or gender expression. However, physicians should do so in a way that encourages healthy gender exploration and does not pressure or externally influence the child's later self-expression.

- Recognize that pubertal suppression, an intervention that was first used in the mid-2000s, shows evidence of mental health benefits in some transgender adolescents, but long-term outcomes are still being studied.

An LGBT- and DSD-Friendly Provider and Practice

It is likely that most providers will need to change their behavior and practice to become more welcoming to LGBT and DSD patients. Again, the AAMC suggests that providers understand that implicit (i.e., automatic or unconscious) bias and assumptions about sexuality, gender, and sex anatomy may adversely affect verbal, nonverbal, and written communication strategies involved in patient care, and that we must engage in effective corrective self-reflection processes to mitigate those effects.

The Institute of Medicine released a report on the Health of Lesbian, Gay, Bisexual and Transgender People in 2011 and along with the AAMC and JCAHO (Joint Commission on Accreditation of Healthcare Organizations) has specific suggestions for **provider** interactions:

- Ask all patients, "How would you prefer that I address you?" and respect the response, including in terms of name, title ("Mr.," "Ms.," "Mrs.," "Dr.," etc.), and pronoun. Use neutral and inclusive language
- Avoid the questions that have gendered assumptions behind them such as, "Do you have a girlfriend?"
- Ask individuals who appear gender nonconforming in a friendly tone, "With which pronoun do you feel most comfortable?"
- Ask every patient when obtaining a sexual history, "Are you sexually attracted to men, women, both, or some alternative gender?"
- Acknowledge and apologize for referring to someone by the wrong pronoun or title or for insensitive responses to a patient's genital or chest anatomy, etc.
- Avoid the use of stigmatizing and outdated terms, e.g. "pseudohermaphrodite," "intersexual," or "homosexual"
- Use "homosexual," "heterosexual," and "transgender" only as adjectives to describe the identities or behaviors of individuals, not as nouns.
- Listen to and reflect patients' choice of language when they describe their own sexual orientation and how they refer to their relationship or partner
- Avoid assumptions about sexual orientation and gender identity
- Facilitate disclosure of sexual orientation and gender identity, but be aware that disclosure or "coming out" is an individual process

The Joint Commission has the following recommendations for making your **practice** more receptive for LGBT and DSD patients:

- Prominently post the hospital's nondiscrimination policy or patient bill of rights
- Create or designate unisex or single-stall restrooms
- Identify opportunities to collect LGBT-relevant data and information during the health care encounter
- Identify a process to document self-reported sexual orientation and gender identity information in the medical record
- Train staff to collect sexual orientation and gender identity data
- Ensure that strong privacy protections for all patient data are in place
- Add information about sexual orientation and gender identity to patient surveys

Practices must modify their intake forms so that they contain inclusive, gender-neutral language that allows for self-identification. As of October 2015, the Centers for Medicare and Medicaid Services and the Office of the National Coordinator for Health Information Technology require electronic health record software certified for Meaningful Use to include sexual orientation and gender identity fields. Providers should also collect sex assigned at birth data as well as current gender identity data. The concern that patients will be unwilling or unable to answer questions about sexual orientation and gender identity are unfounded and studies have shown very high response rates and positive patient experiences with being asked as long as it is done in a sensitive and culturally competent manner.

Conclusion: For too long, the medical community has created a hostile environment for members of the LGBT and DSD communities, which has resulted in fear and avoidance of health care and profound health inequities. It is critical that women's health providers change their practice to accommodate these individuals and become familiar with particular health care risks and needs. There is a concerning lack of LGBT and DSD research.

Well-Woman Care for Obese Women

Background

The global burden of obesity is substantial and is expected to increase dramatically in the next 20 years. Some of the greatest rates of obesity are seen in the United States where it is estimated that 17 percent of US youth are obese. Although all women are at risk of obesity, minority women, low-income women, and women who live in certain geographic regions are at particularly higher risk. In the United States, the South has the highest prevalence of obesity at 30 percent. African American and Hispanic women are twice as likely as their white counterparts to be overweight or obese. Forty-two percent of women with incomes below 130 percent of the poverty level are obese [1].

There is abundant evidence that disparities exist in obesity and related health conditions and there is a complex interplay between socioeconomic status and race/ethnicity. Neighborhood contextual variables that are correlated with race, ethnicity, and socioeconomic status likely account for much of the disparity in obesity. Even the poorest white children live in higher-opportunity neighborhoods than the majority of black or Latino children. Low-income and minority communities often have reduced access to supermarkets or exercise venues, but have an abundance of fast-food outlets and other hazards like crime. Poor dietary intake and physical inactivity are primary risk factors for obesity [2].

Healthy People is a governmental initiative that provides science-based, ten-year national objectives for improving the health of all Americans. Although there seems to have been some modest gains in the fight against obesity especially in childhood, no state or region in the United States met the Healthy People 2010 target to reduce obesity rates to 15 percent.

Obesity is a risk factor for many chronic health conditions including diabetes, hypertension, hyperlipidemia, stroke, heart disease, sleep apnea, arthritis, gastroesophageal reflux, gallbladder disease, and psychiatric illness including depression. As most obese children go on to become obese adults, obese youth are likely at risk for these chronic health conditions also. Obesity drives up health care costs and takes a large toll on the health care system as a whole.

Obesity and Women's Health

There are many women's health implications of obesity. Pregnant obese women are at higher risk for miscarriage, gestational diabetes, preeclampsia, fetal demise, and cesarean delivery. Obese women are also at risk for anovulation and polycystic ovarian syndrome as well as consequent infertility and endometrial cancer. Several contraceptives may be less effective or carry more risk in obese women. In the *well-woman visit*, these risks are addressed in the

topics of contraception and reproductive health and preconception counseling.

There are several American College of Obstetrics and Gynecology (ACOG) publications that address obesity and women's health. It is critical to address weight loss prior to attempting to conceive. Weight loss before pregnancy, achieved by surgical or non-surgical methods, has been shown to be the most effective intervention to improve medical comorbidities. Optimal blood pressure and diabetes control are paramount prior to conception. A careful menstrual history is important. In ovulatory women without risk factors, ACOG recommends endometrial biopsy after age 45 for women with irregular bleeding. Although endometrial cancer in younger women is rare, it increases with age and other risk factors including obesity. Biopsy before the age of 45 should be considered in obese women with a history of amenorrhea or irregular bleeding.

There are practical considerations for seeing obese women in the office setting. Many electric beds have weight limits. Large speculums are necessary as well as excellent mobile lighting. Consideration should also be given to vaginal wall retractors.

There are many national campaigns to combat obesity including the *Let's Move* program, which has five initiatives: create a healthy start for children, empower parents and caregivers, provide healthy food in schools, improve access to healthy, affordable foods, and increase physical activity. Providers for women and children's health care must be advocates for healthier food options and exercise opportunities in poor urban communities.

Well-Woman Care for Women with Disabilities

Individuals with disabilities make up approximately 22 percent of the US population. The 1990 Americans with Disabilities Act (ADA) defined disability as a physical or mental impairment that substantially limits one or more life activities. The World Health Organization utilizes the International Classification of Functioning, Disability, and Health (ICF) to classify changes in body function and structure, activity, participation levels, and environmental factors that affect health. This classification strives to avoid conflating disability with sickness; many women with disabilities (WWD) perceive themselves as healthy, and in the social model of disability, disability is characterized by the restrictions imposed on individuals by the larger society, rather than the limitations an individual has.

We know that disability increases with age; in 2012, 5% of children aged 5–17, 10% of adults aged 18–64, and 36% of adults aged 65 and over were living with a disability. Disabilities can include limitations in basic activities such as mobility and daily function and limitations in complex activities defined by how the individual participates in community life. The most common functional disability is a mobility disability, reported by 1 in 8 adults. Notably, women are more likely to report having a disability compared to men (24.4 percent vs. 19.8 percent). WWD are more economically disadvantaged and socially isolated in comparison to women without disabilities. WWD are less likely to obtain a college degree, less likely to be employed, and more likely to live in poverty. In addition to these vulnerabilities, transportation is a major issue for WWD, most significant of which is lack of or limited public transportation. In general, WWD struggle to have their medical needs met and are less likely to receive routine preventive services, most often due to limited availability of providers and limited provider accessibility.

Providers should be aware of the specific needs of WWD to address their comprehensive health care needs. The ADA prohibits discrimination against individuals with disabilities, including medical services. Federal law requires that health care providers make their services available in an accessible manner. It is recommended to schedule longer appointment times as visits with WWD can take longer; WWD may need additional time for changing and transfers, have more complex medical and psychosocial needs, and need additional time for communication and education. The well-woman exam for WWD should not differ significantly from that of women without disabilities. Given particular vulnerabilities, special attention should be directed to the menstrual history, sexual history, screening for past and present abuse, and previous experiences with the health system, particularly the pelvic examination.

Patient History

Understanding a patient's menstrual pattern and the impact of menstrual bleeding on her life is important, especially for those women who need assistance with hygiene. Additionally, some disability symptoms are exacerbated by menstrual cycling – increased spasticity and catamenial seizures in the premenstrual period, increased neurological symptoms for women with multiple sclerosis, and increased autonomic dysreflexia for women with spinal cord injuries during their menses. Providers should inquire about the effect of bleeding on daily activities and function. Interviewing caregivers, bleeding calendars, and menstrual tracking apps can be used to identify if there is a cyclic nature to symptoms and to characterize the frequency and nature of menses. Tracking bleeding will also identify an abnormal bleeding pattern, which is highly relevant for WWD who have a higher incidence of medical conditions that cause abnormal uterine bleeding, such as thyroid disorders, use of antipsychotic drugs, and obesity.

When seeing a woman with a disability, providers should take a full sexual history as they should for women without disabilities. WWD are often perceived to be "asexual," meaning they are assumed not to be sexually active or interested in sex. Research has shown that most WWD have been sexually active, although they report lower rates of current sexual activity in comparison to women without disabilities. Studies have reported few WWD being asked about their sexuality, low rates of satisfaction with the counseling they received, and few women feeling as if their providers understood their sexual needs. Failure to acknowledge WWD as sexually active can lead to delayed diagnosis of STIs, limited counseling about contraception, and lack of discussion around fertility desires. Health care providers can play an important role in promoting a healthy sexual life for women and can collaborate with the patients to address issues of sexual dysfunction.

Psychosocial Screening

The well-woman exam serves as an opportunity to screen for depression, substance use, and abuse. Clinicians should use validated screening instruments for depression. Providers should be aware that WWD have higher rates of depression than women in general, although the majority of WWD are not depressed. Studies have found that the disability itself is not the reason for depression; it is often the isolation, dependence, low self-esteem, chronic pain, and lack of support that increases the risk for depression for WWD. Interestingly, women with lifelong disabilities have a lower prevalence of depression than those with recently acquired disabilities. Similar to other disparities they experience, WWD with depression are less likely to receive treatment. As for depression, WWD should be screened for substance use, including tobacco use, with the same tools and at the same frequency as all women. Substance use in WWD can increase the risk of impairment, and substance use disorders can exacerbate the vulnerabilities associated with disabilities.

WWD experience a similar prevalence of abuse in comparison to women without disabilities. One striking difference is that WWD experience abuse for a longer period of time, likely because it is more difficult to resolve abuse due to a lack of accessible shelters and programs and potential loss of needed care assistance. Perpetrators of abuse tend to be individuals on whom WWD depend – family members, intimate partners, and personal care attendants. Moreover, WWD are at increased risk for sexual assault; again often the perpetrator is known. Of those women who have been sexually assaulted, approximately half report 10 or more incidents of assault and half experience physical injuries. In the outpatient setting, providers should be mindful of clues of abuse including inconsistent description of an injury, delay in time from injury to treatment, accident-prone history, suicide attempts or depression, and repeated psychosomatic complaints. All women should be asked about abuse using the Abuse Assessment Screen–Disability (AAS-D, see below); this instrument is similar to that used to screen intimate partner violence but addresses the unique vulnerabilities of WWD and has been shown to increase sensitivity in detecting abuse toward women with physical disabilities.

Abuse Assessment Screen–Disability (AAS-D)

1. Within the last year, have you been hit, slapped, kicked, or physically hurt by someone?
2. Within the last year, has anyone forced you to have sexual activities?
3. Within the last year, has anyone prevented you from using a wheelchair, cane, respirator, or other assistive device?
4. Within the last year, has anyone you depended on refused to help you with an important personal need, such as taking your medicine, getting to the bathroom, getting out of bed, bathing, getting, dressed, or getting food and drink?

Exam

Staff should intentionally select the most appropriate exam room, one that can accommodate the patient, her support persons, her assistive devices and transfer equipment if necessary. For those with physical disabilities, an adjustable height examination table should be used. If an office does not have accessible equipment, the ADA mandates that a physician must provide the necessary assistance to access already existent equipment. Preparing the staff for a visit can help facilitate the patient's experience; helpful strategies include eliciting the patients' preferences, providing necessary assistance, and knowing safe transfer techniques. Once a patient has been seen in the clinic, flagging the patient's chart and documenting the important accommodations can expedite care in the future.

Pelvic examinations should be performed only when indicated – to evaluate a symptomatic concern of a patient or to perform recommended health screening. Providers should ask patients about previous pelvic examinations and should specifically inquire about strategies to make the exam easier for patients. Additionally, understanding adverse past experiences can inform a provider's approach. Effort should be taken to avoid injury, minimize discomfort, and preserve dignity for the patient. As stated previously, there should be sufficient time for the examination. In general, patients should not be examined in wheelchairs. Strategies for accomplishing a comfortable pelvic exam include the following:

- Positioning patients in a slow fashion
- Consider alternatives to dorsal lithotomy (Figure 7.2)
- Awareness of impaired balance, weakness, spasticity, skin pressure, and contractures
- Liberal use of blankets and pillows to provide extra padding
- Use of a local anesthetic gel on the speculum or vaginal introitus to decrease discomfort and reduce stimulation
- Consideration of alternatives to foot stirrups – including use of stirrups with knee and leg support or use of two attendants in lieu of stirrups
- Emptying the bladder first in women who require catheterization
- Temporarily reduce spasticity with use of diazepam (first choice) or baclofen

Additionally, providers should be aware of autonomic dysreflexia (ADR), a life-threatening

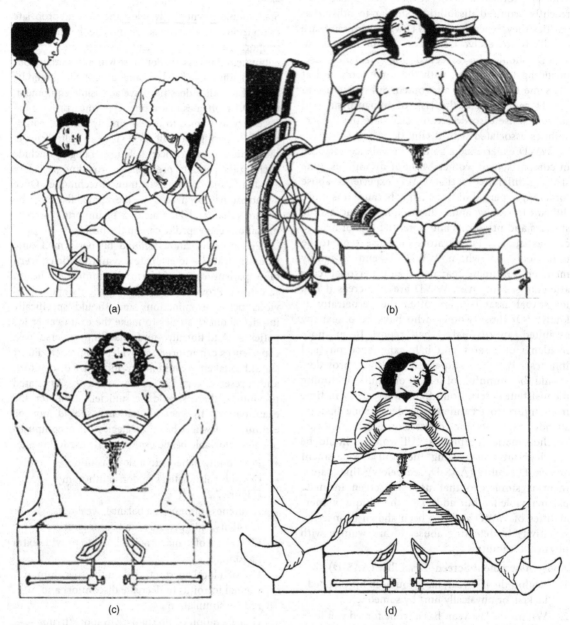

(a)

(b)

(c)

(d)

Figure 7.2 Alternatives to Dorsal Lithotomy. (a) Side-lying knee chest position. (b) Diamond position. (c) M position. (d) V position. Images attributed to Simpson KM. Table manners and beyond: the gynecological exam for women with developmental disabilities and other functional limitations, 2001.

complication in individuals with spinal cord lesions at T6 or above. ADR results from a loss of hypothalamic control of sympathetic spinal reflexes and results in arteriolar vasoconstriction resulting in severely elevated blood pressure followed by bradycardia. ADR

is triggered by noxious stimuli, such as a pelvic examination or bladder distention. Effort should be made to avoid ADR by emptying the bladder prior to the examination, warming the speculum, using anesthetic gel, and proceeding slowly.

For those women who cannot tolerate a pelvic examination, alternatives should be explored such as a pelvic ultrasound to assess for causes of pain or abnormal bleeding, a blind Pap test, or HPV DNA testing. The use of sedation or anesthesia to accomplish a pelvic examination can be considered but requires increased vigilance around the informed consent process. The risk of sedation or anesthesia must be weighed against the benefits of the pelvic examination and the risks of not performing the examination. If possible, it is ideal to coordinate any examination under anesthesia with other indicated health procedures such as colonoscopy or dental work.

If a woman does undergo a pelvic examination, this examination provides an opportunity to assess skin health. Women with mobility impairments and development disabilities are at increased risk for pressure ulcerations given difficulties moving themselves, sensory impairments, incontinence, poor nutrition, vascular disease, smoking, poorly fitted equipment, and inadequate assistant care. Women's health providers should inspect the skin overlying the pubic bones. Any pressure wound or compromise in skin integrity should prompt immediate action.

WWD should be appropriately screened for sexually transmitted infections STIs. Risk factors for STIs in WWD include a lack of education about STIs and their prevention, physical inability to use barrier protection, and sexual abuse. WWD can experience a delay in diagnosis of their STIs as their symptoms are mistaken for urinary tract infections, women cannot visualize discharge or have atypical symptoms, and they are not empowered to disclose sexual abuse. Providers are obligated to inquire about risk for STI and perform regular screenings. If a pelvic examination is difficult, urinary screening with nucleic acid testing is an excellent alternative approach.

Unfortunately, WWD are less likely to have screening for breast and cervical cancer. Their risk of cervical cancer is often underappreciated given presumptions about sexual activity. Compared to the general population, WWD report similar rates of ever being screened for cervical cancer; however, it is notable that they are less likely to be screened within the recommended guidelines. Women with severe functional limitations are least likely to be screened. Women's health care providers must follow standard guidelines around cervical cancer screening. In light of high rates of sexual assault and abuse among girls

and young WWD, HPV vaccination is encouraged and can be administered as early as 9 years old given this increased vulnerability. Similarly, all women should follow the published guidelines for breast cancer screening. Women with contractures or limited movement may necessitate changes in the clinical breast exam. Women with functional limitations may need assistance locating mammogram services that accommodate their wheelchair or difficulty with positioning. It is important to emphasize that there is no evidence to support the use of ultrasound for breast cancer screening.

Counseling

Contraception should be explicitly addressed in the well-woman visit for WWD. There is evidence that WWD are often not asked about contraception and that only half of women are counseled about contraception; this lack of contraceptive counseling and provision has been most notable among women with paralysis or obvious physical impairment. Health care providers should inquire if there is a need for contraception. We know sexual coercion and abuse is more common among women with communication difficulties and development disabilities; thus, providers should be mindful of requests for contraception that come from someone other than the patient and should explore whether a patient has the capability to consent to sexual relations. Contraceptive counseling should be performed on a regular basis and individualized to the needs and desires of the patient. When prescribing contraception, providers need to consider a host of factors including how the method will be administered (or if the patient requires assistance from the partner or caregiver), the side effects of contraception, the effects on menses, pharmacologic interactions with other medications, the patient's care needs, individualized risk for thrombosis and osteoporosis, and the patient's goals for pregnancy. Additionally, all women should be counseled about STI prevention. Table 7.1 provides a summary of the different contraceptive options available and the advantages and disadvantages of those options for WWD.

WWD feel external pressure not to have children; nonetheless, providers should explore pregnancy desires in WWD. Those who desire pregnancy should receive comprehensive preconception counseling which includes genetic counseling (especially if a congenital disability is present), medication review, assessment of potential interactions between

Table 7.1 Contraceptive Considerations in Women with Disabilities

	Advantages	Disadvantages
Condom	• Offers STI prevention • Widely available and cheap in cost	• Requires physical ability to place condom • Need partner participation and agreement • Cognition to understand need for condom use
Combined hormonal contraception (CHC)	• Excellent menstrual control • Decreased cramping • Use in extended cycle (to facilitate menstrual hygiene) • Excellent pregnancy prevention with consistent use	• Potential increased risk of venous thromboembolism (VTE) in patients with lower-extremity mobility impairments • May interact with other medications (including antiepileptic drugs) • Women with Down Syndrome may have increased risk of thrombosis given cardiac or vascular abnormalities
Pill	• see CHC	• May require daily supervision for adherence
Patch	• see CHC	• Needs to be removed and replaced • Can cause skin irritation
Ring	• see CHC	• Difficult to place if mobility impairments
Progestin-only pill	• Option for women in whom estrogen is contraindicated	• Risk of irregular bleeding • Requires timely administration • May interact with other medications
Contraceptive injection (depo-medroxyprogesterone)	• Can achieve excellent menstrual control (amenorrhea) • Requires minimal patient action • Increases seizure threshold • Does not contain estrogen	• Irregular bleeding in initial months • Weight gain due to limited mobility and effect of weight gain on mobility • Administration every 3 months • Implications for bone health in women with mobility impairments
Contraceptive implant	• Long-acting • Excellent pregnancy prevention • Does not require frequent administration • Does not contain estrogen	• Irregular bleeding for duration of implant • Requires a minor invasive procedure
Intrauterine device (IUD)	• Long-acting • Excellent pregnancy prevention • Does not require frequent administration • Does not contain estrogen	• Irregular bleeding in initial months • May necessitate anesthesia for insertion
Copper IUD	• see IUD	• Increase in menstrual bleeding and increased needs around menstrual hygiene
Levonorgestrel IUD	• see IUD • Decrease in menstrual bleeding and potentially amenorrhea	
Permanent sterilization	• Permanent • Nonhormonal	• Permanent • Surgical risks of procedure • Consent issues for women with developmental disabilities

pregnancy and disability, strategies to prevent obstetric and disability considerations, and discussion on the impact of the disability on labor, delivery, and postpartum care.

In summary, WWD warrant similar well-woman care to women without disabilities. Providers should strive to provide humanistic, sensitive, accessible care with increased attention to the vulnerabilities experienced by WWD. Women's health providers can help address the gynecological issues that affect daily function and can explore and address reproductive goals and sexuality.

Well-Woman Care for Women Who Are Homeless

Many assume that most homeless individuals live on the street; in fact, those living on the street are most likely chronically homeless – individuals who have been homeless for at least a year or have had four episodes of homelessness in 3 years. The chronically homeless are more likely to be male and to struggle with mental illness and substance abuse. More commonly, individuals are intermittently homeless – meaning they have multiple short, self-limited episodes of homelessness. Most of those who are intermittently homeless have stayed with friends and family prior to losing their housing; they often regain housing but find that their housing arrangements are tenuous. Homelessness also includes individuals at imminent risk of losing their housing in the next 2 weeks and individuals fleeing domestic violence with insufficient resources to obtain permanent housing. Regardless of the definition, being homeless means to lack stable, adequate, and permanent housing.

The Urban Institute estimates that 2.3–3.5 million individuals are homeless each year. Women make up approximately one-third of the homeless population; families make up approximately 35 percent of the homeless population with the vast majority of homeless families headed by women. Minority racial groups, particularly African Americans, are disproportionately represented among homeless individuals. Notably, domestic violence is the primary cause of homelessness for women. A significant proportion of homeless women report being physically abused within the last year and virtually all have experienced or witnessed violence over the course of their lifetimes. In addition, being homeless can expose women to more trauma. Over the course of 1 year, 30 percent of homeless women are physically assaulted and 10 percent are sexually assaulted.

Homelessness and Poor Health

Homelessness is an extreme form of poverty and has a negative effect on health. In the United States, the mortality rate for homeless individuals is three–four times that of housed, aged-matched controls and this disparity is even greater among homeless youth and young adults. On average, homeless persons die 30 years earlier than housed individuals. Being homeless can lead to new health problems or exacerbate existing ones due to violence, hazardous living conditions, substance abuse, mental illness, inadequate nutrition, and infectious diseases. Homeless individuals have high rates of acute and chronic illness including tuberculosis, hepatitis, STIs, hypertension, and asthma. Finding food and shelter often takes priority over health care. Many homeless individuals do not have a regular source of care. The high rates of substance abuse and mental illness amongst the homeless population further complicate engagement with the health care system. As a result, homeless individuals tend to present later in their disease processes and receive care in acute settings like the emergency room or inpatient settings.

Three-quarters of homeless individuals report an unmet health need – including medical, surgical, mental health, vision, dental, or prescription issues. The current health care system does not often meet the specific needs of the homeless population; moreover, there is evidence that homeless women are less likely to receive preventive care such as prenatal care, pap tests, and mammograms in comparison to women who are housed. Multiple barriers to health care exist for the homeless including lack of insurance, inability to obtain medications, lack of knowledge of where to obtain care, inability to get transportation to medical facilities, and long waiting times. Additionally, homeless individuals have been quite marginalized within the health care system due to stigma around being homeless, lack of insurance, disrespectful treatment, and feeling ignored by providers. Accordingly, they tend to avoid the health care system unless an emergency arises.

Optimizing Medical Care for the Homeless

Medical care for homeless individuals requires flexibility, creativity, and patience to address the patients' primary concerns, to provide the recommended preventive services, and to be mindful of competing priorities. Strategies to encourage patient engagement in care include the adoption of an outreach-based approach (embedding clinical services in places that address more basic needs such as shelters and soup kitchens instead of relying on patients to present to a clinic) and utilization of low-pressure techniques to attract patients (i.e., performing kind gestures like provision of socks or foot soaking/cleansing to convey a service-oriented model of care). All providers should work to build patient trust by showing respect, providing positive reinforcement for seeking care, and adopting a nonjudgmental attitude. In order to encourage longitudinal care with a regular provider, women who are homeless should be encouraged to follow-up frequently. Providers should encourage appointments but allow for drop-in visits and clinic staff should be trained around treating homeless women with kindness and respect.

Guidelines for Clinical Encounters for Homeless Women

The following are recommendation guidelines for clinical encounters for homeless women or women at risk of homelessness:

- Ask patients about their housing status at every visit
  - Ask patients where they stay instead of where do they live
  - If they stay with friends or family, ask how long have they been there and how long do they expect to stay
  - Assess for safety in their current living situation
- Document and update contact information at each visit including emergency contacts
- Be mindful of trauma histories
  - Ask about personal safety and screen for violence
    - Because homeless women may be in nontraditional relationships involving survival sex, ask more broadly than specifically about her partner (i.e., has your partner **or anyone else** ever hit you, hurt you, or threatened you?)
  - Educate staff about personal and emotional boundaries

- Ask for permission to touch and to perform each exam maneuver, particularly a pelvic examination
- Gather history over time to allow patients to guide, pace, and direct initial health interactions
- Perform a physical exam only if necessary
- Strive to understand competing priorities and acknowledge those priorities in treatment plans
- Engage patients in developing treatment plans (often this involves risk reduction as opposed to risk elimination)
- Simplify medication regimens (aim for once daily dosing, minimize side effects, avoid need for medication refrigeration and laboratory monitoring)
- Offer health promotion and disease prevention at each visit (Box 7.1)
- Screen for common conditions among the homeless
  - Substance abuse and mental illness
  - Provide foot care as homeless individuals tend to walk extensively and experience foot problems from ill-fitting shoes, swollen legs, and arthritis
  - Provide referral to dental care
- Provide a brief, portable health record for patients to utilize in other health care settings

Reproductive Health Care for Homeless Women

The increased risks homeless women face result from the complex interplay and power dynamics associated with substance use, mental illness, history of sexual and physical abuse, current trauma, risky sexual behaviors, and survival sex (exchange of sex for protection, food, shelter, and other commodities). Homeless women, in comparison to the general population and to low-income housed women, have:

- Higher rates for STIs
- Higher rates of HIV (three–nine times more prevalent)
- Lower rates of contraceptive use, including condom use
- Higher rates of unplanned pregnancy (twice the national rate for unintended pregnancy)
- Higher rates of adverse birth outcomes including preterm delivery, low-birth-weight infants, and infant mortality

BOX 7.1 Recommended Preventive Health Screening for Homeless Women

Adapted from the Health Care for the Homeless Clinicians' Network
- **Hypertension:** Measure blood pressure
- **Obesity:** Take periodic height and weight measurements, calculate BMI
- **Coronary heart disease:** Periodic measurement of cholesterol
- **Diabetes:** Check fasting blood sugar, Hgb A1c
- **Cervical cancer screening:** Perform pap tests at recommended intervals
- **Breast cancer:** Order screening mammograms as per guidelines
- **Colon cancer:** Assess feasibility of preparation for colonoscopy; consider alternatives such as annual high sensitivity guaiac testing or fecal immunochemical testing
- **Substance abuse:** Utilize standardized screening to assess for tobacco, alcohol, and drug use
- **Intimate partner violence:** Use validated screening tools
- **Sexually transmitted infections:** Screen for chlamydia, gonorrhea, and trichomonas in women with multiple sexual partners, in women using drugs or exchanging sex for commodities. To avoid a pelvic examination, consider urine testing or patient performed vaginal collection for chlamydia and gonorrhea.
- **HIV:** Screen sexually active women with multiple partners and injection drug users
- **Hepatitis C:** Screen those with past or current injection drug use
- **Tuberculosis:** Annual or semi-annual PPD testing for women at increased risk for tuberculosis – those infected with HIV, in close contact with TB-infected individual, individuals with substance use disorders, and those who stay in shelters
- **Immunizations:** Ensure that women are up to date with tetanus, rubella, and influenza vaccinations. Those with certain chronic illnesses should be offered pneumococcal vaccine. Women with high-risk sexual behaviors should be vaccinated against hepatitis A and B.

Some studies have reported that 95 percent of homeless women are sexually active. Notably, three-quarters of pregnancies among homeless women are unintended. Therefore, providers of women's health care must assess a patient's need and desire for contraceptive services. Women should be informed of their contraceptive options; however, it should be acknowledged that contraceptives requiring storage or routine administration – e.g. pills, patch, ring, injection – may have higher failure rates for women who must manage the daily challenges of being homeless. Long-acting reversible contraceptive methods such as the IUD and contraceptive implant have significant advantages for homeless women; they offer excellent protection against pregnancy, do not require storage, frequent follow-up or administration, and are immune to user-based failure. The levonorgestrel IUD offers the added benefit of decreasing or eliminating menses as it can be challenging to attend to menstrual bleeding while living on the streets or in a shelter. The contraceptive implant is an excellent form of contraception that does not require a pelvic examination, a feature that may be helpful for women with histories of trauma and assault.

For all contraceptive methods, women should be offered same day start or insertion; importantly, contraception should not be contingent on participation in preventive care, such as pap tests. Homeless women should be appropriately screened for STIs at the time of IUD insertion. Some providers may hesitate to place an IUD given the higher rates of STIs among the homeless population; however, the US Selected Practice Recommendations for Contraceptive Use (2013) recommend that screening can be performed at the time of IUD insertion for asymptomatic women and that insertion should not be delayed for screening. Absolute contraindications to IUD insertion include women with purulent cervicitis and known chlamydial or gonococcal infection. It should be emphasized that although the risk of pelvic inflammatory disease (PID) is increased in women with STIs at the time of IUD insertion, the overall rate of PID among IUD users is low (0–2 percent in women without an STI at the time of insertion vs. 0–5 percent in women with an STI). In general, all women should be counseled about the use of barrier protection to prevent transmission of STIs.

For pregnant homeless women, providers should deliver nonjudgmental pregnancy options counseling. Health care providers must be incredibly mindful of the stigma and judgment homeless women face, and thus should emphasize that all pregnant women have the choice of abortion (if gestational age appropriate), adoption, and prenatal care. With appropriate services and support, pregnant homeless women can have healthy pregnancies and babies. In fact, pregnancy can offer a window of opportunity to obtain resources and can serve as motivation for change – to stop using drugs or alcohol, to commit to regular health care, and to strive for secure housing.

Securing Housing to Improve Health

In the previous sections, strategies to improve the care homeless patients receive were outlined. Although providers can deliver high-quality, compassionate care to homeless patients, it would be naïve to think that medical providers alone can address the full scope of the needs of homeless patients. Accordingly, the importance of linking patients to community resources must be highlighted. Community-based services and outreach workers may be able to more effectively help patients meet their most basic needs of food, shelter, and clothing. In addition, a multidisciplinary approach involving social workers, mental health professionals, substance abuse counselors, and health care providers can better address the medical and nonmedical issues homeless patients face.

Ultimately, improving the health of homeless individuals requires stable housing. Even the best medical care is not effective if a patient's health is continually compromised by his or her unstable living conditions. Linking services and housing has been shown to reduce use of emergency rooms, hospitalizations, and other public services and to improve overall health through prevention and treatment of acute and chronic disease. Housing First – a strategy that refers to providing housing without preconditions such as sobriety – has been shown to effectively reduce chronic homelessness. Securing housing is critical to realizing better health and well-being.

Well-Woman Care for Incarcerated Women

The United States has the world's highest incarceration rate, with more than 2 million people currently incarcerated. The United States alone accounts for nearly 30 percent of the world's population of incarcerated women. Although women make up less than 10 percent of the prison population, the number of women in prison increased at a rate nearly 1.5 times the rate of men from 1980 to 2011.

Incarcerated women disproportionally come from marginalized communities. They tend to be poor, undereducated, and unemployed. Notably, two-thirds of women in prison in the United States are women of color, a statistic that reflects the stark racial disparities in incarceration. The majority of women prisoners are incarcerated for nonviolent crimes such as drug offenses, fraud, and prostitution.

Coming from disadvantaged environments, women entering correctional settings often have had limited access to health care and often have unmet needs, including reproductive health concerns. In 1976, the Supreme Court in *Estelle* v. *Gamble* established that correctional authorities must treat the serious medical needs of inmates by providing timely access to proper care, in effect stating that individuals in prison have a right to medical care. However, the availability, quality, and access to care in correctional settings are highly variable.

There are no national standards around medical care in prison. Typically, each system – Federal Bureau of Prisons, State Departments of Correction, and local jails – establish their own policies and procedures. Organizations such as the National Commission on Correctional Health Care (NCCHC) do accredit prisons; however their standards only serve as voluntary guidelines.

Previously, medical care was provided on a "sick call" basis, meaning inmates were seen when they had a specific need for medical attention. There has been a shift in care to provide more comprehensive services, and women who are incarcerated have unique, gender-specific health needs. Provision of gynecological services in correctional settings has been consistently described as inadequate with women not receiving gynecological exams on admission or on a regular basis. Moreover, many jails and prisons lack providers trained in obstetrics and gynecology, thus further leading to lower-quality care. ACOG, NCCHC, and the American Public Health Association have each published recommended guidelines for incarcerated women. Fundamentally, the care provided to women in custody should follow the same guidelines as for women not in custody.

Cervical screening and screening mammograms should be performed based on the current screening guidelines. Particular attention should be directed to the increased risk of infectious disease, mental health issues including substance abuse, and reproductive health care.

According to the Centers for Disease Control and Prevention (CDC), prevalence rates for chlamydia and gonorrhea among individuals entering correctional facilities are consistently among the highest observed in any venue. In one study, 27% of incarcerated women had chlamydia and 8% had gonorrhea compared to 0.46% and 0.13% in the general population, respectively. High rates of STIs are likely the result of limited access to STI testing prior to incarceration, the interaction of substance use, unprotected intercourse, and commercial sex work, and of being victims of sexual assault. Additionally, 2 percent of incarcerated women are infected with HIV, a statistic which is notable as outside correctional settings a higher percentage of men are infected with HIV. Thus, screening for chlamydia, gonorrhea, syphilis, and HIV at intake and at recommended intervals offers an opportunity to identify and treat infections, prevent complications, and reduce transmission in the general community. The CDC explicitly recommends opt-out HIV screening, with the test being routinely offered and patients having the option to decline HIV testing if they so desire. Additionally, incarcerated women should be tested for hepatitis and tuberculosis; immunizations against influenza, pneumococcus, meningococcus, and HPV should be provided based on current guidelines.

Additionally, the mental health needs of women in correctional settings cannot be ignored. Seventy-five percent of women in local jails and 73 percent of women in state prisons have mental health problems. Incarceration is a significant risk factor for suicide for adolescent inmates. Leading mental health issues among female inmates include physical and sexual abuse, depression, posttraumatic stress disorder, and substance use disorders. More than half of women in jails and prisons report a history of sexual or physical abuse, and approximately 5 percent of women report sexual victimization by a staff member or another inmate during their time of incarceration. Additionally, 40 percent of women prisoners are under the influence of drugs when they commit their offense and up to 70 percent of women entering jails meet the criteria for substance use disorder. Thus, a thorough mental health assessment should be performed for all incarcerated women and should include:

- Assessment of suicide risk
- Screening for intimate partner violence and abuse
- Counseling to address issues around previous victimization
- Screening for substance use disorders and treatment
- Screening for depression and appropriate counseling and treatment

Stress related to family concerns should also be addressed in the provision of mental health services. Most women in prison are mothers and were the primary, and often sole, caretakers for their children prior to being incarcerated. Incarceration leads to separation of mothers from their children, which in turn leads to high levels of stress and anxiety. NCCHC explicitly recommends the provision of counseling around parenting and child custody issues for female inmates.

Access to contraception is another important component of health care for incarcerated women given that most women in correctional settings are of reproductive age. Research has shown that up to 70 percent of women at risk for pregnancy were not using contraception consistently prior to incarceration and up to 80 percent had a previous unintended pregnancy. In one study, approximately one-third of women had unprotected intercourse within 5 days of incarceration, thus providers should assess the need for emergency contraception. Upon release, many women face competing stressors including food, housing, and family reunification that compete and likely take priority over contraception. Studies show that provision of contraception during incarceration greatly increases the rate of contraception initiation (39 percent vs. 4 percent) compared to making contraception available after release into the community. Women in jails and prisons must be informed about the expected benefits and side effects of contraception. Given the coercive nature of incarceration, family planning services should strive to be patient centered, meaning that care provided is consistent with the patient's reproductive goals and desires. Accordingly, preconception counseling must be provided along with contraceptive services.

Approximately 6–10 percent of incarcerated women are pregnant at any time. All women at risk for pregnancy should be offered a pregnancy test with in 48 hours of admission. All pregnant women should be offered options counseling and access to abortion services or prenatal care. Federal and state courts have upheld that incarcerated women maintain their right to terminate their pregnancy; however, the reality of obtaining abortion care while in a correctional setting is much more complex. Notably, many prisons and jails have no official written policy about how to request an abortion or how the facility must meet the woman's request to obtain an abortion. There have been documented examples of barriers to every aspect of abortion care for incarcerated women with women being denied transportation and women having to use their own resources to pay for transportation, the guards' time, and the procedure itself. In a survey of correctional health providers, 68 percent responded that inmates can obtain elective abortions, suggesting that a considerable percentage of incarcerated women still do not have access to abortion despite their legal right.

Health care providers should strive to provide high-quality and compassionate reproductive care to incarcerated women. Although incarceration has significant repercussions for women, their families, and their communities, it does represent a potential time to provide important health care services to a population that is quite vulnerable and marginalized within our society.

Summary

In general, marginalized and vulnerable populations need to receive routine recommended preventive services. Practitioners should know the particular health risks for these populations and address them appropriately. Attention should be paid to special circumstances of each population that may influence routine care i.e. prescription of different contraception or alternative positions for examinations of disabled women. We must provide evidence-based care and particularly avoid pelvic examinations if unnecessary as many of these individuals have been abused or traumatized in the past. It is critical to acknowledge that these populations have been historically treated poorly by the medical establishment and may avoid care and distrust the system. Culturally appropriate, respectful, and patient-centered care is paramount in providing reproductive health care for marginalized populations.

References

Reproductive Health Care for Lesbian, Gay, Bisexual, Transgender Patients, and Patients with Disorders of Sexual Development

Special recognition to Patricia Robertson MD and Juno Obedin-Maliver MD for their expertise and thoughtful review and editing of this section.

1. Implementing Curricular and Institutional Climate Changes to Improve Health Care for Individuals Who are LGBT, Gender Nonconforming, or Born with DSD. A Resource for Medical Educators. 1st edition. AAMC Advisory Committee on Sexual Orientation, Gender Identity, and Sex Development, 2014. Available at: http://offers.aamc.org/lgbt-dsd-health. Retrieved December 12, 2016.

2. The Institute of Medicine (US) Committee on Lesbian, Gay, Bisexual, and Transgender Health Issues and Research Gaps and Opportunities. *The Health of Lesbian, Gay, Bisexual, and Transgender People: Building a Foundation for Better Understanding, on the Existing Research and Research Gaps on the LGBT Community.* Washington, DC: National Academies Press (US), 2011. www.ncbi.nlm.nih.gov/books/NBK64806/.

3. The Joint Commission. Advancing Effective Communication, Cultural Competence, and Patient- and Family-Centered Care for the Lesbian, Gay, Bisexual, and Transgender Community: A Field Guide. 2011. Available at: https://www.jointcommis sion.org/lgbt/. Retrieved December 29, 2016.

4. Dribble, S.L. and Robertson, P.A., editors. *Lesbian Health 101: A Clinician's Guide.* San Francisco, CA: UCSF Nursing Press, 2010.

Well-Woman Care for Obese Women

5. Centers for Disease Control and Prevention. Available at: www.cdc.gov/obesity. Retrieved December 12, 2016.

6. CDC Health Disparities and Inequalities Report – United States, 2013. *MMWR Suppl.* November 22, 2013, 62:03.

7. US Preventive Services Task Force. Screening for and management of obesity in adults: US Preventive Services Task Force recommendation statement. *Ann Intern Med.* 2012, **157**(5):373–8.

8. US Selected Practice Recommendations for Contraceptive Use, 2013: Adapted from the World Health Organization selected practice recommendations for contraceptive use, 2nd edition. *MMWR Recomm Rep.* 2013, **62**(RR-05):1–60.

Well-Woman Care for Women with Disabilities

9. Interactive site for clinicians for serving women with disabilities. American Congress of Obstetrics and Gynecology. Available at: http://cfweb.acog.org/womenwithdisabilities/index.html.

10. *National Healthcare Disparities Report*. Rockville, MD: Agency for Healthcare Research and Quality, 2013. Available at: www.ahrq.gov/research/findings/nhqrdr/nhdr13/index.html. Retrieved May 2014.

11. Courtney-Long, E.A., Carroll, D.D., Zhang, Q. et al. Prevalence of disability and disability type among adults, United States – 2013. *MMWR Morb Mortal Wkly Rep*. 2015, **64**:777–83.

Well-Woman Care for Women Who Are Homeless

12. Kushel, M. and Jain, S., editors. Care of the homeless patient. In *Medical Management of Vulnerable & Underserved Patients: Principles, Practice, Population*. New York, NY: McGraw-Hill Education, 2007.

13. American College of Obstetricians and Gynecologists. Health care for homeless women. Committee Opinion No. 576. *Obstet Gynecol*. 2013, **122**:936–40.

14. Health Care for the Homeless Clinicians' Network, National Health Care for the Homeless Council. *Healing Hands – Women's Health Care: Show Me the Way to Go Home*. Nashville, TN: NHCHC, August 2000.

15. National Health Care for Homeless Council. *Homelessness & Health: What's the Connection*. Nashville, TN: NHCHC, June 2011.

16. Bonin, E., Brehove, T., Carlson, T. et al. *Adapting Your Practice: General Recommendations for the Care of Homeless Patients*. Nashville, TN: Health Care for the Homeless Clinicians' Network, National Health Care for the Homeless Council, 2010. Available at: www.nhchc.org/wp-content/uploads/2011/09/GenRecsHomeless2010.pdf.

Well-Woman Care for Incarcerated Women

17. American College of Obstetricians and Gynecologists. Reproductive health care for incarcerated women and adolescent females. Committee Opinion No. 535. *Obstet Gynecol*. 2012, **120**:425–9.

18. Sufrin, C.B., Creinin, M.D., and Chang, J.C. Incarcerated women and abortion provision: A survey of correctional health providers. *Perspect Sex Reprod Health*. 2009, **41**:6–11.

19. Clarke, J.G., Rosengard, C., Rose, J.S. et al. Improving birth control service utilization by offering services prerelease vs postincarceration. *Am J Public Health*. 2006, **96**:840–5.

20. Clarke, J.G., Hebert, M.R., Rosengard, C. et al. Reproductive health care and family planning needs among incarcerated women. *Am J Public Health*. 2006, **96**:834–9.

21. National Commission on Correctional Health Care. *Women's Health Care in Correctional Settings Position Statement*. Chicago, IL: NCCHC, 2014. Available at: www.ncchc.org/women's-health-care.

22. Schonberg, D., Bennett, A.H., Sufrin, C., Karasz, A., and Gold, M. What women want: A qualitative study of contraception in jail. *Am J Public Health*. 2015, **105**:2269–74.

Paying for the Well-Woman Visit

Michael S. Policar

Learning Objectives

- List three key features of the Affordable Care Act (ACA) that have had a positive impact on access to women's preventive health services
- Review the four main categories of health insurance that reproductive-aged women are most likely to have and their relative proportions
- List the eight women's preventive services contained in the Institute of Medicine (IOM) recommendations that must be made available without cost sharing
- Review the major contraceptive methods that must be available without cost sharing, except in women with grandfathered health plans or who are beneficiaries of health insurance policies purchased by employers who are exempt from providing contraceptive coverage
- List the preventive service benefits for women enrolled in Medicare

Introduction

In the United States, women who avail themselves of periodic health screening (e.g., well-woman) visits historically have received services from a variety of providers. Insured women visited their obstetrician-gynecologist (OB–GYN), their primary care provider, or both, while women without insurance usually visited a community health center or family planning clinic for their well-woman care.

The design of the Affordable Care Act (ACA) places at its core the critical importance of primary care and preventive services for the dual purposes of improving outcomes and reducing costs. The ACA, as administered by regulations formulated by the US Department of Health and Human Services (HHS), is rich in benefits that are explicitly targeted at women's health. First and foremost is the removal of cost barriers to most preventive services by

guaranteeing "first dollar coverage" ... meaning that, with some exceptions, a woman cannot be charged for specifically defined services with either a co-payment or for partial or full payment until her deductible is met. First dollar coverage is another way of stating that "cost sharing" between the payer and the patient is not permitted and that all costs for specified preventive services must be borne by the payer.

This chapter begins with a review of the major health insurance categories in the United States and how the proportion of women in each category has changed in the years since the enactment of the ACA. The chapter explains the federal regulations that affect payment for the well-woman preventive services detailed in other chapters of this book and uses case study examples to demonstrate their implementation. Since well-woman visits for fertile women of reproductive age include a discussion of reproductive life plans, and most women will request a method of contraception at the well-woman or another visit, the HHS regulations regarding cost sharing for contraceptive services and supplies also will be discussed.

Overview of the Affordable Care Act

The ACA is the health insurance reform legislation passed by Congress and signed into law by President Obama on March 23, 2010. ACA has had an important impact on a variety of features of health insurance in the United States, and in particular, coverage of preventive services for women. It expanded access to coverage to millions of uninsured women, ended discriminatory practices such as gender rating in the insurance market, eliminated exclusions for preexisting conditions, and improved women's access to affordable, necessary care.

The three fundamental objectives of the ACA are to expand access to health insurance, improve quality of care through a focus on prevention and primary care, and stabilize the costs of health care by changing financial incentives through shared risk. The ACA builds upon previously existing health plan and Medicare initiatives to adjust provider payment based upon metrics of quality of care, commonly known as "pay for performance" (P4P).

In turn, the objective of expanding access to health insurance has the following three strategies:

1. Insurers must offer coverage to everyone, regardless of preexisting conditions.

2. To reduce the barrier of the high cost of purchasing health insurance, federal subsidies are available to assist middle-class families to afford coverage, through a direct payment of a share of insurance premiums and tax credits to offset the out-of-pocket costs of co-payments and deductibles.

3. Almost everyone in the United States must have health insurance, a concept that is referred to as the *individual mandate*. This requirement is based on the principle that an insurance risk pool must include both healthy people and those with illnesses, thereby spreading financial risk over a large population of insureds and making premiums more affordable for all. Pragmatically speaking, this is the only way that all individuals with potentially expensive preexisting health conditions can be guaranteed coverage. In the US Supreme Court case that established the constitutionality of the individual mandate, *National Federation of Independent Business et al.* v. *Sebelius*, announced on June 28, 2012, Justice Roberts pointed out that "everyone will become ill at some time and that this compels purchase of coverage that we all will need sooner or later . . . rather than shifting costs to others." In this landmark case, the Supreme Court upheld the constitutionality of the ACA's individual mandate as an exercise of Congress's taxing power. However, the Court held that states cannot be forced to participate in the ACA's Medicaid expansion under penalty of losing their current Medicaid funding. The regulations that apply to the individual mandate are as follows:

- All citizens and legal immigrants aged 18 and older must have health insurance coverage by 2016.
- A tax penalty will be levied if there is no documentation of health insurance coverage which is the higher of $695 per person, up to

three times that amount for a family, or 2.5 percent of household income, whichever is higher.

- Exemptions are granted for undocumented persons, those who have no coverage for less than 3 months, when the lowest cost plan > 8 percent personal income (net of subsidies), religious objection, individuals who are incarcerated, members of Native American tribes, and people who have incomes below the tax-filing threshold ($9,750 for a single and $27,100 for a family of four).

The ACA contains a guarantee of direct access to an OB–GYN without need for a referral from a primary care provider or preauthorization from the woman's health plan. In addition, a health plan cannot restrict a woman's direct access to her OB–GYN to a certain number of visits or types of services. Women in grandfathered plans and Medicaid also may be able to schedule a visit with an OB–GYN without a referral, but policies vary by plan.

Grandfathered plans that were in existence on or before March 23, 2010, and that have continually met certain requirements, are not required to cover any preventive care. Grandfathered plans can lose that status by significantly reducing benefits; adding or tightening annual coverage limits; significantly raising coinsurance, co-pays, deductibles, or employee contributions; or not claiming grandfathered status in policy and benefits materials. Worker enrolment in grandfathered employer-sponsored plans has decreased from 56 percent of covered workers in 2011 to 26 percent in 2014. As more individuals acquire insurance through the state Marketplace (since all Marketplace plans are nongrandfathered) and if more grandfathered plans are discontinued or lose their grandfathered status, within a few years, almost all of the privately insured population will have coverage of preventive services without cost sharing. If a woman (or on her behalf, your office staff) is confused about whether she is enrolled in a grandfathered health insurance policy, she should contact the Member Services Department of her health plan to request her status. Additional resources are listed at the end of this chapter.

Payment for Health Care in the United States

Health insurance coverage is a critical factor in making health care affordable and accessible to women.

According to the Kaiser Family Foundation, most of the 97.5 million women aged 19–64 residing in the United States (87 percent) had some form of coverage in 2014. The vast majority of women aged 65 and older are covered by Medicare. However, gaps in private sector and publicly funded programs left almost one in eight women uninsured [1].

Commercial Insurance

Approximately 57 million women aged 19–64 (58 percent) received their health coverage from their own or their spouse's employer in 2014 [1]. Women are less likely than men to be insured through their own job (34 percent vs. 43 percent, respectively) and more likely to be covered as a dependent (24 percent vs. 16 percent) [2]. Other than the designation of specified preventive health services without cost sharing (discussed below), the most notable modification in coverage for this group as a consequence of the ACA is the ability to include adult children up to age 26 under the coverage of an insured parent.

Individually Purchased Insurance

The ACA expanded access to the individually purchased (nongroup) insurance market by offering premium tax credits to help individuals afford coverage in state-based health insurance exchanges (also known as Marketplaces). It also included many insurance reforms to alleviate some of the long-standing barriers to coverage in the nongroup insurance market, many of which disproportionately affect women. In 2014, about 8 percent of women (approximately 7.7 million women) purchased insurance on their own [1, 2]. This includes women who purchased private policies from the ACA Marketplace in their state, as well as from private insurers that operate outside of Marketplaces. Many of the pre-ACA individually purchased policies did not include coverage for certain women's health services, such as obstetrical care, prescription medications, or treatment for mental health conditions. As a result of the ACA, all direct purchase plans also must cover certain "essential health benefits" (EHBs) that fall under ten different categories, including obstetrical and newborn care, behavioral health, and preventive care.

Medicaid

Medicaid, the state–federal program for low-income individuals, covered 16 percent of nonelderly women in 2014. Traditionally, to qualify for Medicaid, women had to have very low incomes *and* be in one of Medicaid's eligibility categories: pregnant, mothers of children aged 18 and younger, disabled, or over 65. Women (and men) who didn't fall into these categories typically were not eligible regardless of how poor they were. While every state had a traditional Medicaid program before the enactment of the ACA, each state set its own income eligibility level, which often included only financially destitute women. Effective January 2014, the ACA permitted states to eliminate these categorical requirements and broaden Medicaid eligibility to most individuals with incomes less than 138 percent of the Federal Poverty Level (FPL) regardless of their family or disability status or age. However, as of 2016, only 31 states and the District of Columbia have expanded their Medicaid program. In the 19 states that refused to expand Medicaid, women with incomes below 100 percent of FPL are not eligible (and most are too poor) to buy coverage in the state Marketplace, creating what is referred to as the "Medicaid coverage gap" in these states [1]. These women remain uninsured and must rely on local, state, or federal safety net programs for their health care.

Among all sources of coverage, Medicaid disproportionately carries the weight of covering the poorest and sickest population of women. Approximately 70 percent of nonelderly women with Medicaid had incomes below 200 percent of the FPL. And 27 percent of women covered by Medicaid rate their own health as fair or poor, compared to 6 percent of women covered by employer-sponsored insurance and 11 percent of uninsured women.

Medicaid finances nearly half of all births in the United States [3], accounts for 75 percent of all publicly funded family planning services [4], and nearly half (43 percent) of all long-term care spending, which is critical for many frail elderly women [1].

Beneficiaries who are newly eligible for Medicaid through ACA State Medicaid expansion receive coverage through an alternative benefit plan that includes coverage without cost sharing for preventive services recommended by the US Preventive Services Task Force (USPSTF) and Advisory Committee on Immunization Practices (ACIP) and supported by the Healthcare Resources and Services Administration (HRSA) – the same coverage required for nongrandfathered private plans. States must cover certain tobacco cessation services and pregnancy-related care without co-pays or deductibles. Otherwise, states generally are not required to cover preventive care for adult traditional Medicaid beneficiaries and may charge a co-payment. Benefits for adults with traditional Medicaid vary from state to state. In states that have not expanded Medicaid, many lower-income individuals will go without access to affordable preventive services coverage.

Medicare

Medicare is entirely a Federal program, with no state financial contribution, and is managed by the HHS Centers for Medicare and Medicaid Services (CMS). Individuals aged 65 and older who have paid into the program for a certain number of quarters, as well as younger individuals with specific disabilities, such as chronic renal failure, also may be eligible. Medicare coverage of preventive care recommended for non-seniors is important for the millions of Medicare beneficiaries (one in six) who are younger than 65 years. Out-of-pocket costs to beneficiaries include premiums, deductibles, and co-payments. Medicare maintains annual skilled nursing facility (SNF) day limits and a lifetime cap on hospital days. Benefit coverage includes the following categories:

- Part A: hospital care and "skilled need" in SNFs
- Part B: clinician fees, outpatient care, durable medical equipment (DME), and limited preventive care
- Part C: Medicare Advantage Plans, an option available to Medicare beneficiaries in most parts of the country. Most Part C plans are traditional health maintenance organizations (HMOs) although a few are preferred provider organizations. For almost all Part C plans, the beneficiary is required to have a primary care physician, which is not a requirement of standard Medicare
- Part D: prescription drug coverage

Some beneficiaries are dual-eligible, meaning that they qualify for both Medicare and Medicaid. In some states, for those making below a certain income threshold, Medicaid will pay the beneficiaries' Part B premium, as well as some or all of their out-of-pocket medical and hospital expenses.

Other Governmental Programs

Other governmental programs cover 2 percent of women aged 19–64 and include the Veterans Administration Health System, military health care facilities for active duty military and their immediate dependents, and the Tricare insurance system, which is designed pay for care provided to military dependents outside of the military care system. The Indian Health Service (IHS) is an operating division of the HHS and is responsible for providing medical and public health services to members of federally recognized Tribes and Alaska Natives. IHS provides health care to American Indians and Alaska Natives at 33 hospitals, 59 health centers, and 50 health stations.

The benefits of these programs were virtually unchanged as a consequence of the ACA.

Uninsured

Approximately 12.8 million women (13 percent) aged 19–64 were uninsured in 2014. These women often have inadequate access to care, receive a lower standard of care when they are in the health system, and have poorer health outcomes [5]. Compared to women with insurance, uninsured women have lower use of important preventive services such as mammograms and cervical cancer screening and are more likely to forgo medical services due to cost [6]. Uninsured women have a harder time getting in to the health care system. In a survey conducted in Fall 2014, uninsured women were less likely to have a regular source of care compared to women with any form of insurance [7].

Since the passage of the ACA, increasing numbers of women who were previously uninsured have gained coverage, mainly through Medicaid expansion and to a lesser degree, enrolment in commercial insurance through the state Marketplace. However, 29 percent of women remaining uninsured are not eligible for assistance under the ACA because they are undocumented (16 percent) or they fall into the Medicaid coverage gap (13 percent) created by their state's decision not to expand Medicaid. These 3.6 million women lack a pathway to affordable insurance coverage [1].

Barriers to Preventive Services

Barriers to care deter many women from fully realizing the advantages of their newly insured status and optimally utilizing preventive health benefits without cost sharing. Stolp and Fox [8] cite three major barriers in the receipt of preventive services by women.

Access: Access to health care is critical for women to benefit from the preventive service coverage with no out-of-pocket cost provision in the ACA. Accessing a health care location to receive preventive services requires a woman to find a primary care provider who will accept her as a patient and who is part of the patient's insurance network of providers. Successful navigation of these steps can be difficult with the shortage of primary care providers who serve women [9] and use of "narrow networks" in the Marketplace which limited enrolment of primary care providers (PCPs) in a given geographic area. This may also be a challenge for women newly enrolled in a health insurance plan who are not familiar with using health insurance to access primary care services. Assuming a woman is able to locate a primary care provider and schedule a timely appointment, she must still make it to her appointment, which can be challenging for women who work, care for children, provide eldercare, or do a combination of these activities. Making scheduled appointments becomes more difficult if women encounter barriers to transportation, a factor that continues to adversely affect access to health care in the United States. In the end, preventive service coverage alone is not sufficient for women to access preventive care.

Education: A poll conducted in March 2014 found that fewer than half of Americans were aware that the ACA eliminates out-of-pocket costs for select preventive care [10]. A survey found that 20 percent of women aged 18–64 report that they postponed preventive services in the past year due to cost, including 13 percent of insured and 52 percent of uninsured women [11]. Addressing knowledge deficits about recommended preventive care and the health benefits of these services is a key step to increase receipt of preventive care. Recently, a wealth of consumer-facing information about recommended preventive services has been made publicly available online and is listed in the Resources section.

Delivery: Provider factors may also impede receipt of clinical preventive services. One key factor is the limited amount of time a provider has to provide preventive services. Overall, implementing a policy that authorizes nonphysician team members, such as nurses, pharmacists, and community health workers, to support primary care providers in the education or provision of preventive services can be an effective approach to address provider time constraints and increase the provision of preventive services. The movement to improve the quality of care provided also has led to the development of new models of care that hold promise for increasing receipt of recommended services. For example, the National Committee for Quality Assurance Patient-Centered Medical Home (PCMH) Recognition program is the program that HRSA is using to certify HRSA-funded health centers as PCMHs across the nation. It has a "must-pass" standard that requires PCMH-recognized clinics to monitor receipt of preventive care services, chronic care measures, and/or immunization coverage for their patient population. Studies suggest adoption of this PCMH model increases preventive service receipt [12, 13].

Women's Preventive Services and the ACA

The Women's Health Amendment, which was introduced by Senator Barbara Mikulski and added to the ACA, requires that all private health plans cover, with no cost sharing, an identified set of preventive health care services for women. One of the challenges of the ACA was that a *definitive* set of recommendations for preventive services for women did not exist [14]. The amendment was needed to address gaps resulting from the initial ACA's requirement that covered services received a Grade "A" or "B" recommendation from the USPSTF, were part of the Bright Futures recommendations for adolescents from the American Academy of Pediatrics (AAP) in cooperation with HHS, or were vaccinations specified by the Centers for Disease Control and Prevention's (CDC) Advisory Committee on Immunization Practices (ACIP). To address these gaps, the HHS asked the Institute of Medicine (IOM) to develop a comprehensive set of recommended evidence-based preventive services for women. The IOM committee's charge was to identify gaps and opportunities for needed clinical preventive services not already included in the ACA. As a result of the committee's work, the IOM issued a report titled "Clinical Preventive Services for Women: Closing the Gaps," which outlined eight recommendations for clinical services for girls and women aged 10–65 (Table 8.1):

1. Gestational diabetes mellitus screening between 24 and 28 weeks of gestation or at the first prenatal visit for pregnant women identified to be at high risk for diabetes

2. Testing for high-risk human papillomavirus (HPV) DNA for women undergoing cervical cancer screening and HPV testing beginning at

Table 8.1 Women's Preventive Services with No Cost Sharing. The eight additional services contained in "Closing the Gaps" are given in italics. All others are US Preventive Task Force Grade "A" and "B" recommendations.

Reproductive Health	Cancer	Healthy Behaviors	Pregnancy Related	Immunizations	Chronic Conditions
STI and HIV counseling; all sexually active females)	Breast cancer mammography	Alcohol S&C	Alcohol S&C	TdaP, Td booster, MMR, varicella	Hypertension, lipids
Ct, GC, Syphilis screening	Genetic S&C	Tobacco C&I	Tobacco C&I	Influenza	T2DM screen
HIV screening (adults at HR; all sexually active females)	Preventive medication counseling	Diet counseling if CVD risk	Folic acid supplement	Hepatitis A and B Meningococcal	Depression screen
Contraception (women with reproductive capacity)	Cervix: Cytology (21–65) *HPV + cytology (starting at 30)*	*Interpersonal and DV S&C*	*GDM screen* Rh screen Anemia screen	HPV (women 19–26)	Osteoporosis screen
	Colorectal: • FOBT • Colonoscopy • Sigmoidoscopy	*Well-woman visits*	STI screen Bacteriuria screen	Pneumococcal Zoster	Obesity screen; C&I if obese
			Lactation Support and counseling		

S&C: screening and counseling; C&I: counseling and interventions; CVD: cardiovascular disease

Source: IOM. Clinical Preventive Services for Women: Closing the Gaps. Accessed at www.nationalacademies.org/hmd/Reports/2011/Clinical-Preventive-Services-for-Women-Closing-the-Gaps.aspx.

age 30 and every 3 years thereafter for women with normal cytology results

3. Annual counseling on sexually transmitted infections (STIs) for sexually active women and girls

4. Human immunodeficiency virus (HIV) infection counseling and screening on an annual basis for sexually active women and girls

5. Coverage of the full range of US Food and Drug Administration (FDA)-approved contraceptive methods, sterilization procedures, and patient education and counseling for women and girls with reproductive capacity

6. Comprehensive lactation support and counseling and coverage of the costs of renting breast-feeding equipment

7. Interpersonal and domestic violence screening and counseling

8. At least one well-woman preventive care visit annually, including preconception and prenatal care for those interested in having children

On August 1, 2011, DHHS Secretary Kathleen Sebelius recommended that the HRSA accept all of the IOM's recommendations on women's preventive services. Accordingly, all new health plans starting on or after August 1, 2012, are required to include the recommended services without cost sharing.

The specific language in "Closing the Gap" recommendation [15] recognizes the need to extend preventive care over multiple visits for some women:

Recommendation 5.8: The committee recommends for consideration as a preventive service for women: at least one well-woman preventive care visit annually for adult women to obtain the recommended preventive services, including preconception and prenatal care. The committee also recognizes that several visits may be needed to obtain all necessary recommended preventive services, depending on a woman's health status, health needs, and other risk factors.

Although annual preventive case visits are an important part of women's health care, it is difficult in a single visit to elicit a comprehensive medical and social history and to address modifiable behavioral risk factors adequately. The rationale behind the recommendation for coverage of at least one "well-woman" visit per year is partly to enable women to see more than one physician for preventive services in a single year. Under these provisions, a woman could have an annual examination with her primary care clinician, who might provide chronic disease prevention counseling, and in the same year also see her OB–GYN for a preconception counseling visit without a co-payment for either visit [16].

Contraceptive Coverage

The ACA requires that almost all commercial health insurance plans cover all FDA-approved methods of contraception without cost sharing. Specifically [15]:

Recommendation 5.5: The committee recommends for consideration as a preventive service for women: the full range of FDA-approved contraceptive methods, sterilization procedures, and patient education and counseling for women with reproductive capacity.

This requirement applies to most employer-sponsored health insurance plans, unless the plans are grandfathered or if the plan is provided by certain religious institutions. Providing a range of methods is key because women's preferences, values, and medical conditions may vary depending upon their life stage, sexual practices, and health status. Coverage under the ACA allows clinicians to offer women access to a broader range of contraceptive options without preferential or discriminatory practices related to family income or insurance type.

In May 2015, HHS released a frequently asked question (FAQ) document clarifying the contraceptive coverage requirement [17]. For many plans, including most plans purchased in a state Marketplace, the guidance applied beginning on January 1, 2016. The FAQ clarifies that plans must cover at least one form of contraception in each of the 18 method categories as outlined by the FDA with no cost sharing. The 18 categories are as follows: (1) sterilization surgery for women, (2) surgical sterilization implant for women, (3) implantable rod, (4) copper IUD, (5) IUD with progestin, (6) shot/injection, (7) combined oral contraceptives, (8) progestin-only oral contraceptives, (9) extended or continuous use oral contraceptives, (10) contraceptive patch, (11) vaginal contraceptive ring, (12) diaphragm, (13) sponge, (14) cervical cap, (15) female condom, (16) spermicide, (17) levonorgestrel emergency contraception [with a prescription] (Plan B/Plan B One Step/Next Choice), and (18) ulipristal acetate emergency contraception (Ella). In addition to the method itself, "all associated clinical services, including patient education and counseling, needed for provision of the contraceptive method" and "services related to follow-up and management of side effects, counseling for continued adherence, and device removal" must be covered without cost sharing.

Medical management techniques, also known as "utilization controls" in Medicaid, are used by commercial insurers with the goal of controlling costs and promoting efficient delivery of care. Regulations issued by HHS implementing the ACA's preventive services benefit requirements, including contraceptive coverage, allowed health insurance issuers to use "reasonable medical management" techniques when "a recommendation or guidelines does not specify the frequency, method, treatment or setting for the provision of that service." Plans only may use medical management techniques within a contraceptive method category, not between method categories. For example, plans may cover one type of IUD with progestin (e.g., Mirena®) without cost sharing while imposing cost sharing on others (e.g., Skyla®, Liletta®). Conversely, a health plan may not impose cost sharing on the patch or the contraceptive vaginal ring in order to encourage individuals to use oral contraceptives, which are usually lower cost [18].

Plans also may impose cost sharing for brand-name drugs and devices that have a generic equivalent as long as a generic equivalent is covered without cost sharing. A plan cannot, however, have a policy that covers only generic forms of contraception without cost sharing, because some methods (e.g., IUDs) are only available as brand-name devices.

If a plan uses medical management techniques within a specified contraceptive method category, it must have an "expedient exceptions process" so that the patient can access the specific birth control her health care provider determines is medically necessary. Medical necessity is defined in the 2015 FAQ to include such factors as "severity of side effects, differences in permanence and reversibility of contraceptives, and ability to adhere to the appropriate use of the item or service, as determined by the attending provider." The exceptions process must defer to the provider's determination.

The National Family Planning and Reproductive Health Association (NFPRHA) has provided advice in regard to helping a woman who is having trouble accessing her method of choice without cost sharing [18]. First, confirm with the patient's health insurance plan the documentation required for appropriate coverage without cost sharing. In the instance of a plan using "reasonable medical management" techniques within a method category, the plan should be contacted to request an exception (sometimes called a preauthorization or a treatment authorization request). If the previous two actions do not result in appropriate coverage, or if a plan is out of compliance, contact the plan's medical director to voice concerns with barriers to accessing care. In addition, encourage the patient to contact the National Women's Law Center's "CoverHer" hotline (see Resources below). The hotline can help the patient navigate the process to ensure adequate coverage of the method of her choice.

Studies of eligible women performed in 2014–2015 showed that 70 percent were receiving oral contraceptives, the contraceptive patch, and the contraceptive vaginal ring without any out-of-pocket costs, as were 89 percent of women who requested IUDs [19–21].

Even after all plans eventually lose grandfathered status, the proportion of women paying nothing out of pocket will never reach 100 percent. Some women will choose a brand-name drug with a generic equivalent, in which case their health plan could legally ask for a co-payment. Others might choose to receive contraceptive services from an out-of-network provider; cost sharing (or denial of coverage entirely) is allowed in such cases, unless there are no in-network providers for the given service.

By an interim HHS policy specific to contraceptive services, group health plans sponsored by certain religious employers, and group health insurance coverage in connection with such plans, are exempt from the requirement to cover contraceptive services. A "religious employer" is one who has the inculcation of religious values as its purpose, primarily employs persons who share its religious tenets, primarily serves persons who share its religious tenets, and is a non-profit organization under Internal Revenue Code. In addition, HHS specified an additional "accommodation" for religiously-affiliated entities not eligible for the religious exemption, such as educational facilities and health systems. In this case, once an eligible entity requests, and is approved for, the accommodation, the health plan, and not the employer, must cover the cost of contraceptive services. On June 30, 2014, the US Supreme Court issued another decision (*Burwell* v. *Hobby Lobby Stores*) that allows for-profit firms that are "closely held" (defined as more than 50 percent of outstanding stock owned by five or fewer individuals) to opt out of the ACA's contraceptive coverage mandate and become eligible to participate in the accommodation afforded by HHS to religiously affiliated institutions.

Women's Preventive Services in Medicare

Until recently, Medicare did not cover periodic health screening visits, with the exception of cervical cancer screening and breast and pelvic exams [22]. Since January 2011, Medicare reimburses a "Welcome to Medicare" preventive visit, called the Initial Preventive Physical Examination (IPPE), that can be claimed only once only within 12 months of obtaining Part B coverage. This visit includes a review of medical and social history, counseling about preventive services, including certain screenings, immunizations, and referrals for other care, if needed. Afterward, two types of comprehensive wellness visit are covered without cost sharing: the patient's first annual wellness visit (AWV), which is distinct from and must occur at least 12 months after the patient's IPPE visit, and subsequent AWV. Although not required, Medicare also provides coverage without cost sharing for most USPSTF-recommended services and three vaccinations: influenza, hepatitis B, and pneumococcal. Medicare is not required to cover services recommended by the ACIP or women's preventive services supported by the HRSA [23]. There is no cost sharing for the "Welcome to Medicare" preventive visit and the yearly AWV, assuming that the health care provider accepts assignment. However, if a health care provider performs additional tests or services during the same visit that aren't covered under these preventive benefits, coinsurance and the Part B deductible may apply.

ACOG Committee on Coding and Nomenclature believes that it is unlikely that most OB–GYN practices will offer the AWV or IPPE. Correspondingly, clinicians furnishing a preventive medicine Evaluation and Management (E/M) service (i.e., a preventive health visit) that does not meet the requirements for the AWV should continue to report one of the preventive medicine E/M services CPT codes (99381–99397) as appropriate to the patient's circumstances, and these codes will not be covered by Medicare. ACOG has developed a letter template that can be used to help explain to patients that they should seek appointments for these visits with their primary care physicians [22].

Medicare reimburses for collection of a screening Pap smear every 2 years in most cases. This service is reported using HCPCS code Q0091 (Screening Papanicolaou smear; obtaining, preparing, and conveyance of cervical or vaginal smear to laboratory). Both the deductible and co-pay/coinsurance are waived for the laboratory's interpretation of the test.

The collection is reimbursed every year if the patient meets Medicare's criteria for high risk. Following are the only criteria that are accepted by Medicare to indicate a high-risk patient:

- Woman is of childbearing age AND
  - Cervical or vaginal cancer is present (or was present) OR
  - Abnormalities were found within last 3 years OR
  - Is considered high risk (as described below) for developing cervical or vaginal cancer
- Woman is not of childbearing age AND she has at least one of the following:
  - High-risk factors for cervical and vaginal cancer
  - Onset of sexual activity under 16 years of age
  - Five or more sexual partners in a lifetime
  - History of sexually transmitted diseases (STDs; including HPV and/or HIV infection)
  - Fewer than three negative or any Pap smears within previous 7 years
  - Diethylstilbestrol (DES)-exposed daughters of women who took DES during pregnancy

Case Scenarios

1. *Mary is a 60-year-old postmenopausal woman seen by her OB–GYN physician for a well-woman visit. She underwent a vaginal hysterectomy 10 years earlier for uterine prolapse. Both her mother and her father had a history of early heart disease. Physical assessment included assessment of her body mass index (BMI) and blood pressure and a screening breast exam. A screening pelvic exam was offered, but she declined. Because her BMI was 36 kg/m^2, she was advised to schedule an appointment with her primary care provider to be screened for type 2 diabetes and to receive dietary counseling for the purpose of weight loss.*

   Question: Mary is not subject to cost sharing for her well-woman visit. When she visits her PCP, will she need to pay a co-payment for that visit, given that she has already had her annual well-woman visit with her OB–GYN?

   Answer: No. HHS regulations state that "The HRSA Guidelines recommend at least one annual well-woman preventive care visit for adult women to obtain the recommended preventive services that are age- and developmentally appropriate, including preconception and prenatal care [17]. HHS understands that additional well-woman visits, provided without cost sharing, may be needed to obtain all necessary recommended preventive services, depending on a woman's health status, health needs, and other risk factors. If the clinician determines that a patient requires additional well-woman visits for this purpose, then the additional visits must be provided in accordance with the requirements of the interim final regulations (i.e., without cost-sharing and subject to reasonable medical management)."

2. *Georgia is a 25-year-old woman seen for a well-woman visit. Age-appropriate anticipatory guidance, cervical cytology screening, and STD screening tests were performed. When her reproductive life plan was discussed with her, she stated that she had been using the contraceptive patch over the past 3 years, but expressed an interest in having an IUD placed. A front-office staff member checked with her health plan and confirmed that levonorgestrel IUD placement was covered by her health plan. After completing the informed consent process, she had a levonorgestrel IUD inserted during the same office visit.*

   Question: Is any part of this visit subject to cost sharing? Is it appropriate to bill the payer for both the well-woman visit and the IUD insertion procedure on the same date of service?

If Georgia was seen for an episode of irregular vaginal bleeding 3 weeks after the IUD insertion, is that office visit subject to cost sharing?

Answer: All of the services that Georgia received (the well-woman visit, STD screening, cervical cytology, contraceptive counselling, and placement of an IUD) are considered to be women's preventive services that must be available to her without cost sharing. Contraceptive counselling provided within the context of a well-woman visit is considered to be intrinsic to the visit (and not a significant, separately identifiable service). Therefore, the payer should be billed for:

- CPT 58300 (insertion of IUD)
- HCPCS code: J7298 (LN-releasing IUS, 52 mg, 5 years)
- ICD-10 code: Z30.430 (insertion of IUD)
- E/M code: 99395 (preventive medicine visit, established patient, aged 18–39). Modifier -25 is appended to 99395 to indicate that the preventive medicine visit was separate from the IUD insertion.

While some payers might insist that the well-woman visit and the IUD insertion be performed on separate dates of service, this represents unacceptable fragmentation of care, especially since the delay in placing the IUD could result in an unintended pregnancy. For the follow-up visit, Federal regulations state that "services related to follow-up and management of side effects, counselling for continued adherence, and device removal are included under the HRSA Guidelines and required to be covered without cost sharing".

3. *Sally is a 45-year-old uninsured woman, a natural born US citizen, who works part-time as a barista in a small coffee shop. Because her individual income was $19,000 both last year and this, she decided 2 years ago that she would not continue to pay her health insurance premiums and allowed her policy to lapse. She was seen at a community clinic for a well-woman visit 3 weeks ago, and the result of her cervical cytology test was reported as suspicious for squamous cell carcinoma. Colposcopy was performed and biopsies taken, which confirmed a histologic diagnosis of squamous cell cancer.*

Question: Can Sally apply for health insurance immediately in order to receive treatment for her cervical cancer? How can she go about doing that?

Answer: Before January 1, 2014, health plans in the individual and small business markets were permitted to deny an application for coverage based upon the presence of a preexisting health condition. Since January 1, 2014, the practice is illegal in Marketplace health plans, and plans are not permitted to even ask about preexisting conditions in the application for coverage. Since Sally's modified adjusted gross income (MAGI) is between $15,857 and $45,960 for a family of one, she is eligible to choose a Marketplace health plan during the open enrolment period, generally from November through January or February of the following year (specific dates change annually). Sally can visit www.healthcare.gov, enter her state of residence, then will be directed to the website of either her state health insurance exchange or to the section of the federal website that lists the Marketplace plans for her zip code. She will be asked to choose a "metal level" of coverage: Platinum (90 percent), Gold (80 percent), Silver (70 percent), or Bronze (60 percent). Premiums are higher at each level, but out-of-pocket costs are correspondingly lower. The federal subsidy to help Sally pay her premiums will be based upon the average cost of a Silver plan in her state.

If Sally's annual MAGI was below $15,857 and she lived in a Medicaid expansion state, she could easily apply for Medicaid online or through an eligibility worker. Depending upon her state, and in some cases, her county of residence, she will be offered membership in either a Medicaid managed care plan or a state-run Medicaid fee-for-service program.

Finally, if she is unable to enroll in a Marketplace plan because the open enrolment period is closed, CMS allows states to provide full Medicaid benefits to uninsured women under age 65 who are identified through the CDC National Breast and Cervical Cancer Early Detection Program (NBCCEDP) and are in need of treatment for breast or cervical cancer, including precancerous conditions and early-stage cancer. The same is true if she has a low income and lives in a state with the "coverage gap" because of the absence of Medicaid expansion.

Summary

- The ACA has a number of features that enhance access to well-woman visits, including first dollar coverage of a wide range of women's preventive services and the ability to access an OB–GYN without preauthorization

- As a consequence of the ACA, more American women have health insurance, through a combination of women (and their families) enrolling in state Marketplace health plans and Medicaid expansion in about half of the states
- Health plans are required to cover 18 different types of contraceptives without cost sharing, including IUDs and implants. Certain employers are exempt from this requirement
- Medicare covers an initial and annual preventive health visit, but these are more likely to be performed by the woman's primary care provider. Obtaining a cervical cytology sample and performing a screening breast and pelvic examination continue to be benefits payable separately from these preventive health visits.

Additional Resources

http://CoverHer.org
- A program operated by the National Women's Law Center to assist insured women in obtaining contraceptive services without cost sharing. The website offers a "Frequently Asked Questions" section with helpful advice, a "contact us" feature to send messages and questions coverher@nwlc.org, and a direct line at 1–866–745–5487.

http://kff.org/womens-health-policy/
- A website devoted to showcasing the excellent materials developed by the Kaiser Family Foundation on the subject of women's health policy and regulations, including preventive services, contraception, abortion, and current court cases. It is especially helpful in offering interactive maps that assist the user in determining women's health policies in individual states.

www.cdc.gov/prevention/
- The CDC website that provides interactive CDC Prevention Checklists, including information about preventive services with no cost sharing, for nonpregnant and pregnant women, men, and children.

www.healthcare.gov/
- The central federal portal for obtaining health insurance coverage through the Marketplace (state health insurance exchange) in each state.

www.confidentialandcovered.com
- Confidential & Covered is a federally funded research project to help Title X providers (mainly family planning clinics and community clinics) to offer care that is confidential and receive payment that does not breach privacy.

www.nationalfamilyplanning.org/gcfpresources
- Get Covered: Family Planning. ACA patient education materials that have been developed using focus group-tested messages that are geared mainly for use in family planning health centers.

www.medicare.gov/coverage/preventive-visit-and-yearly-wellness-exams.html
- Helpful information about Medicare preventive benefits for women.

References

1. Kaiser Family Foundation. Women's Health Insurance Coverage. Kaiser Family Foundation Fact Sheet. January 2016. Available at: http://kff.org/womens-health-policy/fact-sheet/womens-health-insurance-coverage-fact-sheet/.
2. US Census Bureau. Kaiser Family Foundation Analysis of 2015 Current Population Survey, January 2016. Available at: http://kff.org/health-reform/issue-brief/new-estimates-of-eligibility-for-aca-coverage-among-the-uninsured/. Retrieved May 16, 2016.
3. Markus, A., Andres, E., West, K.D., Garro, N., and Pellegrini, C. Medicaid covered births, 2008 through 2010, in the context of the implementation of health reform. *Women's Health Issues*. 2013, **23**(5): e273–80.
4. Sonfield, A., Alrich, C., and Gold, R.B. Public Funding for Family Planning, Sterilization and Abortion Services, FY 1980–2006. New York, NY: Guttmacher Institute, 2008. Available at: www.guttmacher.org/sites/default/files/pdfs/pubs/2008/01/28/or38.pdf. Retrieved January 30, 2017.
5. Kaiser Commission on Medicaid and the Uninsured. The Uninsured: A Primer. October 2013. Available at: http://files.kff.org/attachment/primer-the-uninsured-a-primer-key-facts-about-health-insurance-and-the-uninsured-in-the-era-of-health-reform. Retrieved January 30, 2017.
6. Kaiser Family Foundation. Women and Health Care in the Early Years of the ACA: Key Findings from the 2013 Kaiser Women's Health Survey, May 2014. Available at: https://kaiserfamilyfoundation.files.wordpress.com/201

4/05/8590-women-and-health-care-in-the-early-years
-of-the-affordable-care-act.pdf. Retrieved January 30,
2017.

7. Kaiser Family Foundation. Analysis of 2014 Survey of
    Low-Income Americans, 2015. Available at: http://kff
    .org/health-reform/issue-brief/adults-who-remained-
    uninsured-at-the-end-of-2014/. Retrieved May 16,
    2016.

8. Stolp, H. and Fox, J. Increasing receipt of women's
    preventive services. *J Women's Health.* 2015, **24:**
    875–81.

9. Xierali, I.M., Puffer, J.C., Tong, S.T., Bazemore, A.W.,
    and Green, L.A. The percentage of family physicians
    attending to women's gender-specific health needs is
    declining. *J Am Board Fam Med.* 2012, **25:**406–7.

10. Hamel, L., Firth, J., and Brodie, M. *Kaiser Health
    Tracking Poll March 2014.* Menlo Park, CA: Henry
    J. Kaiser Family Foundation, 2014.

11. Kaiser Family Foundation. Preventive Services Covered
    by Private Health Plans under the Affordable Care Act.
    Menlo Park, CA: Kaiser Family Foundation, 2014.

12. Ferrante, J.M., Balasubramanian, B.A., Hudson, S.V.,
    and Crabtree, B.F. Principles of the patient-centered
    medical home and preventive services delivery. *Ann
    Fam Med.* 2010, **8:**108–16.

13. Markovitz, A.R., Alexander, J.A., Lantz, P.M., and
    Paustian, M.L. Patient-centered medical home
    implementation and use of preventive services:
    The role of practice socioeconomic context. *JAMA
    Intern Med.* 2015. 175:598–606.

14. Gee, R.E., Brindis, C.D., Diaz, A., et al.
    Recommendations of the IOM Clinical Preventive
    Services for Women Committee: Implications for
    obstetricians and gynecologists. *Curr Opin Obstet
    Gynecol.* 2011, **23:**471–80.

15. IOM. Clinical Preventive Services for Women: Closing
    the Gaps. Available at: www.nationalacademies
    .org/hmd/Reports/2011/Clinical-Preventive-Services-
    for-Women-Closing-the-Gaps.aspx. Retrieved May 16,
    2016.

16. Gee, R.E. Preventive services for women under the
    Affordable Care Act. *Obstet Gynecol.* 2012, **120:**12–14.

17. Affordable Care Act Implementation FAQs – Set 12.
    Available at: www.cms.gov/CCIIO/Resources/Fact-
    Sheets-and-FAQs/aca_implementation_faqs12.html.
    Retrieved May 16, 2016.

18. National Family Planning and Reproductive Health
    Association. Affordable Care Act Contraceptive
    Coverage Requirement: Four Things Providers Should
    Know. December 2015. Available at: www
    .nationalfamilyplanning.org/contraceptive_coverage_
    preventive_services. Retrieved May 16, 2016.

19. Law, A., Wen, L., Lin, J., et al. Are women benefiting
    from the Affordable Care Act? A real world evaluation
    of the impact of the ACA on out-of-pocket costs for
    contraceptives. *Contraception.* 2016, **93**(5):392–7.

20. Finer, L.B., Sonfield, A., and Jones, R.K. Changes in
    out-of-pocket payments for contraception by privately
    insured women during implementation of the federal
    contraceptive coverage requirement. *Contraception.*
    2014, **89:**97–102.

21. Sonfield, A., Taples, A., Jones, R.K., and Finer, L.B.
    Impact of federal contraceptive coverage guarantee on
    out-of-pocket payments for contraceptives: 2014
    update. *Contraception.* 2015, **91:**44–8.

22. ACOG, Medicare Screening Services. 2015. Accessed
    at: www.acog.org/-/media/Departments/Coding/Medi
    care-Preventive-Services-2015.pdf?la=en. Retrieved
    May 16, 2016.

23. Kaiser Family Foundation. Medicare at a glance. 2012.
    Available at: http://kff.org/medicare/fact-sheet/medi
    care-at-a-glance-fact-sheet. Retrieved May 16, 2016.

Suggested Reading

ACOG Committee on Underserved Women. Committee
Opinion 627. Health care for unauthorized immigrants.
Obstet Gynecol. 2015, **125:**755–9.

ACOG Committee on Underserved Women. Committee
Opinion 552. Benefits to women of Medicaid expansion
through the Affordable Care Act. *Obstet Gynecol.* 2013, **121**
(1):223–5.

DiVenere, L. Women's health under the Affordable Care
Act: What is covered? *OBG Manage.* 2012, **24:**46–54.

Gee, R.E. and Rosenbaum, S. The Affordable Care Act.
An overview for obstetricians and gynecologists. *Obstet
Gynecol.* 2012, **120:**1263–6.

Jones, R.K. and Sonfeld, A. Health insurance coverage
among women of reproductive age before and after the
implementation of the ACA. *Contraception.* 2016, **93**(5):
386–91.

Pascale, A., Beal, M.W., and Fitzgerald, T. Rethinking the
well woman visit: A scoping review to identify 8 priority
areas for well woman care in the era of the Affordable Care
Act. *Women's Health Issues.* 2016, **26**(2):135–46.

Weisman, C.S. and Chuang, C.H. Making the most of the
ACA's contraceptive coverage mandate for privately
insured women. *Women's Health Issues.* 2014, **24**(5):465–8.

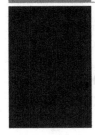

Introduction – Components of the Well-Woman Visit at Different Life Stages

The Well-Woman Task Force (WWTF) organized preventive and screening services by four different age groups. In an online supplement to their report, the WWTF provide tables of recommended components, hyperlinked to their evidence tables. The original WWTF Tables are available at http://links.lww .com/AOG/A676, http://links.lww.com/AOG/A677, http://links.lww.com/AOG/A678, and http://links .lww.com/AOG/A679. We have adapted the tables for use in book form. The tables that follow include the relevant component chapters organized by the four WWTF age groups. We divided several of the especially broad WWTF components into separate chapters and grouped the components into related areas. Readers may either use the tables here or the original online tables depending on their work style and preferred format.

Well-Adolescent (13–18 years) Visit Components – Relevant Chapters

Health Maintenance
   Immunizations
   Visual acuity and glaucoma screening
   Oral hygiene and oral cavity examination
   Injury prevention
   Piercing and tattooing
   Pelvic examination and abdominal examination

Cardiovascular Health
   Dyslipidemia
   Hypertension

Metabolic and Nutritional Health
   Diet and nutrition
   Fitness and exercise
   Obesity
   Metabolic syndrome
   Anemia
   Diabetes

Urinary Tract Assessment
   Bacteriuria

Contraception and Reproductive Health
   Contraception
   Sexual health

Infectious Diseases
   Hepatitis B and C screening
   HIV
   Other sexually transmitted infections

Cancer Screening and Prevention
   Skin cancer
   Cervical cancer
   Genetic screening for cancer

Neurologic, Behavioral, and Psychosocial Health
   Depression
   Domestic and intimate partner violence
   Alcohol misuse
   Tobacco and nicotine use
   Drug use
   Mental health and psychosocial issues, suicide and
      behavioral assessment

Pregnancy
   Breastfeeding
   Neural tube defects
   Postpartum screening of gestational diabetics
   Preconception and interconception care

Well-Woman Visit Components – Relevant Chapters for Reproductive-Aged Women (19–45 Years)

Health Maintenance
   Immunizations
   Visual acuity and glaucoma screening

Hearing
Oral hygiene and oral cavity examination
Injury prevention
Piercing and tattooing
Pelvic examination and abdominal examination

Cardiovascular Health
Dyslipidemia
Hypertension

Metabolic and Nutritional Health
Diet and nutrition
Fitness and exercise
Obesity
Metabolic syndrome
Anemia
Diabetes
Hypothyroidism

Urinary Tract Assessment
Kidney disease
Bacteriuria

Contraception and Reproductive Health
Contraception
Sexual health

Infectious Diseases
Hepatitis B and C screening
HIV
Other sexually transmitted infections

Cancer Screening and Prevention
Skin cancer
Cervical cancer
Colorectal cancer screening and prevention
Ovarian cancer
Breast cancer
Genetic screening for cancer

Neurologic, Behavioral, and Psychosocial Health
Depression
Domestic and intimate partner violence
Alcohol misuse
Tobacco and nicotine use
Drug use
Sleep disorders
Mental health and psychosocial issues, suicide and behavioral assessment

Pregnancy
Breastfeeding

Neural tube defects
Postpartum screening of gestational diabetics
Preconception and interconception care

Well-Woman Visit Components – Relevant Chapters for Mature Women (46–64 Years)

Health Maintenance
Immunizations
Visual acuity and glaucoma screening
Hearing
Oral hygiene and oral cavity examination
Injury prevention
Pelvic examination and abdominal examination

Cardiovascular Health
Dyslipidemia
Hypertension

Metabolic and Nutritional Health
Diet and nutrition
Fitness and exercise
Obesity
Metabolic syndrome
Anemia
Osteoporosis
Diabetes
Hypothyroidism

Urinary Tract Assessment
Kidney disease
Bacteriuria
Pelvic floor disorders

Contraception and Reproductive Health
Contraception
Sexual health

Infectious Diseases
Hepatitis B and C screening
HIV
Other sexually transmitted infections

Cancer Screening and Prevention
Skin cancer
Cervical cancer
Colorectal cancer screening and prevention
Ovarian cancer
Breast cancer

Genetic screening for cancer

Neurologic, Behavioral, and Psychosocial Health
Depression
Domestic and intimate partner violence
Alcohol misuse
Tobacco and nicotine use
Drug use
Sleep disorders
Mental health and psychosocial issues, suicide and behavioral assessment

Well-Woman Visit Components – Relevant Chapters for Women Older than 64 Years

Health Maintenance
Immunizations
Visual acuity and glaucoma screening
Hearing
Oral hygiene and oral cavity examination
Injury prevention
Pelvic examination and abdominal examination

Cardiovascular Health
Dyslipidemia
Hypertension

Metabolic and Nutritional Health
Diet and nutrition
Fitness and exercise
Obesity
Metabolic syndrome
Anemia

Osteoporosis
Diabetes
Hypothyroidism

Urinary Tract Assessment
Kidney disease
Bacteriuria
Pelvic floor disorders

Contraception and Reproductive Health
Sexual health

Infectious Diseases
Hepatitis B and C screening
HIV
Other sexually transmitted infections

Cancer Screening and Prevention
Skin cancer
Cervical cancer
Colorectal cancer screening and prevention
Ovarian cancer
Breast cancer
Genetic screening for cancer

Neurologic, Behavioral, and Psychosocial Health
Depression
Domestic and intimate partner violence
Alcohol misuse
Tobacco and nicotine use
Drug use
Sleep disorders
Mental health and psychosocial issues, suicide and behavioral assessment

Chapter

Immunizations

Regan N. Theiler

Why Vaccinate

Few public health measures in history have been as effective as immunizations in preventing morbidity and mortality. Immunization, or priming of the immune system in advance of exposure to a pathogen, prevents infectious disease in the immunized person. However, additional advantages for the population include herd immunity by reduction of circulating pathogen loads, and in the case of women of reproductive age, passive immunity for neonates. Herd immunity can protect those members of a population who cannot be vaccinated due to allergies to vaccine components, immune compromise, or other contraindications. Effective global immunization programs can even eradicate endemic diseases, as is the case with smallpox.

Rationale for Vaccination

In the United States, most routine vaccines are administered in childhood but adult immunization is also an important part of preventive care. A recent study estimated that vaccination of US seniors aged 65 or older decreased all-cause mortality during influenza season by 16 percent [1]. Despite the proven benefits of immunization, noncompliance is significant in adult women. Immunization for seasonal influenza decreases morbidity and mortality, yet seasonal vaccination rates remain low, despite widespread availability, safety of the vaccine, and a Centers for Disease Control and Prevention (CDC) recommendation for universal immunization. Many strategies to increase vaccine compliance have been studied, but few have been shown to improve adherence to vaccination guidelines [2]. Reminders and discussion at the well-woman visit, as well as immediate administration at that time, are recommended strategies to improve compliance.

The term "vaccine hesitancy" has been used to describe resistance to immunization, and the

phenomenon is now under intense study in an effort to improve vaccination. US adults cannot be legally compelled to accept a vaccine, and whether employers may compel immunization in special settings such as health care facilities remains a topic of much debate [3].

Prevention of late-onset sequelae of chronic infections is relatively new indication for vaccination. For example, the Zostavax is indicated for prevention of shingles in all persons over the age of 60. Human papillomavirus (HPV) vaccines prevent long-term sequelae of HPV infections, including cervical dysplasia, when administered prior to exposure to the virus.

Vaccination can also help prevent infection in the newborn. Additional administration of Tetanus, Diphtheria, acellular Pertussis (Tdap) is recommended for women during each pregnancy to improve passive immunity of the infant. Because of high rates of nasopharyngeal carriage of *Bordetella pertussis* among adults, cocooning, or clustering of adult Tdap boosters of close family members and infant caregivers, can help protect the neonate during times of increased pertussis activity. Ensuring that each family member has obtained one adult Tdap vaccination is adequate for this strategy.

Factors that Affect Vaccination

Age: Advisory Committee on Immunization Practices (ACIP) different age groups are susceptible to different infections, so immunization guidelines vary by age, with recommendations changing at 19, 22, 27, 50, 60, and 65 years.

Pregnancy: Pregnancy is a contraindication to live, attenuated vaccines except in the most emergent circumstances [4]. Influenza can cause particularly severe infection in pregnancy, and administration of Tdap helps give infants passive immunity to pertussis.

Health conditions: Medical conditions including asplenia, diabetes, cardiovascular disease, liver disease, lung disease, renal disease, and immune compromise alter disease susceptibility and influence vaccine recommendations.

Profession: Health care workers may need additional immunizations to protect them against occupational exposure to infections like hepatitis B, and prevent transmission of infections like pertussis and influenza to patients.

International travel: Patients traveling to other countries may need protection against infection endemic to their destination, including Yellow Fever, Hepatitis A, Meningococcus, and Typhoid.

Recommended Guidelines and How to Find Them

The WWTF recommends immunization according to the schedule and protocols outlined by ACIP. These schedules are updated yearly and are published and available online as the Adult Immunization Schedule [a]. There are several useful resources. Updated vaccine schedules, clinical guidance for US practice, and vaccine information statements can be found on the ACIP website (www.cdc.gov/vaccines/acip/). Adult schedules apply to those 19 and older. ACIP recommendations, practice tools, smartphone apps, and downloadable immunization schedules are available at www.cdc.gov/vaccines/schedules/index.html. Patient-level information, Vaccine Information Statements (VIS), foreign-language translations, and CDC-approved vaccine eligibility screening tools may be obtained from the Immunization Action Coalition (www.vaccineinformation.org/). The American College of Obstetrics and Gynecology (ACOG) has information specifically for women on their website (immunizationforwomen.org).

For non-US practices, the World Health Organization (WHO) publishes recommended routine immunization schedules to guide the development of more specific country-level vaccine schedules (www.who.int/immunization/policy/immunization_tables/en/). Each country develops individual recommendations based on this framework, and contacting the relevant national health authority is recommended.

Advice about vaccinations for US residents planning foreign travel may be found on the CDC website. Refer to www.cdc.gov/travel/ where visitors can get advice for travel to foreign countries, even tailored to the type of travel and age or pregnancy status of the traveler. Some countries require proof of vaccination for visa issuance, so checking the country-specific information far in advance of travel is of paramount importance.

How to Vaccinate

ACIP recommends the following treatment standards for adult immunization practices.

1. ASSESS immunization status of all your patients at every clinical encounter.
2. Strongly RECOMMEND vaccines that patients need.
3. ADMINISTER needed vaccines or REFER your patients to a vaccination provider
4. DOCUMENT vaccines received by your patients.

After initial documentation of adequate childhood immunizations, the women's health provider will typically monitor the adequacy of immunity to a limited number of relevant pathogens (Table 9.1) and update immunizations based on the ACIP recommendations. ACIP also provides guidance on frequently encountered problems like completing vaccine series that are off schedule. Increasingly, adolescent patients have received a complete course of three HPV immunizations with their pediatric provider, and this should be documented on entry to care. Women up to age 26 are eligible for catch-up vaccination and should be offered completion of partial HPV vaccine series as needed. Similar complete vaccination status will be frequently encountered for Hepatitis B and the Measles, Mumps, Rubella (MMR) vaccine. For older women and patients with immune compromise or respiratory conditions, pneumococcal polysaccharide vaccine may be indicated at the well-woman visit for prevention of pneumococcal pneumonia, and the indications for this should be reviewed regularly.

Most vaccines require refrigeration with frequent temperature logging and recording of lot numbers and expiration dates. Designated staff at each clinical site should be familiar with the specific storage, administration, and reporting compliance requirements of state and federal regulatory agencies.

The US National Vaccine Childhood Injury Act requires that all patients receive the Vaccine Information Sheet (VIS) (available at www.immunize.org/vis/) at the time of each immunization, and

Table 9.1 Adolescent and Adult Routine Vaccines. Light gray shading indicates immunizations to assess annually. Dark gray shading indicates immunizations to be documented for new adult patients. For timing of administration, refer to ACIP Immunization schedule.

Name	Pathogen(s)/Disease	Vaccine Type	Dosing
Hepatitis A	Hepatitis A	Inactivated virus	Two doses
Hepatitis B	Hepatitis B	Inactivated virus	Series of 3
Hepatitis A/B (Twinrix)	Hepatitis A and B	Inactivated virus	Series of 3
Bivalent HPV (Cervarix*)	Human papillomavirus (HPV) 16, 18	Noninfectious virus-like particle	Series of 3 before age 26**
Quadrivalent HPV (Gardasil)	HPV 6, 11, 16, 18	Noninfectious virus-like particle	Series of 3 before age 26**
9-Valent HPV (Gardasil 9)	HPV 6, 11, 16, 18, 31, 33, 45, 52, 58	Noninfectious virus-like particle	Series of 3 before age 26**
Influenza	Influenza seasonal serotypes	Multiple.	Annually
MMR	Measles, mumps, rubella	Live attenuated virus	One time
Meningococcal	*N. meningitidis*	Quadrivalent polysaccharide conjugate	One time
Pneumococcus-13 conjugate (Prevnar-13)	*S. pneumonia*, 13 types	Polysaccharide conjugate	One time, >65 years of age or risk factors
Pneumococcus-23 conjugate (Pneumovax- 23)	*S. pneumoniae*, 23 types	Polysaccharide conjugate	One time, >65 years for age or risk factors
Td	Tetanus, Diptheria	Inactivated bacterial toxoids	Every 10 years. Substitute Tdap booster for one dose
Tdap (Adacel/Boostrix)	Tetanus, Diptheria, and Pertussis	Inactivated bacteria	One-time adult booster and once every pregnancy
Varivax	Varicella	Live attenuated virus	Two doses
Zostavax	Varicella – shingles	Live attenuated virus	One time, >60 years of age

* Licensed only for females in the United States
** Second dose 1–2 months after first dose, third dose at least 6 months after first dose

patients should be prescreened for vaccine-specific contraindications prior to administration. State vaccine programs provide vaccines free of charge to practitioners, and the available offerings and compliance rules differ by state. Contact your state health authorities for assistance. The Vaccines for Children program (www.cdc.gov/vaccines/programs/vfc) is a federally funded program that provides ACIP-recommended vaccines at no cost to children who are unable to pay.

Serious adverse reactions and deaths from vaccination are exceedingly rare, and in the setting of ongoing infectious threats the risk of infection far outweighs the risk of vaccine-associated adverse events (VAEs). If a VAE is suspected after administration of any vaccine, it should be reported through the national Vaccine Adverse Events Reporting System (VAERS). Additional information is available at http://vaers.hhs.gov [5].

New Developments Likely to Affect Future Recommendations

Creation and expansion of vaccine coverage continues to develop. Pneumococcus vaccine administration guidelines have changed due to inclusion of additional serotypes, and evolution of pneumococcus and HPV subtype combination vaccines is likely to continue [6]. Pregnancy vaccination recommendations for neonatal immune protections are also evolving, with strong recommendations for influenza and Tdap vaccines during every pregnancy. Research efforts are ongoing to develop a maternal vaccine against group B streptococcus (GBS) for neonatal protection.

Perhaps the most exciting areas of research involve vaccinomics, or the study of individual variation in the immune response to vaccines. It is well known that individual responses to the rubella vaccine result in waning immunity or lack of protection for subsets of the population. Researchers are working to understand genetic and immunologic diversity in the context of antigenicity, with the potential for future individualization of vaccine recommendations based on human leukocyte antigen (HLA) subtypes, adjuvant effectiveness, and other personal characteristics.

Billing

Under ICD-10, coding for vaccine administration has been simplified with the use of a single diagnosis code for all immunization encounters. Use ICD-10 code Z23 for administration of immunization or vaccination (all vaccine types), along with the vaccine-specific CPT code and the administration code. Each vaccine has a unique CPT code assigned to it, to be used for reimbursement when the clinic has purchased the vaccine. An additional set of generic CPT codes is designated for administration of vaccines, assigned by route (injection vs. oral) and whether it is the first administration or additional administration at the same visit. For state-supplied or other free vaccines, providers cannot charge for the vaccine but may charge for counseling and immunization administration.

Illustrative Cases

An 18 year-old nulligravid patient presents for her well-woman visit. She has a history of sickle-cell disease with anemia and functional asplenia. Her childhood vaccines were administered by her local pediatrician, and she is transferring to your care. Because it is

November, you inquire about her influenza vaccination status. She received her influenza vaccine last week at a community health fair. However, she has never received a pneumococcal vaccine.

Administration of pneumococcal polysaccharide vaccine is indicated because of her chronic disease. She will first need a single dose of pneumococcus-13 conjugate (PCV13) vaccine with a subsequent visit for pneumococcus-23 conjugate (PPSV23) vaccine 6–12 months from now, as they may not be given concomitantly [7, 8]. The ACIP guidelines provide details for sequential vaccine scheduling [8].

Immunize now? Yes

Next immunization: 6–12 months

A 21-year-old nulligravid woman presents in November for her well-woman examination. She has had two male sexual partners and is currently using combined oral contraceptives for contraception. She last saw her pediatrician at age 18, and she believes she received at least one injection of HPV vaccine. She does not recall having additional injections in the series, and she does not know which vaccine she received. She has been away at college and has not received routine care. You obtain records from her pediatrician's office, confirming she received her Tdap at age 18, as well as her MMR booster and one dose of bivalent HPV vaccine. Her routine childhood immunizations were administered on schedule, including the hepatitis B series.

This is the beginning of flu season; therefore you recommend influenza vaccination today.

You encourage completion of her HPV vaccine series. However, your office has only the new 9-valent HPV vaccine. Completion of the series with the available vaccine is indicated. Instruct her to ask her 20-year-old sexual partner about his immunization status and refer him for the series as needed. You bill with **ICD-10 code Z23** for diagnosis of needed vaccination and the **CPT codes 90471** for administration of the first vaccine and **90472** for administration of the second vaccine. Because your vaccine supply is state-supplied, you cannot use CPT code 90686 (for adult administration of quadrivalent influenza vaccine) or CPT code 90651 (for the 9-valent HPV vaccine) [9].

Immunize today? Yes (9-valent HPV vaccine)

Next immunization: 4 months

A 36-year-old G3P1021 patient presents for her well-woman examination. The patient has a history of herpes simplex virus type 2 genital infection with frequent recurrences, for which she takes valacyclovir prophylaxis. The patient mentions that during her pregnancy 2 years ago, someone told her she that was not immune to chicken pox. You review her chart to find her varicella IgG result to be "not detected." She has no recollection of childhood infection, and her daughter has recently been vaccinated with the first dose of the series. She is wondering whether she should receive the vaccine.

Administration of the two-dose varicella vaccine series is indicated. She should have a negative pregnancy test and be using reliable contraception. Because her valacyclovir could reduce the efficacy of the live attenuated virus vaccine, it would be preferable for the patient return for the vaccine at least 24 hours after her last valacyclovir dose, and to refrain from using the medication for 14 days after the live vaccine is administered [10].

Immunize now? No

Next immunization: ≥24 hours after her last valacyclovir dose

Guideline

a. Kim, D.K., Bridges, C.B., and Harriman, K.H. Advisory Committee on Immunization Practices. Advisory Committee on Immunization Practices recommended immunization schedule for adults aged 19 years or older: United States, 2016. *Ann Intern Med.* 2016, **164**:184–94. Available at: www.cdc.gov/vaccines/schedules/hcp/adul t.html retrieved 5/29/16.

References

1. Castilla, J. et al. Enhanced estimates of the influenza vaccination effect in preventing mortality: A prospective Cohort Study. *Medicine (Baltimore).* 2015, **94**(30):e1240.

2. Armstrong, C. ACIP releases recommendations for influenza vaccination, 2015–2016. *Am Fam Physician.* 2015, **92**(8):732–40.

3. Jarrett, C. et al. Strategies for addressing vaccine hesitancy – A systematic review. *Vaccine.* 2015, **33**(34):4180–90.

4. Fox, K.A. and Theiler, R. Vaccination in pregnancy. *Curr Pharm Biotechnol.* 2011, **12**(5):789–96.

5. Miller, E.R. et al. Deaths following vaccination: What does the evidence show? *Vaccine.* 2015, **33**(29):3288–92.

6. Tomczyk, S. et al. Use of 13-valent pneumococcal conjugate vaccine and 23-valent pneumococcal polysaccharide vaccine among adults aged >/=65 years: recommendations of the Advisory Committee on Immunization Practices (ACIP). *Morb Mortal Wkly Rep.* 2014, **63**(37):822–5.

7. Kobayashi, M. et al. Intervals between PCV13 and PPSV23 vaccines: Recommendations of the Advisory Committee on Immunization Practices (ACIP). *Morb Mortal Wkly Rep.* 2015, **64**(34):944–7.

8. Centers for Disease Control and Prevention. Use of 13-valent pneumococcal conjugate vaccine and 23-valent pneumococcal polysaccharide vaccine for adults with immunocompromising conditions: Recommendations of the Advisory Committee on Immunization Practices (ACIP). *Morb Mortal Wkly Rep.* 2012, **61**(40):816–9.

9. Petrosky, E. Use of 9-valent human papillomavirus (HPV) vaccine: Updated HPV vaccination recommendations of the advisory committee on immunization practices. *Morb Mortal Wkly Rep.* 2015, **64**(11):300–4.

10. Kroger, A.T., Sumaya, C.V., Pickering, L.K., and Atkinson, W.L. General recommendations on immunization. Recommendations of the Advisory Committee on Immunization Practices (ACIP). *Morb Mortal Wkly Rep.* 2011, **60**:1–60.

Visual Acuity and Glaucoma

Melanie D. Altizer

Why Screen?

Impairment of vision is a serious public health problem in older adults [a]. A number of conditions of the eye can result in impairment of visual acuity including macular degeneration, cataracts, diabetic retinopathy, and refractive errors. The prevalence in adults older than 60 years is approximately 9 percent [1]. The prevalence of visual impairment in 12–19-year olds is similar at 9.7 percent [1].

Glaucoma is a term that collectively refers to a group of eye disorders that lead to progressive damage of the optic nerve. It is characterized by loss of nerve tissue around the optic disc that ultimately leads to vision loss. There are many forms of glaucoma, with the most common being primary open-angle glaucoma (POAG). POAG affects 2.5 million Americans and is the single leading cause of visual impairment or loss of peripheral vision and blindness [b]. In the United States alone, POAG is thought to affect 1.9 percent of people over the age of 40 [b]. Glaucoma is second only to cataracts as the leading cause of blindness in the world [2]. It remains a leading cause of irreversible blindness and is the leading cause of blindness in certain patient populations such as African Americans and Hispanics [3]. Glaucoma poses a huge threat to quality of life worldwide and also places a large economic burden on society. In addition to the cost to society, glaucoma has been associated with diminished daily function including falls, motor vehicle accidents, and other difficulty driving [3, 4].

Rationale for Screening

There is convincing evidence that screening with a visual acuity test identifies persons with refractive error [a]. Evidence suggests that screening questions are not as accurate as visual acuity testing for assessing visual acuity [a]. However, visual acuity testing alone does not accurately identify early age-related macular degeneration (AMD) [a].

POAG is generally asymptomatic and most cases are found incidentally on ophthalmologic exam. There is no universally accepted test to screen for glaucoma. While there is no direct evidence that screening is harmful, treatment for glaucoma can result in numerous harms including cataract formation secondary to local eye irritation from medications and the risks of complications from surgery [b]. There are no studies that confirm that early diagnosis reduces impaired vision or improves quality of life [b].

The American Academy of Pediatrics (AAP) states that "eye examinations and vision assessments are critical for the detection of conditions that often result in visual impairment, signify serious systemic disease, lead to problems with school performance, and, in some cases, threaten the child's life" [c]. Most of these problems happen in younger children.

Factors That Affect Screening

Age: Conditions causing visual impairment including glaucoma worsen with age. Most refractive visual acuity problems are evident by the end of adolescence.

Race: African Americans and nonwhite Hispanics are at increased risk for glaucoma.

Family history: Family history influences glaucoma risk likely through inherited and environmental influences.

Medical conditions: Medical conditions such as hypertension, coronary artery disease, and diabetes can increase risk for the development of glaucoma.

Recommended Guidelines and How to Find Them

The Well-Woman Task Force (WWTF) derived its recommendations for adults from the recommendations of the US Preventive Services Task Force (USPSTF). The USPSTF concludes that the current evidence is insufficient to assess the balance of benefits and harms of screening for impaired visual acuity in older adults [a]. The USPSTF also concludes that the current evidence is insufficient to assess the balance of benefits and harms of screening for POAG in adults [b]. The USPSTF did acknowledge that some patients were at increased risk for glaucoma. They suggest that "patients at increased risk, especially African Americans and older adults, talk to their primary care clinician or eye care specialist for advice about glaucoma screening."

The Bright Futures Guidelines [c] make recommendations for visual acuity screening in adolescents. The guidelines include guidance on timing of examinations [d] and procedures [e].

How to Screen

In adults, no visual acuity or glaucoma screening is recommended for asymptomatic patients. Patients with problems with vision noted on review of systems or who exhibit clear signs of visual difficulty during their examination should be evaluated.

In adolescents, screening with a Snellen eye chart is recommended once in early adolescence (younger than 15 years) and once in late adolescence (15–18 years). Patients with any abnormality or suspicion of abnormality should be referred to an optometrist or ophthalmologist. In addition, the following may be indicative of myopia, and should prompt additional screening [5]:

- Complaint that the classroom blackboard has become difficult to see
- Failure to pass a school vision screening test
- Holds toys or books close to the eyes
- Difficulty recognizing faces at a distance
- Tends to squint

New Developments Likely to Affect Future Guidelines

Additional research is needed to better understand the national progression of vision disorders, specifically glaucoma, and determine if screening and early treatment may have a positive impact on patient outcome, daily level of functioning, independence, and overall quality of life. Studies identifying subgroups of patients who benefit from glaucoma screening could change the current guidelines.

Billing

Medicare provides coverage for an annual glaucoma screening for all beneficiaries who fall into one or more of the following high-risk categories [6] (CMS 2011):

- Diabetes mellitus
- Family history of glaucoma
- African Americans 50 or older
- Hispanic Americans 65 or older

Coverage for screening includes a dilated eye examination with an intraocular pressure measurement or a direct slit-lamp biomicroscopic examination (CMS 2011).

Illustrative Cases

A 65-year-old African American woman presents to your office for a well-woman visit. Her medical history is significant for hypertension that is well controlled with medication. There is a family history of glaucoma in her mother. The patient denies any symptoms of visual impairment, but asks if she should be screened for glaucoma.

According to the USPSTF, increased intraocular pressure, family history of glaucoma, older age, and African American race increase a patient's risk of glaucoma. Older African American patients have a higher incidence of glaucoma than Caucasians and may have a more rapid progression of disease.

Screen now? The WWTF and USPSTF do not recommend screening. The USPSTF acknowledges the risk factors and lack of evidence, and suggests the patient discuss screening with the provider.

Next screen: If symptoms develop

A 45-year-old Caucasian patient presents for a well-woman visit. She denies a personal or family history of vision problems.

No screening is recommended in the absence of symptoms.

Screen now? No

Next screen: If symptoms develop

Guidelines

a. US Preventive Services Task Force. Impaired visual acuity in older adults: Screening. US Preventive Services Task Force Recommendation Statement. *Ann Intern Med.* 2009, **151**:37–43. Available at: www.uspreventiveservicestaskforce.org/Page/Docum

ent/UpdateSummaryFinal/impaired-visual-acuity-in-older-adults-screening. Retrieved May 30, 2016.

b. Moyer, V.A. Screening for glaucoma. U.S. Preventive Services Task Force Recommendation Statement. *Ann Int Med.* 2013, **59**:484–9. Available at: www.uspreventiveservicestaskforce.org/Page/Document/UpdateSummaryFinal/glaucoma-screening. Retrieved May 30, 2016.

c. American Academy of Pediatrics. *Recommendations for Preventive Pediatric Health Care.* Elk Grove Village: AAP, 2014. Available at: www.aap.org/en-us/Documents/periodicity_schedule.pdf. Retrieved May 30, 2016.

d. Committee on Practice and Ambulatory Medicine. Section on Ophthalmology. American Association of Certified Orthoptists. American Association for Pediatric Ophthalmology and Strabismus, American Academy of Ophthalmology. Visual system assessment in infants, children, and young adults by pediatricians. Available at: http://pediatrics.aappublications.org/content/137/1/1.51. Retrieved May 30, 2016.

e. Committee on Practice and Ambulatory Medicine. Section on Ophthalmology. American Association of Certified Orthoptists. American Association for Pediatric Ophthalmology and Strabismus, American Academy of Ophthalmology. Procedures for the evaluation of the visual system by pediatricians.

Available at: http://pediatrics.aappublications.org/content/137/1/1.52. Retrieved May 30, 2016.

References

1. Vitale, S., Cotch, M.F., and Sperduto, R.D. Prevalence of visual impairment in the United States. *JAMA.* 2006, **295**:2158–63.

2. Distelhorst, J.S. and Hughes, G.M. Open-angle glaucoma. *Am Fam Physician.* 2003, **67**:1937.

3. Tham, Y.C., Li, X., Wong, T.Y. et al. Global prevalence of glaucoma and projections of glaucoma burden through 2040: A systematic review and meta-analysis. *Ophthalmology.* 2014, **121**:2081.

4. Sommer, A., Tielsch, J.M., Katz, J. et al. Racial differences in the cause specific prevalence of blindness in east Baltimore. *N Engl J Med.* 1991, **325**:1412.

5. Bright Futures: Guidelines for health supervision of infants, children, and adolescents. Rationale and evidence. Available at: https://brightfutures.aap.org/Bright%20Futures%20Documents/13-Rationale_and_Evidence-1.pdf. Retrieved May 30, 2016.

6. Center for Medicare and Medicaid Services. Your Medicare Coverage – Glaucoma Tests. Available at: www.medicare.gov/coverage/glaucoma-tests.html. Retrieved May 30, 2016.

Hearing Screening for the Well-Woman Visit

Efua Leke

Why Screen?

In adults older than 65, hearing loss is the third most common condition and some population studies suggest prevalence of up to 20–40 percent in adults older than 50 [1]. In people affected by hearing loss, the ability to communicate can significantly affect their daily activities and contribute to a poor quality of life. Since patients with hearing loss could promptly benefit from management such as hearing aids, identification of these patients is important.

Rationale for Screening

The most common cause of hearing loss in older adults is age-related hearing loss or presbycusis, a sensorineural hearing loss caused by cellular degeneration with increasing age. Other factors contributing to hearing loss include systemic disease such as diabetes, genetic factors, and exposure to toxic agents [2].

The prevalence of hearing loss in adults over the age of 65 allows targeting of a specific age range for heightened awareness and possible screening at a well-woman visit. The impact of poor communication from hearing loss can have widespread consequences including functional decline, psychological implications, and social isolation. People with hearing loss are known to have a higher prevalence of depression, dementia, and poor ability to self-manage over the long term [3]. Additionally, older adults may not recognize or report their hearing loss symptoms due to other conditions such as cognitive impairment.

Reports suggest that fewer than 20 percent of people with hearing loss who would benefit from measures such as hearing aids are actually using them [4]. Additional reports indicate that there is a 7–10-year delay between identification of hearing loss and treatment for it [5]. Depending on the type of hearing loss, there are other measures which could significantly alter quality of life in these patients, such as speech reading training, information packages, and coping training. To be able to recommend these measures, hearing loss must be appropriately diagnosed.

There are several potential barriers to screening. Physician-related barriers include involvement with other clinical issues that appear more pressing, having a patient population that is younger with lower prevalence of hearing loss, lack of experience with screening, lack of time, and lack of reimbursement [6].

In determining if there was insufficient evidence to make a recommendation, the US Preventive Services Task Force (USPSTF) recognized the potential benefits, but in their evidence review found "a paucity of directly applicable trials" [a]. The only randomized controlled trial they identified [7] found increased hearing aid use with screening, but only in patients who self-perceived hearing loss at baseline, not in patients who were asymptomatic. There is also no evidence that the course of the hearing loss is changed by early intervention.

Factors That Affect Screening

Age: Age is the most significant risk factor for hearing loss. The hearing loss associated with presbycusis is typically gradual, progressive, and bilateral and increases with age.

Race: Studies suggest 70 percent lower rates of hearing loss in black subjects compared to white subjects [8].

Exposure to loud noise: Occupation typically plays a part, as service workers with chronic exposures to high decibel noises are more likely to develop hearing loss.

Comorbid conditions: Smoking, hypertension, and diabetes are associated with higher risk of hearing loss.

Recommended Guidelines and How to Find Them

The Well-Women Task Force concluded "hearing screening in adults who show no signs or symptoms of hearing loss is not recommended." This recommendation was derived from the USPTF guidelines [b], which were adopted by the American Academy of Family Physicians (AAFP). Their guidelines state: There is insufficient evidence to assess the benefits or harms of screening for hearing loss in asymptomatic adults aged 50 and older who show no signs or symptoms of hearing loss.

The American Speech-Language-Hearing Association recommends screening adults at least every decade through age 50 and at 3-year intervals thereafter [c]. Two other relevant organizations, the American Geriatrics Society and the American Academy of Otolaryngology Head and Neck Surgery, do not have specific recommendations.

How to Screen

Asymptomatic women should not be screened. The focus of the well-woman visit should be to detect signs and symptoms. Patients who report hearing difficulty during their review of symptoms or have obvious difficulty hearing or problems with their communication skills during the visit should be referred for formal audiometric testing to establish the diagnosis of hearing loss. The cost and required training for audiometric testing typically precludes its use in the primary care setting. To assess for symptoms, a question such as "do you have trouble or difficulty with hearing?" should be used as a starting point. Simple clinical tests such as assessing whether the patient can hear a finger rub or a whispered voice from a distance can then be employed. The most commonly used screening questionnaire is called the Hearing Handicap Inventory for the Elderly-Screening (HHIE-S). This 2-minute questionnaire evaluates the social and emotional aspects of hearing loss. Patients in whom the initial examination suggests hearing loss should have this questionnaire administered. The questionnaire can be found at: www.uspreventiveservicestaskforce.org/Home/GetFileByID/231.

Billing

Screening for hearing loss is covered under the ICD-10 code Z01.10, encounter for examination of ears and hearing without abnormal findings. However, in the preventive care setting, age-appropriate counseling constitutes part of the preventive medicine service. Unless there are specific problems diagnosed, this screening would be included in the general well-woman visit and would fall under the code Z01.419, encounter for gynecological examination without abnormal findings.

Illustrative Cases

A 65-year-old woman presents for a well-woman visit. Your introduction draws a blank stare until she asks you to speak louder.

This patient falls in the age group with the most concern for hearing loss. This preliminary response should prompt screening. If hearing loss is suggested by the examination, she should be referred for formal audiologic evaluation.

Screen now: Yes

Next screen: Not indicated if formal diagnosis and treatment have been established

A 28-year-old woman presents to you for a well-woman visit. Her review of systems is negative and she appears responsive and appropriate.

This case exemplifies the more typical well-adult patient, for whom screening is not necessary

Screen now: No

Next screen: Not indicated

A 69-year-old woman is seeing you for her well-woman visit. She asks you to speak louder as she forgot her hearing aids.

This patient already has a diagnosis of hearing loss and has hearing aids prescribed. Screening is no longer necessary. Given the low rates of actual usage of hearing aids, it would be prudent to inquire about her usage pattern and encourage her to use her aids more frequently.

Screen now: No

Next screen: Not indicated as she already has a diagnosis

Guidelines

a. American Academy of Family Physicians. *Hearing: Clinical Preventive Service Recommendation.* Leawood, KS: AAFP, 2015. Available at: www.aafp.org/patient-care/clinical-recommendations/all/hearing.html. Retrieved May 24, 2016.

b. Moyer, V.A. Screening for hearing loss in older adults: US preventive services task force recommendation statement. *Ann Intern Med.* 2012, **157**(9):655–61.

c. American Speech-Language-Hearing Association. *Hearing Screening and Testing.* February 8, 2011. Rockville, MD: American Speech-Language-Hearing Association. Available at: www.asha.org/policy/GL1997-00199/#sec1.11.3. Retrieved May 24, 2016.

References

1. Cruickshanks, K.J., Wiley, T.L., Tweed, T.S. et al. Prevalence of hearing loss in older adults in Beaver Dam, Wisconsin. The Epidemiology of Hearing Loss Study. *Am J Epidemiol.* 1998, **148**(9):879–86.

2. Gates, G.A. and Mills, J.H. Presbycusis. *Lancet.* 2005, **366**(9491):1111–20.

3. Saito, H., Nishiwaki, Y., Michikawa, T. et al. Hearing handicap predicts the development of depressive symptoms after three years in older community-dwelling Japanese. *J Am Geriat Soc.* 2010, **58**(1):93–7.

4. Kochkin, S. Subjective measures of satisfaction and benefit: Establishing norms. *Sem Hear.* 1997b, **18**:37–48.

5. Kochkin, S., Beck, D.L., Christensen, L.A., Compton-Conley, C. et al. MarkeTrak VIII: The impact of the hearing healthcare professional on hearing aid user success. *Hearing Review.* 2010, **17**(4):12–34.

6. Bogardus, S.T. Jr., Yueh, B., and Shekelle, P.G. Screening and management of adult hearing loss in primary care: Clinical applications. *JAMA.* 2003, **289**(15):1986–90.

7. Yueh, B., Collins, M.P., Souza, P.E. et al. Long-term effectiveness of screening for hearing loss: The screening for auditory impairment – Which Hearing Assessment-Test (SAI-WHAT) randomized trial. *J Am Geriatr Soc.* 2010, **58**:427–34.

8. Agrawal, Y., Platz, E.A., and Niparko, J.K. Prevalence of hearing loss and differences by demographic characteristics among US adults: Data from the National Health and Nutrition Examination Survey, 1999–2004. *Arch Intern Med.* 2008, **168**:1522–30.

Oral Hygiene and Oral Cavity Examination

C. Nathan Webb

Why Screen?

Oral Cavity Examination

In the United States, over 12,000 women were diagnosed with either oral or pharyngeal cancer in 2012, and 2,661 women died from these cancers [1]. The majority were squamous cell carcinomas. Most were diagnosed in later stages, which carries a poorer prognosis than those diagnosed at earlier stages.

Oral Hygiene

Dental caries remains the most common oral disease of children in the United States and is a significant source of morbidity in adolescents and adults. The anticariogenic effect of fluoride from systemic exposure during secondary tooth development and topical exposure at the time of primary tooth eruption and into adulthood is well established.

Rationale for Screening

Oral Cavity Examination

About 90 percent of oral cavity cancers are squamous cell carcinomas. The remainders are minor salivary gland carcinomas and lymphomas. Tobacco and alcohol use account for up to 75 percent of oral cancers in the United States. Over half of these cancers have regional or distant metastases at the time of diagnosis. The 5-year survival rates vary by stage at the time of diagnosis, 82.4 percent for locally advanced disease compared to 33.2 percent with distant metastases [2]. Pharyngeal cancers involving the posterior third of the tongue and oropharynx have a strong association with oral human papillomavirus (HPV) infection, particularly HPV-16. These cancers are typically diagnosed about 5 years earlier than non-HPV-associated cancers and have a better prognosis.

Although there is a plausible benefit for screening for oral cancer, there is currently insufficient evidence to support the accuracy of oral cavity examination by nondental providers in detecting malignant and premalignant disease, nor is there data to support the benefit of early detection on disease-specific mortality. One randomized controlled trial involving over 190,000 individuals performed in India examined the impact of community-based screening on asymptomatic adults and showed no difference in oral cancer mortality between the intervention group and controls after 15 years of follow-up [3]. However, a subgroup analysis of participants who used tobacco or alcohol did find a significant reduction in mortality. Screened participants were diagnosed with oral cancer at earlier stages and had greater 5-year survival rates. The study had methodological limitations, including probable length and lead-time biases.

Oral Hygiene

Dental caries is an infectious disease. Acids produced by bacterial fermentation of carbohydrates demineralize the tooth enamel surfaces and may result in structural erosion and tooth loss, pain from exposed dental pulp, and potential systemic infection. Although appropriate oral hygiene and dietary practices may help prevent formation of dental caries, fluoride use remains the most effective intervention. Topical applications via tooth pastes, mouth rinses, and varnishes aid in prevention of decay and promote remineralization of damaged tooth surfaces [5].

Despite possible benefit from screening examination and risk assessment for dental caries, there remains a lack of evidence to support recommendations for performing either of these by nondental primary care providers.

Factors That Affect Screening

Oral Cavity Examination

HPV-16: The incidence of HPV-associated squamous cell carcinomas of the oropharynx is increasing. Over 85 percent of HPV-positive oropharyngeal cancers are associated with HPV-16. Risk factors for oral HPV infection include increasing age, number of sex partners, and number of cigarettes smoked per day.

Tobacco and alcohol use: The most significant risk factors for oral cancer are tobacco use and heavy alcohol consumption. For women, this is generally considered an average of more than one drink daily.

Other factors: Other risk factors include older age, ultraviolet light exposure (for labial cancer), oral infection with *Candida* or bacterial flora (*Candidal leukoplakia* and *Syphilitic leukoplakia*), and immunocompromise.

Oral Hygiene

Socioeconomic status: Dental caries disproportionately affects racial and ethnic minorities.

Other factors: Additional risk factors include frequent sugar exposure, low level of parental education, history of caries in other family members or caregivers, wearing of dental prostheses, and reduced salivary flow from medication, radiation treatment, or disease.

Recommended Guidelines and How to Find Them

Oral Cavity Examination

For women of all ages, an oral cavity examination may be performed as part of a routine health assessment, but is done so at the discretion of the clinician. The US Preventive Services Task Force (USPSTF) found no evidence that oral cancer screening led to improved outcomes and no evidence establishing harms of screening or benefits to early treatment of oral cancer [a]. The American Academy of Family Practitioners similarly concluded there is insufficient evidence to assess the balance of benefits and harms for oral cancer screening in asymptomatic adults [b]. The American Cancer Society recommends adults aged 20 or older who get periodic health exams receive health counseling and undergo an oral cavity examination to assess for cancer [c]. The American Dental Association recommends clinicians remain alert for signs of potentially malignant lesions or early-stage cancers while performing routine visual and tactile examinations in all patients, but particularly in those who use tobacco or are heavy consumers of alcohol. For woman, they define this as greater than one drink per day [d]. Each of these guidelines can be found on the associated organization's website.

Oral Hygiene

The USPSTF has inactivated prior guidelines pertaining to counseling for adult dental caries and periodontal disease. Current guidelines focus on children and find insufficient evidence to recommend routine oral screening examinations of preschool children by primary care physicians for the prevention of dental disease. The USPSTF recommends oral fluoride supplementation for children aged 6 months to 5 years living in areas with inadequate fluoride content in their drinking water (less than 0.6 ppm F). They also recommend application of fluoride varnish to primary teeth, starting at the time of tooth eruption and continued to age 5, which may also be considered for adolescents considered high risk for dental caries [e]. The American Academy of Family Practitioners has adopted these guidelines for children and has no recommendations for adults [f]. The American Academy of Pediatrics (AAP) recommends periodic oral health risk assessments, dietary counseling, and supervised use of fluoride toothpaste for all children with teeth. They differ from the USPSTF guidelines in that they recommend fluoride varnish only for those patients with significant risk of dental caries who are unable to establish a dental home [g]. The American College of Obstetrics and Gynecology (ACOG) guidelines urge counseling on fluoride supplementation and dental hygiene for adolescents and counseling on hygiene, including dental hygiene, for all ages, but no specific guidance is given on content [h]. Caries risk assessment is not supported by the literature for any age group.

The USPSTF recommend all adults be screened for tobacco use and either receive counseling to prevent initiation of tobacco use or cessation interventions for those that currently use tobacco products [i]. Similar recommendations have been made by the AAP for children and adolescents [j]. The USPSTF also recommends assessing for alcohol abuse and provision of behavioral counseling interventions as needed [k].

How to Screen

Oral Cavity Examination

Routine oral cavity examination is not recommended. The decision of whether or not to perform an oral cavity examination rests with the judgment of the clinician and may be based on the presence of risk factors. An oral cancer screening examination may be performed on adults aged 18 and older and includes a systematic visual inspection of the face, neck, lips, and oral surfaces. The oral surfaces include the labial and buccal mucosa, gingiva, floor of the mouth, the tongue, hard and soft palate, tonsils and oropharynx. The examination can also include palpation of the tongue, floor of the mouth, and the submental and submandibular, pre- and postauricular, occipital and cervical chains of lymph nodes [a]. Clinical features concerning for malignancy include induration, persistent ulceration with size >1 cm, tissue proliferation or destruction, red and white color variegation (erythroplakia and leukoplakia), loss of mucosal tissue mobility, dysesthesia, paresthesia, or lymphadenopathy [b]. When abnormalities are identified, the exam should be repeated in 1–2 weeks and if a suspect lesion persists, it should be evaluated and biopsied, most appropriately by a dental provider [b].

Oral Hygiene

Patients of all ages should be counseled to brush their teeth daily with fluoride toothpaste and clean between their teeth with dental floss to promote dental health. For children aged 6 months to 5 years, fluoride content of their primary water supply should be assessed and prescription of oral fluoride supplements provided if the level falls below 0.6 ppm F. A fluoride varnish may be periodically applied to the teeth in all children from the time of primary tooth eruption to age 5 and in adolescents at high risk for dental caries [f].

Inquiries about tobacco use and smoke exposure should be performed for women of all ages at every well-woman visit. Adolescents who do not use tobacco should be warned about its harmful effects to discourage initiation. For those who currently use tobacco products, cessation interventions should be provided [h]. Women aged 18 and older should receive periodic screens for alcohol misuse

and, brief behavioral counseling interventions should be provided for those that exhibit risky or dangerous drinking patterns [i].

New Developments Likely to Affect Future Guidelines

Oral Cavity Examination

Adjunctive screening aids are available but have not been evaluated yet in the primary care, nondental setting and are not recommended at this time. These aids include tissue staining, brush cytology, and several illuminating devices that aid in the detection of abnormal lesions based on tissue reflectance and autofluorescence [4]. Given the growing incidence of HPV-associated pharyngeal cancer, screening tests for oral HPV infection may play some future role, but at present none are approved by the US Food and Drug Administration (FDA) and there are no current recommendations for their use [1]. Hopefully, with the introduction of HPV vaccines, the incidence of these cancers may decline with time but there are presently no studies evaluating the impact of HPV vaccines against oral cancers.

Oral Hygiene

Xylitol, a nonfermentable sugar alcohol, holds some promise as another means of reducing the risk of dental caries when used in the form of dental wipes or chewing gum. There is presently inadequate evidence to make a recommendation as the existing data is conflicting [e].

Billing

An oral cavity examination may be billed under the ICD-10 code Z12.81, *screening for cancer of the oral cavity*, or code Z13.84, *encounter for screening for dental disorder*.

For many state-run Medicaid and Children's Health Insurance Programs, there are reimbursement policies in place for preventive oral health services for children and adolescents provided by primary care physicians. These may include oral health risk assessment and counseling, billed under code Z13.84, *encounter for screening for dental disorder*, and covered under CPT codes for well-child or well-adolescent visits. These programs also cover the provision of fluoride varnish, which would be billed under the

ICD-10 code Z41.8, *Encounter for other procedures for purposes other than remedying health state (topical fluoride application)*, and CPT code 99188, *application of topical fluoride varnish by a physician or other qualified health care professional*. Most states require the practitioner to complete a training program for varnish application before considering reimbursement claims.

Illustrative Cases

A 17-year-old is seen for an initial well-adolescent visit. She is from a rural part of the state and drinks well water. She is a nonsmoker.

Screen now? No. Oral examination is not recommended. It is important to assess for tobacco use or tobacco smoke exposure. Time should be taken to make recommendations against initiating tobacco use. Inquiry into oral hygiene is recommended and recommendations should be made for routine flossing and brushing. Particularly as she may live in an area without a community water fluoridation program, she will benefit from routine topical fluoride use via fluoridated mouth rinses and toothpastes.

Next screening? There are no recommendations for oral hygiene or oral cancer screening intervals. The decision should be individualized based on symptoms or concerns.

A 32-year-old is seen for her well-woman visit. She is a former smoker, has one sex partner, and occasionally uses alcohol.

Screen now? She lacks risk factors for oral cancer and caries. Clinicians may perform an oral examination at their discretion. She should be discouraged about tobacco use and advised on routine oral hygiene, including use of fluoride.

Next screening? There are no recommendations for oral hygiene or oral cancer screening intervals. The decision should be individualized based on symptoms or concerns.

A 48-year-old presents for a well-woman visit. Smokes 15 cigarettes daily, drinks over eight drinks per week, and has had over 20 lifetime sex partners.

Screen now? This patient has a number of risk factors for oral cancer, which may prompt an oral cavity examination. At the very least, she should be provided counseling and assistance with tobacco use cessation, and behavioral counseling interventions for alcohol misuse. Counseling on routine oral hygiene, including use of fluoride, should also be provided.

Next screening? There are no recommendations for oral hygiene or oral cancer screening intervals. The decision should be individualized based on symptoms or concerns.

A 60-year-old presents for her well-woman visit and complains of a "bump" on her tongue and hoarseness for several months. She is a former smoker and currently drinks "several glasses of wine" per week.

Screen now? As the patient is symptomatic, she needs evaluation rather than a screening exam. An oral cavity examination is indicated. If a discrete lesion or abnormality is observed, she should be reevaluated within 2 weeks and, if the lesion persists, a biopsy of the area should be obtained. If the clinician is uncomfortable with or inexperienced in obtaining a biopsy of oral tissue, the patient should be referred to a dental provider for further evaluation.

Guidelines

a. US Preventive Services Task Force. Screening for oral cancer: US Preventive Services Task Force recommendation statement. *Ann Intern Med.* 2014, **160** (1):55–60.

b. American Academy of Family Physicians. *Oral Cancer.* Leawood, KS: American Academy of Family Physicians, 2004. Available at: www .aafp.org/patient-care/clinical-recommendations/all/ oral-cancer.html.

c. American Cancer Society. *American Cancer Society Guidelines for the Early Detection of Cancer.* Atlanta: American Cancer Society, 2013. Available at: www.can cer.org/healthy/findcancerearly/cancerscreeningguide lines/american-cancer-society-guidelines-for-the-early-detection-of-cancer.

d. Rethman, M.P., Carpenter, W., Cohen, E.E. et al. Evidence-based clinical recommendations regarding screening for oral squamous cell carcinomas. *J Am Dent Assoc.* 2010, **141**(5): 509–20.

e. Moyer, V.A. Prevention of dental caries in children from birth through age 5 years: US Preventive Task Force recommendation statement. *Pediatrics.* 2014, **133** (6):1102–11.

f. American Academy of Family Physicians. Dental caries: Clinical preventive service recommendation. *AAFP,* 2015. Available at: www .aafp.org/patient-care/clinical-recommendations/all/de ntal-caries.html. Retrieved February 23, 2016.

g. American Academy of Pediatrics Section on Pediatric Dentistry and Oral Health. Preventive oral health intervention for pediatricians. *Pediatrics*. 2003, **122** (6):1387–94.

h. American College of Obstetricians and Gynecologists. *Well-woman Recommendations*. Washington, DC: American College of Obstetricians and Gynecologists, 2015. Available at: www.acog.org/About-ACOG/AC OG-Departments/Annual-Womens-Health-Care/Wel l-Woman-Recommendations. Retrieved February 23, 2016.

i. US Preventive Services Task Force. Counseling and interventions to prevent tobacco use and tobacco-caused disease in adults and pregnant women: US Preventive Services Task Force reaffirmation recommendation statement. *Ann Intern Med*. 2009, 150:551–5.

j. Sims, T.H. and Committee on Substance Abuse. Technical report – Tobacco as a substance of abuse. *Pediatrics*. 2009, 124(5):e1045–53.

k. Moyer, V.A. and US Preventive Services Task Force. Screening and behavioral counseling interventions in primary care to reduce alcohol misuse: US Preventive Services Task Force recommendation statement. *Ann Intern Med*. 2013, 159:210–8.

References

1. US Cancer Statistics Working Group. *United States Cancer Statistics: 1999–2012 Incidence and Mortality Web-Based Report*. Atlanta: US Department of Health and Human Services, Centers for Disease Control and Prevention and National Cancer Institute, 2015. Available at: www.cdc.gov/uscs. Retrieved December 15, 2015.

2. American Cancer Society. Cancer Statistics Center. Available at: http://cancerstatisticscenter.cancer.org. Retrieved February 21, 2016.

3. Sankaranarayanan, R., Ramadas, K., Thomas, G. et al. Effect of screening on oral cancer mortality in Kerala, India: A cluster-randomised controlled trial. *Lancet*. 2005, **365**(9475):1927–33.

4. American College of Obstetricians and Gynecologists. Committee Opinion No. 460. The initial reproductive health visit. *Obstet Gynecol*. 2010, **116**:240–3.

5. Recommendations for using fluoride to prevent and control dental caries in the United States. Centers for Disease Control and Prevention. *MMWR Recomm Rep*. August 17, 2001, **50**(RR-14):1–42.

Chapter

13

Injury Prevention

Aaron Goldberg

Why Counsel?

Unintentional injuries are the number one cause of death in girls and women under age 35. According to the Centers for Disease Control and Prevention (CDC), more children and adolescents are killed by motor vehicle accidents (MVAs) than any other cause. In addition, MVAs represent the leading cause of death from injury among all age groups, leading to more than 32,000 deaths in the United States annually and millions of emergency room visits [1,2]. Unintentional falls represent the number one cause of injury and death in women aged 65 and older, with over 25,000 deaths in 2013 alone according to the CDC. Hip fractures represent one of the most serious injuries resulting from falls. Hip fractures are associated with significant morbidity and mortality, leading to 250,000 hospitalizations annually in those over 65 years old, with women accounting for more than three-quarters of this group [3]. Older women are more likely than men to experience a fall and are more likely to experience a fracture from a fall given their increased risk of osteoporosis.

Rationale for Counseling

MVA-related injuries can be prevented by not driving while impaired by drugs or alcohol and by not riding in a vehicle with an impaired driver. Daily exercise or physical therapy and vitamin D supplementation can reduce the fall risk for community-dwelling people over 65 years old [4].

Factors That Affect Counseling

Age: MVAs are a leading cause of death in adolescents, whereas falls are a leading cause of morbidity and mortality in women aged 65 or older.

Fall risk: Older women vary considerably in their fall risk, making risk factor identification

important to guide counseling. Muscle weakness, balance and gait problems, low blood pressure, sensory problems, polypharmacy, confusion, or visual problems increase fall risk, and osteoporosis increases fracture risk if there is a fall.

Recommended Guidelines and How to Find Them

The Well-Woman Task Force considered two key resources in developing its recommendations for injury prevention. The American Academy of Pediatrics' *Bright Futures: Guidelines for Health and Supervision of Infants, Children, and Adolescents* represents a comprehensive set of guidelines put forth by the Bright Futures National Center for the care of children and adolescents. It is available at the American Academy of Pediatrics (AAP) website [a]. In addition, the AAP provides an app available for download to help with identifying recommendations for screening and counseling children and adolescents. Recommendations regarding fall prevention put forth by the US Preventive Services Task Force (USPSTF) are similarly found on the USPSTF website [b].

The WWTF recommends counseling adolescents age 13–18 regarding injury prevention as part of every well-child visit. Adolescent counseling should be part of a broader discussion of healthy lifestyle choices, especially the avoidance of alcohol, tobacco, or other drug use. The Task Force recommends exercise or physical therapy and vitamin D supplementation in community-dwelling adults over the age of 65 who are at increased risk of falls. Generalized in-depth risk assessment and comprehensive management of identified risks to prevent falls in community-dwelling adults over the age of 65 is not recommended.

How to Counsel

No specific guidelines exist regarding how injury prevention counseling should be conducted. AAP's *Bright Futures: Guidelines for Health Supervision of Infants, Children and Adolescents* provides suggestions for "anticipatory guidance" to help clinicians in their counseling efforts for children of all ages and their parents. Accordingly, children and adolescents should be counseled about safety belt use in cars and wearing helmets when biking, skating, or engaging in water sports, should develop strategies to avoid being a passenger in a car with a driver impaired by alcohol or other drugs, and should be counseled about managing anger and conflict, dating violence, bullying, and fighting. For those aged 18–21, Bright Futures recommends removal of guns from the homes of those with aggressive or violent behaviors, suicide attempts, or depression. Counseling about prevention of unintentional injury into counseling about an overall healthy lifestyle, including avoidance of well as avoiding alcohol, tobacco, and other drugs.

For preventing falls in the elderly, the CDC's "Stopping Elderly Accidents, Death & Injuries (STEADI)" initiative provides information to help clinicians identify those at risk of falls as well as to identify modifiable risk factors and other interventions [5]. STEADI initiative provides a simple three-step intervention to help identify and counsel patients aged 65 and older who are at risk of falls:

- ASK patients if they've fallen in the past year, feel unsteady, or worry about falling.
- REVIEW medications and stop, switch, or reduce dosage of drugs that increase fall risk.
- RECOMMEND vitamin D supplements of at least 800 international units per day with calcium.

In addition, the American Geriatrics Society (AGS), in conjunction with the British Geriatrics Society, has published recommendations on specific interventions to help reduce fall risk [6].

The routine use of clinical tests of mobility, such as the timed up-and-go test, is not beneficial in helping prevent falls in healthy elderly women. However, this test may be helpful in evaluating those who have already experienced a fall [7].

New Developments Likely to Affect Future Recommendations

The appropriate amount of vitamin D supplementation and whether to include calcium supplementation remains uncertain. The USPSTF currently recommends all adults between 51 and 70 years old take 600 international units of vitamin D daily, and those over 70 years old take 800 international units of vitamin D daily, but finds insufficient evidence to recommend calcium supplementation as well. Conversely, the AGS 2013 recommendations regarding vitamin D supplementation to prevent falls involve 1,000 international units of vitamin D combined with calcium daily [8]. Future recommendations may provide clearer guidance on vitamin D supplementation and calcium supplementation for prevention of falls and fractures.

Recommendations to counsel adolescents regarding safety belt use, violence prevention, and avoidance of tobacco, alcohol, and drugs are unlikely to change in the near future.

Billing

Counseling for injury prevention should generally be included with the ICD-10 codes for routine preventive care visits. Examples are listed as follows:

Z01.419 – Encounter for routine gynecologic examination without abnormalities

Z01.411 – Encounter for routine gynecologic examination with abnormalities

Z00.129 – Encounter for child health examination without abnormal findings

Z00.121 – Encounter for child health examination with abnormal findings

Z00.00 – General adult medical exam without abnormal findings

Z00.01 – General adult medical exam with abnormal findings

In addition, Medicare requires HCPCS codes for billing preventive care services. Relevant codes include those for the annual wellness visit, G0438 and G0439.

Illustrative Cases

A healthy 17-year-old female presents to your office for a well-adolescent visit. She complains of foul smelling vaginal discharge.

In addition to evaluating her discharge and risk factors for sexually transmitted infections, this patient should be counseled regarding lifestyle choices to prevent injuries. Counseling should include avoidance of tobacco, alcohol, and other drugs, as well as counseling not to ride in a car being driven by a person impaired by drugs of alcohol. The patient should also be counseled about safety belt use in cars and wearing helmets when biking, skating, or engaging in water sports, as well as managing anger and conflict, dating violence, bullying, and fighting.

Counsel now? Yes

Next counseling? Counsel annually through age 18

A 77-year-old-female presents to your office for a well-woman visit. She is recovering from knee surgery several months ago and states she has been slow to regain her normal strength. She is otherwise without complaints. She takes multiple medications to treat medical problems including diabetes, hypertension, and depression.

Poorly controlled diabetes may lead to sensory impairment, which, in conjunction with her reduced mobility while recovering from knee surgery, increases the patient's fall risk. In conjunction with the other required elements of the well-woman visit, this patient should be counseled to engage in regular physical activity or physical therapy and take 800 international units of vitamin D orally daily. The STEADI ASK/REVIEW/RECOMMEND intervention can be used by clinicians as a helpful tool for decreasing fall risk in patients aged 65 and older.

Counsel now? Yes

Next counseling? Counsel with each well-woman visit

Guidelines

a. American Academy of Pediatrics. Bright Futures: Guidelines for Health Supervision of Infants, Children and Adolescents. Available at: https://brightfutures.aap.org. Retrieved January 31, 2016.

b. US Preventive Services Task Force. Falls Prevention in Older Adults: Counseling and Preventive Medication. May 2012. Available at: www.uspreventiveservicestaskforce.org/Page/Document/RecommendationStatementFinal/falls-prevention-in-older-adults-counseling-and-preventive-medication. Retrieved January 31, 2016.

References

1. Traffic Safety Facts 2012. National Highway Traffic Safety Administration. Available at: www.nhtsa.gov. Retrieved January 31, 2016.

2. Web-Based Injury Statistics Query and Reporting System (WISQARS). *Fatal Injury Reports*. Atlanta, GA: Centers for Disease Control and Prevention. Available at: www.cdc.gov/injury/wisqars/. Retrieved January 31, 2016.

3. Jordan, K.M. and Cooper, C. Epidemiology of osteoporosis. *Best Pract Res Clin Rheumatol.* 2002, **16**(5):705–806.

4. Moyer, V.A. Preventions of falls in community-dwelling older adults. US Preventive Services Task Force recommendation statement. *Ann Intern Med.* 2012, **157**:197–204.

5. STEADI: Stopping Elderly Accidents, Deaths & Injuries. Available at: www.cdc.gov/steadi/index.html. Retrieved February 11, 2016.

6. Summary of the Updated American Geriatrics Society/ British Geriatrics Society Clinical Practice Guideline for prevention of falls in older persons. *J Am Geriatric Soc.* 2011, **59**(1):148–57.

7. Schoene D., Wu SM, Mikolaizak AS, Menant JC, Smith ST, Delbaere K, and Lord SR. Discriminative ability and predictive validity of the timed up and go test in identifying older people who fall: Systemic review and meta-analysis. *J Am Geriatrics Soc.* 2013, **61**(2):202–8.

8. Judge J, Birge S, Gloth F, Heaney RP, Hollis BW, Kenny A, Kiel DP, Saliba D, Schnieder DL, and Vieth R. Recommendations abstracted from the American Geriatrics Society Consensus statement on vitamin D for prevention of falls and their consequences. *J Am Geriatric Soc.* 2014, **62**:147–52.

Piercing and Tattooing

Margaret Boozer

Why Counsel?

Body art, which refers to the elective practice of piercing or tattooing, has become increasingly prevalent, especially in adolescent and young adult patients. Although the prevalence of piercing and tattooing varies according to the population surveyed, estimates of body art in the United States range from 10 percent to nearly 50 percent. The age groups most likely to obtain body art are adolescents and individuals aged 18–29 [1,2]. Both piercing and tattooing can result in complications and there is a significant risk of later regret.

Rationale for Counseling

Body piercing is the piercing of any body part with a decorative object, such as stud, ring, or pin, for the purpose of cosmetic outcome. Commonly pierced sites include the ear, nose, tongue, lip, nipple, navel, and genitals. Time required for healing varies according to the site pierced, ranging from several weeks to several months. Tattooing entails the introduction of exogenous pigments or dyes into the dermis using varied numbers of solid needles with puncture depth ranging 1–4 mm. The inks are usually of synthetic origin, and contain azo pigments, black carbon compounds, or polycyclic aromatic hydrocarbons (PAH). Generally, tattoos are obtained in commercial studios, but may be applied in home settings, unregulated tattoo parlors, or prisons. The commercial entity, the tattoo artist, and the inks themselves are often poorly and inconsistently regulated, with the potential for complications resulting from substerile technique.

While not clearly risk factors for adverse health outcomes, piercing and tattooing have been associated with greater risk-taking behaviors, including eating disorders, drug use, high-risk sexual activity, and suicide. This relationship is stronger in patients with greater numbers of piercings or tattoos and in patients with nipple or genital piercings [3]. As many as 16–21 percent of individuals either regret obtaining body art or desire removal [4]. Complication rates from piercing range from 17 percent to 31 percent, and vary depending on piercing site, material used, degree of sterile technique, and aftercare. Complication rates from tattooing range from 6 percent for persistent effects to as high as 22 percent for acute complications. Complications are more frequent when the tattoo is obtained in a nonprofessional setting [4,5].

Infections at the body art site are common. Acute localized infection is the most common complication. Superficial infection may present as folliculitis, cellulitis, impetigo, or vesicular or pustular eruption. Abscesses may develop. Rare case reports of necrotizing fasciitis and sepsis have been reported [6,7]. Both piercing and tattooing also can cause local skin reactions, including allergic reactions or scarring, as well as granulomatous-type reactions associated with tattooing. Allergic reactions to piercings are due to metal sensitization, especially to nickel. Risk of sensitization increases with increasing number of piercings [6]. Allergic reactions to tattoos are thought to be associated with the inks and their frequent impurities. Adverse reactions are more likely to occur with use of colored inks, especially red, and are more likely to involve tattoos on the extremities. Reactions may occur acutely within days of application or may develop years later as a delayed-type hypersensitivity reaction. Both piercing and tattooing can trigger scarring. The scarring may take the form of hyperpigmentation, hypertrophic scarring, or keloid formation. Tattoos may cause foreign body type or sarcoidal granulomatous reaction. Sarcoidal reaction may be the initial presentation of systemic sarcoid, so any tattoo-associated granuloma should prompt further evaluation for sarcoid. Normal healing after tattooing can include aseptic inflammation, superficial crusting, and "sterile edema," and should not be confused with a granulomatous reaction.

Because piercing and tattooing involve puncture of the dermis with needles or a foreign body, transmission of systemic infection can occur. Comparison to injection drug use (IDU) raises the concern for transmission of HIV, Hepatitis B (HBV), and Hepatitis C (HCV). Multiple studies and systematic reviews have not shown increased risk of HIV transmission [5,6]. In contrast, there are studies with equivocal results and some positive findings suggesting piercing and tattooing may increase risk of HBV and HCV. These studies are complicated by other confounding risk factors, especially IDU, incarceration, and high-risk sexual activities. Odds ratios (ORs) from studies of HCV associated with tattooing range from 2.0 to 8.9. The risk was greater when tattoos were obtained in a nonprofessional setting, especially prisons, but also in unregulated shops and home settings [8]. Rather than focusing on incidence of HCV in patients with body art, Carney et al. looked at an HCV-positive population and found that HCV-positive patients were significantly more likely to have one or more tattoos (OR 5.17), establishing a clear association between HCV infection and tattooing [9]. A meta-analysis of studies examining the association of tattooing and HBV showed increased risk, with a pooled OR of 1.48. Again, the association was stronger in high-risk populations [10]. Piercing has also been associated with an increased risk of viral hepatitis, but with a lower OR of 1.83 [8].

Site-specific complications can occur with piercing. Significant bleeding at time of piercing is generally uncommon. The likelihood is increased with tongue or genital piercings. Oral piercings can cause pain, abnormal tooth wear, and dental defects. Nipple piercings have a longer healing time and are 20 percent more likely to become infected, with possible development of a subareolar abscess. Infection may involve breast implants in patients who have undergone breast augmentation. Nipple piercings may also cause galactorrhea due to excess stimulation and resultant hyperprolactinemia. Generally, galactorrhea will resolve with removal of the jewelry. Nipple piercing may interfere with lactation. Intraductal scarring may occur, interfering with latching or causing leakage of milk despite successful latch. Nipple piercings should be removed prior to nursing in order to avoid a choking hazard [6]. Piercings placed at the clitoris, clitoral hood, or labia may interfere with barrier contraception by damaging the device. Piercings in the clitoral region are also prone to painful sensitivity,

irritation, and numbness. They can cause tearing or extended injury during the second stage of labor due to surrounding tissue edema. Patients should remove genital piercings prior to labor [6].

Factors That Affect Counseling

Age: The highest prevalence of tattooing and piercing is in adolescents and young adults.

Keloid scarring: Patients with a history of keloid reaction are at increased risk of complications with both piercing and tattooing.

Other medical problems: Immunosuppression and congenital heart disease may place those undergoing piercing or tattooing at risk for more involved infection and infective endocarditis. Individuals on chronic anticoagulation should avoid piercings, especially of the tongue or genitals. Patients with breast implants should avoid nipple piercings.

Recommended Guidelines and How to Find Them

The Well-Woman Task Force (WWTF) recommends "annual evaluation and counseling adolescents about concerns associated with piercing and tattooing." These guidelines are derived from recommendations from the American College of Obstetrics and Gynecology (ACOG) and the American Academy of Pediatric Dentistry (AAPD). ACOG includes educating adolescents about concerns associated with piercing and tattooing as part of the recommendations for evaluation and counseling for adolescents aged 13–18 [a].

The AAPD strongly opposed the practicing of piercing intraoral and perioral tissues [b]. They have guidelines recommending providing anticipatory guidance/counseling about intraoral/perioral piercing. They include initiating counseling in their recommendations starting for patients aged 6–12, and reinforcing during subsequent health visits.

How to Counsel

While the WWTF, ACOG, and the AAPD all provide recommendations for counseling, none provides detailed recommendations for the content of the counseling. Questions should be asked about the patient's interest in piercing and tattooing. Where appropriate, further counseling should be done about risks and permanence of the body art. If the patient indicates interest in specific types of body art, counseling should include issues relevant to the patient's interest. For patients contemplating oral piercings, the AADP discussion notes complications that "range from pain, infection, and tooth fracture to life-threatening conditions of bleeding, edema, and airway obstruction." Providers should convey that tattoos should be considered permanent. ACOG [a] suggests several questions an adolescent should ask before getting a tattoo:

"How will I feel about this tattoo in 5 years?"
"Will I still want this name or picture on my body?"
"Will I be embarrassed if other people can see it?"

Including information about the expense and difficulty of removing tattoos and the need to cover tattoos in many places of employment should be shared. Suggesting wearing a temporary tattoo may also help an adolescent make her decision [a]. Complications should be reviewed including minor and serious local infections, allergies to piercings, transmission of systemic infections, and scarring. Patients should be informed that risks can be minimized by having piercings and tattoos placed at professional facilities following appropriate infection control procedures, and if the patient chooses to proceed, she should go to a place that is licensed and regulated.

Given their association with other high-risk behaviors, patients with piercings and tattoos should also have careful age-appropriate counseling and screening about injury prevention, STD prevention, high-risk sexual behaviors, and drugs and alcohol.

Patients with medical problems should be counseled about specific risks. Patients with congenital heart disease may have associated endocarditis risk. Patients with coagulopathies or on anticoagulation may have bleeding risk. Patients with histories of keloid scars will have risk of keloid with piercing and tattooing.

New Developments Likely to Affect Future Guidelines

Further evidence of increased risk of viral hepatitis associated with piercing and tattooing would likely impact recommended screening in patients with body art. Recommendations to expand screening for sexually transmitted and systemic infections in high-risk groups, such as injection drug users, could possibly include patients with body art. If an additional risk like tumorigenicity of tattoo inks is established, then guidelines around surveillance of patients with tattoos may be developed.

Billing

Piercing and tattooing counseling and screening are recommended parts of the well-adolescent visit. Billing for these services would fall under preventive codes for adolescent well-child exam or well-woman exam. A preventive health code for counseling might also be used.

Illustrative Cases

A healthy 17-year-old presents for a well-adolescent visit. She has been sexually active since age 15, and states that she uses condoms regularly. Some of her friends are planning on getting piercings before graduation. She asks your advice. What counseling will you provide?

Both ACOG and the AAPD recommend counseling adolescents regarding the risks associated with piercing and tattooing. Site-specific concerns for piercing, including oral piercings, should be addressed. Emphasis should also be placed on the importance of obtaining body art in a professional setting with sterile conditions. She should also be encouraged to avoid risk-taking behaviors, to practice safe sex, and to use effective contraception.

Counsel now? Yes
Next counseling? Next well-adolescent visit

A 28-year-old female returns to clinic for a well-woman visit. She reports being in a new relationship and wants birth control. On performing her pelvic examination, you notice a tattoo on her lower abdomen, which is new since her last visit. What related counseling and testing should you provide?

She should be counseled regarding the possible increased risk of HBV and HCV depending on the setting where the tattoo was applied.

Counsel now? Yes
Next counseling? Piercing and tattooing counseling is not specifically recommended after adolescence, but may be appropriate in the setting of new body art applied between visits or questions from the patient.

A 32-year-old female presents for a routine new OB visit. She has multiple piercings including her nipple, navel, and genitals. During counseling, she inquires whether these piercings could complicate her pregnancy. What guidance do you offer?

Nipple piercing – may be associated with increased risk of mastitis, even in the absence of pregnancy and lactation. If she wishes to breastfeed, her infant may encounter difficulty latching or leakage outside of his or her latch. Milk production and release may be affected by intraductal scarring. The piercing should be removed prior to nursing.

Navel piercing – may migrate out of place or be rejected as the gravid abdomen expands.

Genital piercing – may cause further injury during labor due to genital edema and trauma. The piercing should be removed prior to labor.

Counsel now? Yes

Next counseling? Piercing and tattooing counseling is not specifically recommended after adolescence, but may be appropriate in the setting of new body art applied between visits or questions from the patient.

Guidelines

a. American College of Obstetricians and Gynecologists. *Guidelines for Adolescent Health Care*, 2nd edition. Washington, DC: American College of Obstetricians and Gynecologists, 2011. Available at: www.acog.org/Resources-And-Publications/Guidelines-for-Adolescent-Health-Care/Guidelines-for-Adolescent-Health-Care. Retrieved May 28, 2016.

b. American Academy of Pediatric Dentistry. Policy on intraoral/perioral piercing and oral jewelry/accessories. *Pediatr Dent.* 2012, **34**(special issue):65–6. Available at: www.aapd.org/media/Policies_Guidelines/G_Periodicity.pdf. Retrieved May 28, 2016.

c. American Academy of Pediatric Dentistry. Guideline on periodicity of examination, preventive dental services, anticipatory guidance/counseling, and oral treatment for infants, children, and adolescents. In *2014–15 Reference Manual: Definitions, Oral Health Policies, and Clinical Guidelines.* Chicago, IL: AAPD, 2014. pp. 118–25. Available at: www.aapd.org/media/Policies_Guidelines/G_Periodicity.pdf. Retrieved May 26, 2016.

References

1. Laumann, A.E. and Derick, A.J. Tattoos and body piercings in the United States: A national data set. *J Am Acad Dermatol.* 2006, **55**(3):413–21.

2. Mayers, L.B., Judelson, D.A., Moriarty, B.W., and Rundell, K.W. Prevalence of body art (body piercing and tattooing) in university undergraduates and incidence of medical complications. *Mayo Clin Proc.* 2002, **77**(1):29–34.

3. Koch, J.R., Roberts, A.E., Armstrong, M.L., and Owe, D.C. Body art, deviance, and American college students. *Soc Sci J.* 2010, **106**:467.

4. Liszewski, W., Kream, E., Helland, S., et al. The demographics and rates of tattoo complications, regret, and unsafe tattooing practices: A cross-sectional study. *Dermatol Surg.* 2015, **41**(11): 1283–9.

5. Wenzel, S.M., Rittmann, I., Landthaler, M., and Baumler, W. Adverse reactions after tattooing: Review of the literature and comparison to results of a survey. *Dermatology.* 2013, **226**(2):138–47.

6. Holbrook, J., Minocha, J., and Laumann, A. Body piercing: complications and prevention of health risks. *Am J Clin Dermatol.* 2012, **13**(1):1–17.

7. Kluger, N. Acute complications of tattooing presenting in the ED. *Am J Emerg Med.* 2012, **30**(9):2055–63.

8. Tohme, R.A. and Holmberg, S.D. Transmission of hepatitis C virus infection through tattooing and piercing: A critical review. *Clin Infect Dis.* 2012, **54**(8): 1167–78.

9. Carney, K., Dhalla, S., Aytaman, A., Tenner, C.T., and Francois, F. Association of tattooing and hepatitis C virus infection: A multicenter case–control study. *Hepatology.* 2013, **57**(6):2117–23.

10. Jafari, S., Buxton, J.A., Afshar, K., Copes, R., and Baharlou, S. Tattooing and risk of hepatitis B: A systematic review and meta-analysis. *Can J Public Health.* 2012, **103**(3):207–12.

Abdominal and Pelvic Examinations

Hope Ricciotti

Why Screen?

The abdominal and pelvic examinations have histori-cally been part of a well-woman visit. Potential bene-fits include detection of abdominal and pelvic pathology, as well as an opportunity to advance con-versations about reproductive health that may improve quality of life. With revisions in cervical cancer screening schedules, as well as the availability of methods of screening for sexually transmitted infections that do not require a pelvic examination, some professional groups are changing recommenda-tions for the pelvic examination, which is time con-suming for the health care provider and distressing to some patients [1].

Rationale for Screening

Recommendations for the abdominal and pelvic examinations as part of a well-woman visit differ among professional organizations. There is a paucity of data about the effectiveness of the abdominal and pelvic examinations in reducing all-cause mortality, cancer- and disease-specific morbidity and mortality (including ovarian cancer), and in improving quality of life. There is also some concern about the adverse effects of screening for gynecological conditions with the pelvic examination [2,3].

Factors That Affect Screening

Age: Problems detectable by speculum or bimanual examination are rare in asymptomatic adolescents and young women, and many are frightened of the pelvic examination. Screening does not make sense when a woman's age or health would lead her to refuse medical intervention for conditions detected during the examination.

Hysterectomy: Surgical removal of uterus and ovaries significantly decreases the risk of many gynecological problems that could potentially be detected on examination.

Recommended Guidelines and How to Find Them

The need for an abdominal and pelvic examination in the asymptomatic well woman is controversial, and recommendations differ among professional organi-zations. Currently, there is no clear evidence that abdominal and pelvic examinations reduce all-cause mortality or cancer- and disease-specific morbidity and mortality, or improve quality of life. There is also concern about the adverse effects of screening for gynecological conditions with the pelvic examina-tion. Groups including Well-Woman Task Force (WWTF), the American College of Obstetrics and Gynecology (ACOG) [1–3], the American College of Physicians (ACP) [4], and the US Preventive Services Task Force (USPSTF) [5–8] have made recommenda-tions regarding the abdominal and pelvic examina-tions as part of a well-woman visit.

The WWTF and ACOG consider an abdominal examination an appropriate part of routine care for women of all ages.

ACOG currently recommends pelvic examina-tions be performed on an annual basis in all women aged 21 and older, only when indicated by the medical history for patients younger than 21 years, and they be discontinued when a woman's age or health would lead her to refuse medical intervention for conditions detected [1–3]. While acknowledging that no current scientific evidence supports or refutes an annual pelvic examination for an asymptomatic, low-risk patient, ACOG states that pelvic examinations allow gynecologists an opportunity to recognize issues such as incontinence and sexual dysfunction [3]. In contrast, the ACP and the USPSTF do not recom-mend pelvic or abdominal examinations as part of routine care. The USPSTF does not recommend the abdominal examination because it is not a good screening test for abdominal aortic aneurysm or for pancreatic cancer screening [7,8]. Both the USPSTF and the ACP guidelines recommend against performing screening pelvic examination in asymptomatic, nonpregnant, adult women [4,6].

The WWTF took a middle ground between these groups on the pelvic examination, emphasizing shared, informed decision-making between patient and provider.

How to Screen

The WWTF recommends speculum or bimanual examination for all symptomatic patients and in asymptomatic patients with specific indications (e.g., intrauterine device placement and cervical cancer screening). External examinations may be performed annually in healthy patients.

In asymptomatic patients without specific indications for a pelvic examination, the WWTF recommends a "shared, informed decision between patient and provider" in making a decision about performing a pelvic examination. Open communication can elucidate the patient's values and concerns to determine if the findings on the pelvic examination may enhance quality of life, such as by assessing issues related to sexuality, continence, or other sensitive or potentially embarrassing questions that a patient may be reluctant to spontaneously bring forward. For some women, education about normal findings is helpful in alleviating anxiety or concerns, which in turn can enhance quality of life. Women have very different goals in a well-woman visit, and their views about risks they want to take and questions they may need to have answered about their bodies, coupled with how difficult the experience of pelvic examination is to them, can help determine if it adds helpful information or if the benefits are not worth the discomfort it may cause. This needs to be balanced with the risks of overtreatment and an understanding of the limits of the pelvic examination.

For patients younger than 21 years, the WWTF recommends pelvic examinations be performed only when indicated by the medical history [1,3]. ACOG currently recommends the decision to receive an internal examination be left to the patient if she is asymptomatic and has undergone a total hysterectomy and bilateral salpingo-oophorectomy for benign indications and has no history of vulvar intraepithelial neoplasia, cervical intraepithelial neoplasia 2 or 3, or

cancer; is not HIV infected; is not immunocompromised; and was not exposed to diethylstilbestrol (DES) in utero [2,3]. Annual examination of the external genitalia should continue. Also, when a woman's age or health would lead her to refuse medical intervention for conditions detected during routine examination, pelvic examinations may be discontinued, particularly if she is discontinuing other routine health care maintenance assessments [2,3].

Both the World Health Organization and ACOG have published recommendations explicitly stating that routine pelvic examinations are not required prior to initiating hormonal contraception for healthy asymptomatic women [4]. Pelvic examination is no longer necessary for testing for cervicitis. Urine nucleic acid amplification tests (NAATs) are at least as sensitive as specimens collected from the endocervix [5,6].

New Developments Likely to Affect Future Guidelines

In response to a topic nomination from the public, the USPSTF has commissioned a review of the evidence on the benefits and harms of performing routine periodic pelvic examinations to screen for gynecological conditions. The review will focus on nonpregnant, asymptomatic women aged 18 and older who are at average risk for these conditions. The aim is to determine the effectiveness of screening with the pelvic examination in reducing all-cause mortality and cancer- and disease-specific morbidity and mortality, and in improving quality of life, as well as determining the adverse effects of screening for gynecological conditions with the pelvic examination.

Billing

In an asymptomatic patient, the pelvic and abdominal examinations are part of a well-woman examination and cannot be billed separately. The well-woman visit is covered under the ICD-10 code Z01.419, encounter for gynecological examination (general) (routine) without abnormal findings. Other possible codes include Z01.411, encounter for gynecological examination (general) (routine) with abnormal findings. The visit should be billed under the age-appropriate preventive visit CPT code (new patients 99384–99387 and established patients 00394–99397).

Medicare does not cover comprehensive preventive visits, but will reimburse for a screening pelvic examination (HCPCS code G0101, pelvic and clinical breast examination) as well as for collection of cervical cancer screening (HCPCS code Q0091, cervical or vaginal cancer screening) every 2 years. If the patient meets Medicare's criteria for high risk, then the pelvic examination and cervical cancer screening are reimbursed every year.

Medicare Criteria for High Risk
Cervical High-Risk Factors

- Early onset of sexual activity (younger than 16 years)
- Multiple sexual partners (five or more in a lifetime)
- History of a sexually transmitted disease (including HIV infection)
- Fewer than three negative pap smears within the previous 7 years

Vaginal Cancer High-Risk Factors: DES-exposed daughters of women who took DES during pregnancy.

Personal History of Health Hazards (V15.89 diagnosis) and the appropriate health history hazard (e.g., V10.3 History of Breast Malignancy). Any V15.89 diagnosis is considered high risk and makes the patient eligible for the yearly G0101 and Q0091.

A screening pelvic examination (HCPCS code G0101) should include documentation of at least 7 of the following 11 elements:

- Inspection and palpation of breasts for masses or lumps, tenderness, symmetry, or nipple discharge
- Digital rectal examination including sphincter tone, presence of hemorrhoids, and rectal masses
- External genitalia (e.g., general appearance, hair distribution, or lesions)
- Urethral meatus (e.g., size, location, lesions, or prolapse)
- Urethra (e.g., masses, tenderness, or scarring)
- Bladder (e.g., fullness, masses, or tenderness)
- Vagina (e.g., general appearance, estrogen effect, discharge, lesions, pelvic support, cystocele, or rectocele)
- Cervix (e.g., general appearance, lesions, or discharge)
- Uterus (e.g., size, contour, position, mobility, tenderness, consistency, descent, or support)
- Adnexa/parametria (e.g., masses, tenderness, organomegaly, or nodularity)
- Anus and perineum

Illustrative Cases

An 18-year-old presents for contraceptive counseling and sexually transmitted infection screening. She recently began to have sexual intercourse with her boyfriend. She uses condoms. She is asymptomatic. She would like to be started on oral contraceptive pills, but does not want a pelvic examination.

Guidelines from all major groups, including ACOG, do not include pelvic examination for women younger than 21 years, unless indicated by symptoms or medical history. Urine can be used to test for cervical infection. Hormonal contraception can be initiated in healthy, asymptomatic women without a pelvic examination.

Abdominal or pelvic exam now? Abdominal examination: yes; Pelvic examination: no.

Next screening: Pelvic examination at age 21 with initiation of cervical cancer screening, or if she develops symptoms that need evaluation in the interim.

A 25-year-old G1P1 presents for a well-woman visit. She is asymptomatic. Her last well-woman visit was 1 year ago. She is due for an annual well-woman visit. She is in a new relationship with a male partner. She has no questions or concerns.

Abdominal or pelvic exam now? Abdominal examination: yes; Pelvic examination: decision made with shared decision-making. If the history reveals that the patient is comfortable in her relationship and with sexuality, the health care provider can ask this patient if a normal pelvic examination would alleviate any anxiety or worries, in which case it may be included, since a normal examination may improve quality of life through reassurance. Conversely, if the examination is painful or stressful, the pelvic examination can be excluded.

Next screening: Annual well-woman visit in 1 year.

A 55-year-old postmenopausal woman presents for a well-woman visit. She is overweight, and has type II diabetes. She is asymptomatic. Her last pelvic examination was 5 years ago when she had cervical cancer screening done. She wonders if she needs a bimanual examination at the time of her cytology and human papillomavirus (HPV) specimen collection today. Her friend was just diagnosed with ovarian cancer.

Abdominal or pelvic exam now? Abdominal examination: yes; Pelvic examination: decision made with shared decision-making.

This patient's last cervical cancer screening was 5 years ago, so she requires cervical cancer screening, which should consist of cytology and HPV co-testing. She should be informed that a pelvic examination is not an effective screening method for ovarian cancer, and once she understands this limitation, she can make an informed decision.

Next screening: Annual well-woman examination in 1 year.

A 60-year-old presents for annual well-woman visit after recently moving to the area. She brings all of her prior medical records. She had a total abdominal hysterectomy for painful fibroids 10 years ago. She is asymptomatic. She has never had an abnormal cervical cancer screening test, and her gynecologist stopped doing them after her hysterectomy. She is not sexually active, and finds pelvic examinations uncomfortable.

Abdominal or pelvic exam now? Abdominal examination: yes; Pelvic examination: decision made with shared decision-making.

In this patient who finds examinations uncomfortable, one can educate the patient about the limitations of the pelvic examination for screening for cancer or other pelvic pathology, and reassure her that it is acceptable to not perform a pelvic examination, especially since she finds them uncomfortable.

Next screening: Annual well-woman examination in 1 year.

An 80-year-old woman is in poor health from complications of cardiac disease. She and her primary care physician have made a decision to discontinue mammograms.

It is reasonable to stop performing pelvic examinations when a woman's age or other health issues reach a point where the woman would not choose to intervene on conditions detected during the routine examination, particularly if she is discontinuing her other routine health care maintenance assessments. The abdominal examination may be less intrusive to some patients.

Abdominal or pelvic exam now? Abdominal examination: yes; Pelvic examination: no.

Next screening: No further pelvic examinations.

Guidelines

a. American College of Obstetricians and Gynecologists. The initial reproductive health visit. Committee Opinion No. 460. *Obstet Gynecol.* 2010, **116**:240–3. Available at: www.acog.org/Resources-And-Publications/Committee-Opinions/Committee-on-

Adolescent-Health-Care/The-Initial-Reproductive-Health-Visit.

b. American College of Obstetricians and Gynecologists. Well-woman visit. Committee Opinion No. 534. *Obstet Gynecol.* 2012, **120**:421–4. Available at: www.acog.org/Resources-And-Publications/Committee-Opinions/Committee-on-Gynecologic-Practice/Well-Woman-Visit.

c. American College of Obstetrics and Gynecology. *Practice Advisory on Annual Pelvic Examination Recommendations.* Washington, DC, 2014 [updated June 30, 2014]. Available at: www.acog.org/About-ACOG/News-Room/Practice-Advisories/ACOG-Practice-Advisory-on-Annual-Pelvic-Examination-Recommendations.

d. Qaseem, A., Humphrey, L.L., Harris, R., Starkey, M., and Denberg, T.D.; Clinical Guidelines Committee of the American College of Physicians. Screening pelvic examination in adult women: A clinical practice guideline from the American College of Physicians. *Ann Intern Med.* 2014, **161**:67–72.

e. Moyer, V.A.; US Preventive Services Task Force. Screening for ovarian cancer: US Preventive Services Task Force reaffirmation recommendation statement. *Ann Intern Med.* 2012, **157**(12):900–4.

f. US Preventive Services Task Force *Final Update Summary: Ovarian Cancer: Screening.* July 2015. Available at: www.uspreventiveservicestaskforce.org/Page/Document/UpdateSummaryFinal/ovarian-cancer-screening.

g. US Preventive Services Task Force *Final Update Summary: Abdominal Aortic Aneurysm: Screening.* July 2015. Available at: www.uspreventiveservicestaskforce.org/Page/Document/UpdateSummaryFinal/abdominal-aortic-aneurysm-screening.

h. US Preventive Services Task Force *Final Update Summary: Pancreatic Cancer: Screening.* July 2015. Available at: www.uspreventiveservicestaskforce.org/Page/Document/UpdateSummaryFinal/pancreatic-cancer-screening.

References

1. Bloomfield, H.E. and Wilt, T.J. *Evidence Brief: Role of the Annual Comprehensive Physical Examination in the Asymptomatic Adult,* VA-ESP Project #09–009., Washington, DC: Department of Veterans Affairs *US, 2011 https://www.ncbi.nlm.nih.gov/books/NBK82767/.

2. Jacobs, I., Stabile, I., Bridges, J., et al. Multimodal approach to screening for ovarian cancer. *Lancet.* 1988, 1:268–71.

3. Adonakis, G.L., Paraskevaidis, E., Tsiga, S., Seferiadis, K., and Lolis, D.E. A combined approach for the early detection of ovarian cancer in asymptomatic women. *Eur J Obstet Gynecol Reprod Biol.* 1996, **65**: 221–5.

4. Stewart, F.H., Harper, C.C., Ellertson, C.E., et al. Clinical breast and pelvic examination requirements for hormonal contraception: Current practice vs evidence. *JAMA*. 2001, **285**(17):2232–9.

5. Centers for Disease Control and Prevention. Recommendations for the laboratory-based detection of *Chlamydia trachomatis* and *Neisseria gonorrhoeae* – 2014. *MMWR Recomm Rep*. 2014, **63**:1–19.

6. Nelson, H.D., Cantor, A., Zakher, B., Fraenkel, M., and Pappas, M. *Screening for Gonorrhea and Chlamydia: Systematic Review to Update the U.S. Preventive Services Task Force*. Recommendations. Evidence Synthesis No. 115. AHRQ Publication No. 13-05184-EF-1. Rockville, MD: Agency for Healthcare Research and Quality, 2014.

Chapter

16

Dyslipidemia

Sangini S. Sheth

Why Screen?

Cardiovascular disease (CVD) is the leading cause of death in women, accounting for 1 in 4 deaths annually among females of all ages in the United States [1]. CVD includes coronary heart disease (CHD), cerebrovascular disease, peripheral artery disease, and aortic atherosclerosis and thoracic/abdominal aortic aneurysm. Dyslipidemia, which includes elevations of total cholesterol, low-density lipoprotein (LDL), or triglycerides, or deficiencies in high-density lipoprotein (HDL), is a key risk factor for CVD. CHD events and mortality increase with increasing levels of total cholesterol and LDL and decreasing levels of HDL [a]. Screening for dyslipidemia as part of the well-woman visit provides an important opportunity for treating lipid abnormalities and for identifying women at increased risk for CVD who would benefit from CVD risk reduction efforts to decrease associated morbidity and mortality.

Rational for Screening

Although awareness of CVD in women is growing, only 54 percent of women recognize heart disease as their number one killer [2]. Unfortunately, nearly two-thirds of women who die from sudden CHD have no previous symptoms, so identifying women with risk factors for CVD is critical to reduce CVD morbidity and mortality [3]. The preventable fraction of CVD mortality among women aged 45–79 associated with modifiable risk factors such as elevated cholesterol, diabetes, hypertension, obesity, and smoking is about 50 percent [4] and the presence of multiple risk factors is at least additive. Screening for dyslipidemia aids in assessing overall CVD risk and provides an opportunity for identifying women who would benefit from primary prevention interventions.

Dyslipidemia contributes to CVD risk through atherosclerosis or plaque buildup within arteries. Plaques are made up of cholesterol, fat, calcium, and other substances found in blood. As the plaque builds, arteries become narrowed and oxygenated blood flow to the heart is reduced. Coronary events occur when atherosclerotic plaque ruptures and leads to thrombotic occlusion of coronary vessels.

Dyslipidemia is asymptomatic and requires screening for detection. Screening is performed through serum lipid tests with complete lipoprotein analysis including total cholesterol, HDL, triglycerides, and LDL. Measuring total cholesterol alone for screening is acceptable but total cholesterol and HDL on nonfasting or fasting samples is preferred due to increased sensitivity and specificity for assessing CVD risk [a]. The relationship between increasing total and LDL cholesterol levels and reduced HDL cholesterol level and CVD risk is well established.

Once lipid abnormalities known to be associated with increased CVD risk are detected, effective treatment strategies through lifestyle modification (weight loss, diet, exercise) and lipid-lowering pharmacologic therapy are available. Counseling on diet and exercise in adults with cardiovascular risk factors reduces total cholesterol levels, LDL levels, blood pressure, fasting glucose, and diabetes incidence [5]. A Cochrane review showed statins, the first-line medical management for patients with lipid abnormalities, to be effective for primary prevention with reduction in all-cause mortality (odds ratio 0.86, 95% CI 0.79–0.94), combined fatal and nonfatal CVD (relative risk (RR) 0.75, 95% CI 0.70–0.81), combined fatal and nonfatal CHD events (RR 0.73, 95% CI 0.67–0.80), and combined fatal and nonfatal stroke (RR 0.78, 95% CI 0. 68–0.89) [6].

Factors That Affect Screening

Age: Cardiovascular risk and the presence of dyslipidemia increases with age. Over 45 percent of adult women aged 20 and older in the United States have borderline high total cholesterol level (≥200 mg/dL); 16 percent of the adult female population has an elevated total cholesterol (>240 mg/dL) [7]. With an increasing proportion of obese children, dyslipidemia among young girls and adolescents is also growing and this places them at risk for accelerated early atherosclerosis. Assessing for risk based on family history alone may miss 30–60 percent of children with dyslipidemia.

- **Additional CVD risk factors**: The 10-year risk for CHD is lowest in young women without additional risk factors, even in the presence of abnormal lipids. Based on general US population data from the National Health and Nutrition Examination Survey (NHANES) III, among women <40 years who do not smoke and do not have hypertension or diabetes, no combination of lipid and blood pressure levels would lead to a 10-year major CVD event risk of more than 10 percent, a threshold often used in determining initiation of pharmacologic lipid-lowering therapy with statins [8]. The presence of multiple risk factors such as obesity, diabetes, tobacco use, hypertension, personal history of CHD or atherosclerosis, or family history of CVD leads to at least an additive increased risk [a]. Diabetes, tobacco use, hypertension, personal history of CHD or noncoronary atherosclerosis, and family history of CVD before age 50 in male relatives or age 60 in female relatives are also significant factors associated with CHD mortality.

Recommended Guidelines and How to Find Them

The US Preventive Services Task Force (USPSTF) recommendations [a] have been adopted by the American Academy of Family Physicians [b] as well as the Well-Woman Task Force (WWTF). They specifically recommend:

The USPSTF strongly recommends screening women aged 45 and older for lipid disorders if they are at increased risk for CHD.

The USPSTF recommends screening women aged 20–45 for lipid disorders if they are at increased risk for CHD.

Dyslipidemia screening guidelines for children and adolescents have been issued by National Heart, Lung, and Blood Institute (NHLBI) [c], endorsed by American Academy of Pediatrics (AAP) [d], and adopted by WWTF. Dyslipidemia screening is recommended once between ages 17 and 21 years, and in younger adolescents with risk factors. The guidelines are included in the *Bright Futures Guidelines for Health Supervision of Infants, Children and Adolescents*, 3rd edition [e], and on AAP's online schedule of screenings and health assessments (http://pediatrics.aappublications.org/content/133/3/568).

Guidelines for the treatment of abnormal blood cholesterol are available from the American College of Cardiology (ACC) and the American Heart Association (AHA) [f].

How to Screen

Women aged 20 and older should be screened for dyslipidemia if they are at increased risk for CHD. The USPSTF [a] defines increased risk as the presence of one or more risk factors (Box 16.1). Adolescents should be screened once in late adolescence (17–21 years of age) regardless of risk factors [d, c], and earlier if risk factors are present (Box 16.2). Risk factor assessment should be performed as part of well-woman care, as should measurement of body mass index (BMI). Counseling should address modifiable risk factors, particularly exercise, weight loss, diet, and smoking cessation.

Dyslipidemia screening is performed using serum lipid profile testing. Lipid profiles can be performed in the fasting or nonfasting state. Preferred screening tests for dyslipidemia are total cholesterol and HDL on fasting or nonfasting specimens, although total cholesterol level alone is acceptable if reliable HDL measurements cannot be obtained [a]. Total cholesterol with HDL provides a more sensitive and specific assessment of CHD risk. LDL can also be evaluated, but requires a fasting lipid profile. Among children and adolescents, nonfasting or fasting lipid profiles for screening are also recommended [d, c]. The NHLBI guidelines strongly support the use of non-HDL cholesterol level (total cholesterol – HDL cholesterol = non-HDL cholesterol) which is a significant predictor of atherosclerosis; non-HDL cholesterol can be calculated from a nonfasting lipid profile. On fasting lipid profile samples, guidelines are available for interpreting LDL and triglyceride levels as well [c]. Current treatment recommendations [f] rely on interpretation of total cholesterol and HDL results in conjunction with other risk factors

---

BOX 16.1 Risk Factors for Coronary Heart Disease in Adults

- Obesity (BMI ≥30 kg/m²)
- Diabetes
- Tobacco use
- Hypertension
- Personal history of CHD or noncoronary atherosclerosis*
- Family history of CVD before age 50 in male relatives or age 60 in female relatives

* Abdominal aortic aneurysm, peripheral artery disease, and carotid artery stenosis.
Source: *Final Recommendation Statement: Lipid Disorders in Adults (Cholesterol, Dyslipidemia): Screening.* US Preventive Services Task Force, June 2008.

BOX 16.2 Risk Factors for Lipid Screening for Adolescents Younger Than 20 Years

- Parent or grandparent (men <55 years, women <65 years) with
  - Coronary artery disease
  - Myocardial infarction
  - Angina
  - Stroke
  - Sudden cardiac death
- Parent with total cholesterol ≥240 or known dyslipidemia
- BMI ≥85th percentile for age
- Diabetes
- Hypertension
- Smokes cigarettes
- Other moderate or high-risk special condition*

* Listed in tables 9–7 of NHLBI report.
Source: Adapted from: Table 9.5 of Expert panel on integrated guidelines for cardiovascular health and risk reduction in children and adolescents: Summary report. *Pediatrics.* 2011,(Suppl 5):S213–56.

---

calculated with a Risk Calculator based on Pooled Cohort Equations available at http://professional .heart.org/professional/GuidelinesStatements/Preven tionGuidelines/UCM_457698_Prevention-Guideline s.jsp.

Among women aged 20 and older meeting criteria for dyslipidemia screening, an optimal screening interval has not been established; the USPSTF supports screening every 5 years as a reasonable option with shorter intervals for women whose lipid levels may be close to warranting therapy and longer intervals for women who are not at increased risk for a CHD event and who have repeatedly normal levels [a]. Screening cessation guidelines have also not been established; however, the USPSTF supports screening older women who have never previously been screened. They comment that repeated screening in women over 65 years old is less necessary as lipid levels are unlikely to rise in this population, but they stand to gain greater benefit from screening because they have a higher baseline risk for CHD [a].

Discussion of management of abnormal screens is beyond the scope of the chapter, but they are covered in detail in recommendations by the ACC and the AHA [f].

New Developments Likely to Affect Future Recommendations

In 2013, the ACC/AHA issued new statin therapy guidelines which included the Pooled Cohort Equations CV Risk Calculator for evaluation of CVD risk [9]. This calculator is intended to predict major cardiovascular events that can be reduced by lipid-lowering pharmacologic therapy and incorporates several variables including total and HDL cholesterol levels. Although this calculator is the only US-based CVD risk prediction tool with published external validation among other US populations and can provide sex- and race-specific risk estimates, it is still under review by the USPSTF [10] and there remain concerns about its accuracy. Adoption of the ACC/AHA guidelines on the use of statins for primary prevention of CVD in adults and incorporation of the risk calculator into USPSTF recommendations is currently being considered and could lead to universal lipid screening in adults aged 40–75 in the future. An update of the USPSTF guidelines is currently in progress.

Billing

Dyslipidemia screening is typically covered under ICD-10 code Z13.6, encounter for screening for cardiovascular disorders. Medicare covers three clinical laboratory tests under this code: total cholesterol, HDL, and triglycerides. These tests are covered once every 5 years as individual tests or as a combination panel. The lipid screening test is reported as 80061 for the lipid panel or individual codes for each test in the panel: 82465, 83718, and 84478.

Illustrative Cases

A 15-year-old presents for her well-adolescent visit. Her BMI is elevated (>85th percentile for age). She has never been screened for lipid abnormalities.

AAP guidelines recommend universal lipid screening for all adolescents once between 17 and 21 years, and earlier if risk factors (Box 16.2) are present. This patient has never been screened before and has a risk factor of obesity. Screening for dyslipidemia is recommended for patients with elevated BMI.

Screen now? Yes

Next screen if normal: Between ages 17 and 21. Approximately age 20 would be preferred given the generally accepted screening interval of 5 years.

A 19-year-old presents for her well-woman visit. She asks what screening tests she needs as she has not had health care in 2 years.

NHLBI/AAP guidelines recommend universal lipid screening for all patients once between 17 and 21 years. This patient has not been to a provider in 2 years and has likely not yet been screened for dyslipidemia in her late adolescence. Regardless of risk factors, she should be screened. As she has probably not

fasted before for the visit, a nonfasting lipid profile can be obtained to assess risk.

Screen now? Yes

Next screen if normal: In 5 years (age 24) *if* she is still at increased risk for CHD (Box 16.2)

A 35-year-old smoker with hypertension presents for her well-woman visit. She says her cholesterol was normal 7 years ago and she has lost weight since then.

USPSTF and WWTF guidelines recommend screening women aged 20–45 for dyslipidemia who are at increased CHD risk. Although there is not clear evidence to guide screening intervals, every 5 years is considered reasonable. This patient meets criteria for being at increased CHD risk based on her smoking and hypertension history and she was last screened 7 years ago.

Screen now? Yes

Next screen if normal: Age 40

A 53-year-old healthy woman with asthma and no significant family history presents for a well-woman visit and asks about cholesterol screening.

USPSTF and WWTF guidelines recommend screening women aged 45 and older who are at increased CHD risk for dyslipidemia. This patient is not at increased CHD risk and therefore is unlikely to gain benefit from lipid-lowering statin therapy, even in the presence of dyslipidemia alone. She should be counseled on the benefits of maintaining a healthy diet, engaging in regular physical activity, avoiding tobacco use, and maintaining a healthy weight.

Screen now? No

Next screening? Reassess annually whether she is at increased risk for CHD by the presence of one or more risk factor (Box 16.1). Screen for dyslipidemia if one or more criteria are met.

Guidelines

a. *Final Recommendation Statement: Lipid Disorders in Adults (Cholesterol, Dyslipidemia): Screening.* US Preventive Services Task Force, June 2008. Available at: www.uspreventiveservicestaskforce.org/Page/Document/RecommendationStatementFinal/lipid-disorders-in-adults-cholesterol-dyslipidemia-screening. Retrieved May 22, 2016.

b. American Academy of Family Physicians. Clinical practice guideline manual: Lipid disorders. Available at: www.aafp.org/patient-care/clinical-recommendations/all/lipid-disorders.html. Retrieved May 22, 2016.

c. Expert panel on integrated guidelines for cardiovascular health and risk reduction in children and adolescents: Summary report. *Pediatrics*. 2011 (Suppl 5):S213–56. Available at: http://pediatrics.aappublications.org.proxy .library.vcu.edu/content/128/Supplement_5/S213.long. Retrieved May 22, 2016.

d. Geoffrey R.S., Baker C., Barden III G.A. et al. 2014 recommendations for pediatric preventive health care. *Pediatrics*. 2014, 133:568–70. Available at: http://pediatrics.aappublications.org.proxy.library .vcu.edu/content/133/3/568.long. Retrieved May 22, 2016.

e. Hagan J.F., Shaw J.S., Duncan P., editors. 2008. *Bright Futures: Guidelines for Health Supervision of Infants, Children, and Adolescents*, 3rd edition. Elk Grove Village, IL: American Academy of Pediatrics. Available at: https://brightfutures.aap.org/materials-and-tools/gu idelines-and-pocket-guide/Pages/default.aspx. Retrieved May 22, 2016.

f. Stone N.J., Robinson J.G., Lichtenstein A.H. et al. 2013 ACC/AHA guideline on the treatment of blood cholesterol to reduce atherosclerotic cardiovascular risk in adults. *Circulation*. 2014, 129:S1–45. Available at: htt p://circ.ahajournals.org/content/129/25_suppl_2/S1. Retrieved May 22, 2016.

References

1. Kochanek, K.D. et al. Deaths: Final data for 2009. *Natl Vital Stat Rep*. 2011, **60**:1–116.

2. Mosca, L. et al., Twelve-year follow-up of American women's awareness of cardiovascular disease risk and barriers to heart health. *Circ Cardiovasc Qual Outcomes*. 2010, **3**:120–7.

3. Roger, V.L. et al. Heart disease and stroke statistics – 2012 update: A report from the American Heart Association. *Circulation*. 2012, **125**:e2–e220.

4. Patel, S.A. et al. Cardiovascular mortality associated with 5 leading risk factors: National and state preventable fractions estimated from survey data. *Ann Intern Med*. 2015, **163**:245–53.

5. Lin, J.S., O'Connor, E., Evans, C.V. et al. Behavioral counseling to promote a healthy lifestyle in persons with cardiovascular risk factors: A systematic review for the US Preventive Services Task Force. *Ann Intern Med*. 2014, **161**:568–78.

6. Taylor, F., Huffman, M.D., Macedo, A.F. et al. Statins for the primary prevention of cardiovascular disease. *Cochrane Database Syst Rev*. 2013 (1):CD004816. doi: 10.1002/14651858.CD004816.pub5.

7. Writing Group, M. et al. Heart disease and stroke statistics – 2012 update: A report from the American Heart Association. *Circulation*. 2012, **125**: e2–e220.

8. Helfand, M. and Carson, S. *Screening for Lipid Disorders in Adults: Selective Update of 2001 U.S. Preventive Services Task Force Review. Evidence Synthesis No. 49*. Rockville, MD: Agency for Healthcare Research and Quality.

9. Goff, D.C. Jr. et al., 2013 ACC/AHA guideline on the assessment of cardiovascular risk: A report of the American College of Cardiology/American Heart Association Task Force on Practice Guidelines. *Circulation*. 2014, **129**:S49–73.

10. *Draft Recommendation Statement: Statin Use for the Primary Prevention of Cardiovascular Disease in Adults: Preventive Medication*. US Preventive Services Task Force.

Hypertension

Christine R. Isaacs

Why Screen?

Heart disease remains the number one cause of death in the US population [1]. Hypertension or high blood pressure now affects over 73 million Americans, of which over 38 million are women [2]. The relationship between high blood pressure and risk of cardiovascular disease is continuous, consistent, and independent of other risk factors. Higher blood pressure values are associated with a greater chance of heart attack, heart failure, stroke, and kidney disease [3].

Rationale for Screening

Hypertension is a "silent disease" with few warning signs to alert a patient until late in the disease process. Early identification with blood pressure screening and intervention is important. Effective management and control of hypertension can reduce the risks of heart failure by 50%, reduce myocardial infarctions by 20%–25%, and reduce strokes by 35%–40% [4]. Because hypertension is a modifiable risk factor for cardiovascular disease and premature mortality, evidence-based interventions and counseling are key components of the well-woman visit.

Factors That Affect Screening

Age: Hypertension can be present at any age. It is uncommon in childhood and adolescence, and there are limited data to assess benefits and harms of screening in this group. Prevalence increases with age, leading to recommendations for increased frequency of screening with increasing age.

Prehypertension: Patients with blood pressures of 130–139/85–89 on prior screens are at increased risk of developing hypertension.

Weight: Patients who are overweight and obese have increased risk of hypertension and merit more frequent screening.

Race/ethnicity: Hypertension risk varies with race and is highest in African Americans.

Recommended Guidelines and How to Find Them

The Well-Woman Task Force (WWTF) endorses blood pressure screening for all ages and notes "routine blood pressure screening is recommended." They categorize this as a strong recommendation, "based on evidence based or evidence informed guidelines" [a]. The WWTF recommendations are based on the US Preventive Services Task Force (USPSTF) guidelines, which can be accessed through the USPSTF website at: www.uspreventiveservicestaskforce.org/P age/Document/UpdateSummaryFinal/high-blood-pr essure-in-adults-screening [b]. The USPSTF recommends beginning blood pressure screening every 3–5 years beginning at age 18. Women aged 40 or older, or those with risk factors including prehypertension, overweight, obesity, and African American ethnicity should be screened annually. The USPSTF recommends obtaining measurements outside of the clinical setting for diagnostic confirmation before starting treatment.

How to Screen

The Joint National Committee on Prevention, Detection, Evaluation and Treatment of High Blood Pressure (JNC 7) report [4] provides guidelines for measuring blood pressure and includes the following options:

1. **Blood pressure measurement in the office**. The auscultatory method should be used with a properly calibrated and validated instrument. Patients should be seated quietly in a chair (not the exam table) for at least 5 minutes with feet on the floor and the arm supported at heart level. An appropriate size cuff where the cuff bladder

encircles at least 80 percent of the arm should be used. At least two measurements should be recorded several minutes apart.

2. **Ambulatory blood pressure monitoring (ABPM).** ABPM devices are fully automated devices that can be comfortably worn by the patient for 24 hours and allow for blood pressure monitoring throughout the day and night at preset automatic intervals that are recorded. This method can help identify "white coat" hypertension as it allows the collection of multiple data points throughout the day and night.

3. **Self-measurement of blood pressure.** The option of home blood pressure monitoring requires appropriate patient training and equipment to ensure accurate home blood pressure recordings. Patients should use an automated, validated device to perform measurements in a quiet room after 5 minutes of rest in the seated position with the back and arm supported. At least 12–14

measurements should be obtained (both morning and evening) throughout a 1 week period. Home measurement devices should be checked regularly for accuracy.

All these methods require a validated, calibrated instrument to accurately measure blood pressure [4]. The USPSTF recommends obtaining measurements outside of the clinical setting for diagnostic confirmation before starting treatment for hypertension.

The JNC 7 report introduced a classification system to help guide care providers with the clinical diagnosis and management of hypertension (Table 17.1). When prehypertension or any further stage of hypertension is identified, lifestyle modifications should be initiated to reduce blood pressure (Table 17.2). These interventions include weight reduction to a normal body mass index (BMI) as well as adopting a Dietary Approaches to Stop Hypertension (DASH) diet, which includes a focus on fruits, vegetables, low-fat dairy, and reduced

Table 17.1 Classification and Management of Blood Pressure for Adults*

BP Classification	SBP* (mm Hg)	DBP* (mm Hg)	Lifestyle Modification	Initial Drug Therapy Without Compelling Indication^	Initial Drug Therapy With Compelling Indications
Normal	<120	<80	Encourage	No antihypertensive drug indicated	Drug(s) for compelling indications‡
Prehypertension	120–139	80–89	Yes		
Stage 1 hypertension	140–159	90–99	Yes	Thiazide-type diuretics for most. May consider ACEI, ARB, BB, CCB, or combination	Drug(s) for the compelling indications‡ Other antihypertensive drugs (diuretics, ACEI, ARB, BB, CCB) as needed
Stage 2 hypertension	≥160	≥100	Yes	Two-drug combination for most† (usually thiazide-type diuretic and ACEI or ARB or BB or CCB)	

BP: blood pressure; DBP: diastolic blood pressure; SBP: systolic blood pressure; ACEI: angiotensin converting enzyme inhibitor; ARB: angiotensin receptor blocker; BB: β-blocker; CCB: calcium channel blocker

* Treatment determined by highest BP category

^ Compelling indications include heart failure, postmyocardial infarction, high coronary disease risk, diabetes, chronic kidney disease, and recurrent stroke prevention

† Initial combined therapy should be used cautiously in those at risk for orthostatic hypotension

‡ Treat patients with chronic kidney disease or diabetes to BP goal of <130/80 mm HgSource: Modified from the JNC 7 [4]

Table 17.2 Lifestyle Modifications to Manage Prehypertension and Hypertension*†

Modification	Recommendation	Approximate SBP Reduction (Range)
Weight reduction	Maintain normal body weight (body mass index 18.5–24.9 kg/m^2)	5–20 mm Hg/10 kg weight loss
Adopt DASH eating plan	Consume a diet rich in fruits, vegetables, and low-fat dairy products with a reduced content of saturated and total fat	8–14 mm Hg
Dietary sodium reduction	Reduce dietary sodium intake to no more than 100 mmol per day (2.4 g sodium or 6 g sodium chloride)	2–8 mm Hg
Physical activity	Engage in regular aerobic physical activity such as brisk walking (at least 30 min per day, most days of the week)	4–9 mm Hg
Moderation of alcohol consumption	Limit consumption to no more than 2 drinks (1 oz or 30 mL ethanol; e.g., 24 oz beer, 10 oz wine, or 3 oz 80-proof whiskey) per day in most men and to no more than 1 drink per day in women and lighter weight persons	2–4 mm Hg

DASH: Dietary Approaches to Stop Hypertension; SBP: systolic blood pressure
* For overall cardiovascular risk reduction, stop smoking
† The effects of implementing these modifications are dose and time dependent, and could be greater for some individuals
Source: Modified from the JNC 7 [4]

saturated and total fat intakes. In addition, dietary sodium reduction, exercise, and moderation of alcohol consumption (≤1 drink/day in women) can also lead to a significant reduction in systolic blood pressure. Stages 1 and 2 hypertension warrant drug therapy in addition to lifestyle modification to optimize blood pressure, with the main objective of treatment being to attain and maintain goal blood pressure. If the target blood pressure is not reached within a month of treatment, drug dosing should be increased or a second drug class should be added [5].

New Developments Likely to Affect Future Recommendations

The JNC 7 endorsed the American Public Health Association resolution that food manufacturers and restaurants reduce sodium in the food supply by 50 percent over the next decade. Public health interventions and national campaigns aimed at good nutrition, exercise, and obesity management are becoming an attractive strategy to interrupt and prevent the continuing costly cycle of managing hypertension and its disease burden [5]. While these efforts may not ultimately influence hypertension screening guidelines, the importance of hypertension

prevention, diagnosis, and early management is a public health priority.

In February 2014, the Eighth Joint National Committee (JNC 8) updated the JNC 7 report with nine evidence-based recommendations. This update principally served to address blood pressure *goals* rather than being a revision of the JNC 7. The first five of the nine recommendations address the threshold of blood pressure levels at which treatment should be started in specific populations and age groups, as well as the target blood pressure to be achieved with such treatment. The remaining recommendations directed specific pharmacologic choices and guide management when goal blood pressure is not reached within a month of treatment. These recommendations were designed to aid both the clinician and the patient in their management expectations and provide guidance to optimize treatment regimens as well as referral to a hypertension specialist when the recommended strategies were unsuccessful [5]. At the time of writing this chapter, the JNC 8 has not yet been endorsed by the National Heart, Lung, and Blood Institute, the American College of Cardiology, the American Heart Association, the American Society of Nephrology, or the American College of Obstetricians and Gynecologists.

Billing

Blood pressure screening is typically incorporated into the ICD-10 code Z01.419, the encounter for a gynecological examination (general) (routine) without abnormal findings.

Other possible codes include:

Z01.30, Encounter for examination of blood pressure without abnormal findings.

Z01.31, Encounter for examination of blood pressure with abnormal findings (additional codes to be used to identify the abnormal findings).

Illustrative Cases

A healthy 19-year-old Caucasian female presents for her well-woman examination requesting a refill on her combined hormonal contraceptive pills. Her blood pressure is 118/78. Her BMI is 23.

The patient should have her blood pressure results reviewed and she should be provided reassurance that her blood pressure is normal. Healthy lifestyle activities should be encouraged and the focus of her encounter directed to other health topics.

Screen now? Yes

Next screen? At future clinical encounters, and certainly at her next annual well-woman exam. As contraceptive medical eligibility criteria are influenced by hypertension, blood pressure screening should be part of continued contraceptive surveillance.

A 41-year-old G2P2 who has had a tubal ligation presents for her well-woman visit without complaints. Her blood pressure is 139/89 and 135/88 when repeated 5 minutes later. Her BMI is 33.

The patient has prehypertension suggested by the current encounter. Lifestyle modifications should be reviewed and recommendations for modifications made. These modifications should include weight reduction to a normal BMI, adopting a DASH diet plan, reducing dietary sodium, engaging in regular aerobic physical activity (such as brisk walking for 30 or more minutes per day), and limiting alcohol consumption. Focused expectations should be outlined. The patient should be encouraged to initiate home blood pressure monitoring for continued surveillance. Follow-up blood pressure screening should be monitored at least annually.

Screen now? Yes

Next screen? Annually and with future clinical encounters

A 55-year-old postmenopausal woman presents for her well-woman visit with complaints of fatigue and depression after the death of her husband. She has no active gynecological complaints. Her blood pressure is 180/99 on intake and is 175/95 when repeated. Her BMI is 25. Upon reviewing her vital signs from her last examination 1 year ago, her blood pressure was noted to be 150/90.

The patient has stage 2 hypertension and had stage 1 hypertension 1 year prior. While she has no severe active complaints, blood pressure management should be an immediate priority. An antihypertensive should be initiated.

Screen now? Yes

Next screen? Patient has been diagnosed with hypertension. Further screening is no longer appropriate. Patient now needs ongoing hypertension management.

Guidelines

a. Conry, J.A. and Brown, H. Well-Woman Task Force: Components of the Well-Woman Visit. *Obstet Gynecol.* 2015, **126**(4):697–701. Appendices 2–5, Available at: http://links.lww.com/AOG/A676, http://links.lww.com/AOG/A677, http://links.lww.com/AOG/A678, http://links.lww.com/AOG/A679. Retrieved December 9, 2015.

b. Siu, A.L. US Preventive Services Task Force. Clinical guideline: Screening for high blood pressure in adults: US Preventive Services Task Force recommendation statement. *Ann Int Med.* 2015, **163**(10):778–86. Available at: www.uspreventiveservicestaskforce.org/Page/Document/UpdateSummaryFinal/high-blood-pressure-in-adults-screening. Retrieved December 9, 2015.

References

1. Centers for Disease Control and Prevention. Leading causes of death. Available at: www.cdc.gov/nchs/fastats/leading-causes-of-death.hem. Retrieved December 7, 2015.

2. Schmitz, P.G. and Nguyen, T. Hypertension. *Clinical updates in women's health care.* January 2016, **XV**(1). Available at: www.clinicalupdates.org/viewIssue.cfm?issue=cuwhc-v15n1.

3. Centers for Disease Control and Prevention. High blood pressure. Available at: www.cdc.gov/bloodpressure/. Retrieved December 2, 2015.

4. US Department of Health and Human Services, National Institutes of Health, and National Heart, Lung, and Blood Institute. *JNC 7 Express: The Seventh Report of the Joint National Committee on Prevention, Detection, Evaluation, and Treatment of High Blood Pressure.* NIH Publication No. 03-5233. Bethesda, MD: US Department of Health and Human Services, 2003.

5. James, P.A., Oparil, S., Carter, BL. et al. Evidence-based guideline for the management of high blood pressure in adults: Report from the panel members appointed to the Eighth Joint National Committee (JNC8). *JAMA.* 2014, **311**(5):507–20.

Diet and Nutrition

Margaret L. Dow

Why Screen and Counsel?

Poor diet and nutrition are responsible for a large burden of disease in women. In 2012, 34.9 percent of US adults were obese (body mass index [BMI] >30) [a]. In reproductive-aged women, obesity is associated with infertility, and if pregnancy is achieved, with neural tube defects, miscarriage, stillbirth, and pregnancy complications. In addition to complications like preeclampsia, gestational diabetes, and liver disease, obese gravidas are far more likely to require cesarean delivery and have increased risk of perioperative complications thereof, including embolic events and wound complications. In middle and older age, obesity carries additional risk. Most leading causes of death – heart disease, stroke, hypercholesterolemia, hypertension, diabetes, and some cancers (breast, colon, and endometrial) – are related to obesity [1]. It is, therefore, incumbent upon providers to assess nutrition and weight status during well-woman visits at every age in order to identify and support healthy diet and nutrition. Evidence supports many diet approaches, although underlying mechanisms for success, including factors such as genetic predisposition and metabolism differences, are unclear.

Rationale for Screening and Counseling

Interest in diet and nutrition is high; 42 percent of working adults routinely read nutrition labels [2] and new diet programs debut daily. The well-woman visit is a prime opportunity to identify and augment self-directed efforts at better health. Counseling women with poor diet improves their nutritional status, facilitates weight loss, and improves a wide range of health outcomes. The goal of counseling is reduction of obesity-related diseases. Correcting abnormal BMI leads to important health benefits. Underweight is

associated with nutrient deficiency disorders, including anemia and osteoporosis. Underweight women may also suffer from infertility and ovulatory dysfunction. Obesity is associated with increased risk of all-cause mortality [b]. In normal-weight women, limited evidence suggests early counseling on healthy diet and physical activity can reduce type 2 diabetes risk [3].

Factors That Affect Screening and Counseling

Age: While US Department of Agriculture (USDA) and Institute of Medicine (IOM) guidelines [c] recommend global attention to potassium, fiber, calcium, and vitamin D intake, the goals of additional dietary screening vary somewhat by age group. Reproductive-aged women require at least 400 mcg of folic acid daily to prevent neural tube defects in their offspring. Women over age 50 benefit from attention to B12 intake. Recommended calcium intake increases from 1,000 to 1,200 mg daily in women over 50.

Vegetarian and vegan diets: Iron and B12 stores are affected by vegetarian and vegan diets, and are important to address at the well-woman visit. Vegetable and legume iron sources are less bioavailable, and vegetable-source iron absorption is improved by concomitant vitamin C intake [c].

Recommended Guidelines and Where to Find Them

For adolescent and adult women, the American College of Obstetrics and Gynecology (ACOG) Well-Woman Task Force (WWTF) recommends regular assessment of BMI, with concomitant evaluation of diet, nutrition, and physical activity in women with abnormal BMIs and/or risks for obesity-related diseases (diabetes, dyslipidemia, hypertension, coronary artery disease, breast, colon, and endometrial cancers) [d]. The WWTF reviewed guidelines from the USPSTF, IOM, Academy of Nutrition and Dietetics, and the National Heart, Lung, and Blood Institute (NHLBI) while forming its recommendations. Each set of guidelines differs somewhat, and the NHLBI and IOM guidelines have been revised since publication of the WWTF recommendations [a, c]. The IOM guidelines focus on specific nutrients, with minimum and maximum intake recommendations [c]. The USPSTF recommendations focus on a lack of data for efficacy of general nutrition counseling in low-risk populations [e]. The NHLBI recommendations focus on identification of obesity and weight loss, addressed elsewhere. The new USDA recommendations provide a comprehensive interactive website for patients and providers focused on a healthy lifestyle [b]. The prevailing message is one of healthy eating over the life span rather than endorsing any particular diet or specifying daily macro- or micronutrient intake.

How to Screen and Counsel

The first step in screening nutritional status is assessment of BMI, which is weight in kilograms divided by height in centimeters squared. Patients' BMIs should be recorded each visit. In women with risk factors for diet-related chronic disease or abnormal BMI (<19 or >25) diet, nutritional status, and physical activity should be investigated, followed by education, counseling, and behavior interventions. Chapters on related topics provide more detailed information on screening for *Obesity, Fitness & Exercise*, and *Diabetes* as well as *Promoting Lifestyle Modification and Behavior Change*.

Assessing diet and nutrition may be done by asking patients to describe their daily food intake, number of meals eaten out weekly, frequency of label reading, and favorite foods. Counseling and behavioral interventions are directed at adjusting calorie intake to maintain a healthy weight, correcting nutritional deficiencies, and increasing physical activity. The USPSTF has advised that counseling and evaluation in low-risk populations (women with normal BMI and no comorbidities) does not have a measurable effect on health outcomes and, in fact, may preclude adequate visit time to address other health-related issues [e].

Overweight and obese patients should reduce calories to 1,200–1,500 per day and increase their physical activity, with a goal of losing 1–2 pounds per week. Virtually all of the popular diet modifications of macronutrients (protein, carbohydrates, and fats) result in comparable weight loss and confer benefits in reversing associated morbidity. Diets that advocate complete avoidance of particular food groups do not confer benefit to most patients. For example, gluten-free diets are not shown to confer any benefit except to patients with true celiac disease and may decrease fiber intake, a nutrient deficient in many Americans' diets. While lactose intolerance is common in adults, elimination of dairy products is ill-advised, as calcium and vitamin D are often deficient in American diets. Use of lactase supplements may be helpful in this setting.

The new USDA 2015 Dietary Guidelines [c], released after the WWTF report, simplify diet recommendations and include an easily navigable online resource for patients and providers. These guidelines reflect a major shift in approach to diet, with an emphasis on variety and balance and a move away from indemnifying or vilifying any particular foods. Weight loss and nutrition myths are debunked at: www.niddk.nih.gov/health-information/health-topics/weight-control/myths/Documents/Myths.pdf.

Up to 82 percent of US adults cited that a desire not to give up foods they enjoy was a major obstacle to weight loss; by advocating a broader approach to a healthy diet, these perceived barriers may be transcended [4]. Maintaining a focus on nutrient density, that is consuming foods that contain multiple micro- and macronutrients required for health, focusing on variety of foods, and ensuring appropriate serving portions, is the major message therein. Furthermore, obtaining balanced nutrition from food rather than supplements or processed products is emphasized. Ample intake of vegetables and fruits, supplemented by lean protein, whole grains, and low-fat dairy are the mainstays. Overall cautions fall into a few major categories:

- Added sugar should comprise no more than 10% of daily calories
- Saturated fats should comprise no more than 10% of daily calories
- Daily sodium intake should be less than 2,300 mg
- Alcohol consumption should be moderate, up to 1 drink daily for women

Additional recommendations include increasing intake of calcium, vitamin D, folic acid (particularly in women of childbearing age), iron, and fiber. The IOM recommends 14 g of fiber per 1,000 calories of intake daily.

Several agencies maintain easily accessible, evidence-based resources for providers and patients. The NHLBI recently updated the 1998 obesity guidelines [a]. The USDA compiles a wealth of reference material including the 2015 Dietary Guidelines, an easily navigable, comprehensive guide to nutrition, diet, and counseling [b]. The USDA calculators and other calorie counting guides may be found at http://fnic.nal.usda.gov/dietary-guidance/interactive-tools/calculators-and-counters. The IOM nutrient recommendations, as well as links to data on fraud and nutrition misinformation, may be accessed at http://fnic.nal.usda.gov/dietary-guidance/dietary-reference-intakes. ChooseMyPlate.gov provides an interactive visual aid to creating healthy meals. The Centers for Disease Control and Prevention (CDC) maintains multiple visual aids, including obesity maps and other high-impact tools for education, as well as a page of reliable healthy eating guidelines and apps for patient use (www.cdc.gov/healthyweight/).

Group weight loss programs including Weight Watchers and applications such as www.MyFitnessPal.com or www.Supertracker.usda.gov have also been shown to fulfill the need for ongoing intervention.

New Developments Likely to Affect Future Recommendations

Future recommendations are likely to be informed by advances in knowledge regarding weight loss and maintenance, including differences by gender, race, and age. Underlying genetic and endocrine mediation of weight homeostasis, appetite, and satiety are just becoming understood. Few data exist regarding cost-effective strategies for identifying patients likely to benefit from office-initiated treatment of obesity. Newer medications have entered the marketplace but have no long-term data yet.

Billing

While obesity-related medical costs topped $130 billion in 2006 [5], billing opportunities for nutrition and obesity-related interventions has lagged. The Affordable Care Act mandates coverage of health-promoting care, including intensive counseling; Medicaid and most private insurers cover these services without co-pay. Fifteen-minute follow-up visits can be reimbursed but cannot be billed for services other than obesity counseling. It is incumbent upon the provider and patient to clarify beforehand what services particular carriers cover. Billing codes differ by BMI and range from Z68.25 through Z68.45. The Academy of Nutrition and Dietetics maintains a website of commonly used ICD-10 codes, news regarding Center for Medicare and Medicaid Services (CMS) coverage for obesity-related services, and tips on billing (www.eatrightpro.org/resources/practice/getting-paid).

Illustrative Cases

A healthy 17-year-old G0 presents for a well-woman care. Her BMI is noted to be 16.4. She is a high school runner. She rarely menstruates and wonders if she is at risk for becoming pregnant.

This young woman should be counseled that her low BMI likely contributes to her oligomenorrhea and that there may be related health risks. Brief evaluation of her dietary approach, including usual daily intake, may elucidate an underlying eating disorder. If her food intake is reasonable but does not meet her nutritional needs due to her high activity level, she should be counseled to increase her total caloric intake by increasing densely nutritious foods rather than added sugars. Involving a dietician would be helpful. If she is sexually active, she should be counseled that weight gain may help regulate her menses and improve her fertility, increasing the chance of undesired pregnancy if she is not using contraception.

Screen and counsel now? Yes

Next screening and counseling: Annually

A 31-year-old G0 presents to your office for a well-women visit after being told by her infertility doctor that she must lose 30 pounds before undergoing in vitro fertilization (IVF). Her current BMI is 43. Blood pressure is 142/94 and remains elevated on recheck. Records show a recent hemoglobin A1c was 6.6 percent. The patient has attempted dieting and exercising for 7 years with minimal success.

Gathering a brief history of diet and activity habits may quickly elucidate targets for change, and basic nutrition and weight loss teaching can be addressed in the office. A review of number of meals eaten outside the home, frequency of label reading, and normal daily food diary can quickly identify appropriate areas for intervention. Encouraging this patient to create a calorie deficit by modestly cutting calories, reducing sugar and saturated fats, and increasing exercise can be accomplished in just a few minutes, with guidance to websites and other resources to help choose healthier foods. Visual aids, such as ChooseMyPlate.gov, may be helpful in illustrating appropriate meal plans and website recommendations are easy to compile.

Screen and counsel now? Yes

Next screening and counseling: Annually

A 28-year-old G3P3 comes to your office for a well-woman visit. Her BMI is 23, and her blood pressure is normal. Family history is significant only for colon cancer in her maternal grandmother.

While the available anthropomorphic data are normal, her family history of colon cancer translates into a heightened need to continue her healthy trajectory. A very brief inquiry into diet habits to ensure adequate vegetable, fruit, and fiber intake would suffice in this setting, with a reminder of IOM recommendations for intake of 14 g of fiber per 1,000 calories consumed daily.

Screen and counsel now? Yes

Next screening and counseling: Annually

A 50-year-old G2P2 presents for a well-woman visit. She is concerned about her overall health, as she is aware she is perimenopausal. Her blood pressure is normal; she recently had a screening test for diabetes that was normal. Her BMI is 26. She is concerned that losing a small amount of weight would be risky at her age.

While the risks of weight loss may be higher than the benefits in women over 65, and certainly over 80, this particular patient may benefit from judicious weight loss. She should pay attention to maintaining adequate intake of calcium and vitamin D and should be certain to incorporate exercise into her plan.

Screen and counsel now? Yes

Next screening and counseling: Annually

Guidelines

a. American College of Cardiology/American Heart Association Task Force on Practice Guidelines, Obesity Expert Panel, 2013. Expert panel report:

Guidelines (2013) for the management of overweight and obesity in adults. *Obesity.* 2014, July 22 (Suppl 2): S41–410.

b. US Department of Agriculture and US Department of Health and Human Services. Dietary Guidelines for Americans, 2015–2020. January 2016. Available at: http://health.gov/dietaryguidelines/2015/guidelines/. Retrieved January 18, 2016.

c. Institute of Medicine. Dietary Reference Intakes Essential Guide Nutrient Requirements. September 15, 2006. Available at: www.nap.edu/catalog/11537/dietary-reference-intakes-the-essential-guide-to-nutrient-requirements. Retrieved December 20, 2015.

d. American College of Obstetricians and Gynecologists. Guidelines for Woman's Health Care: A Resource Manual (4th edition). Ebook. Available at: www.acog.org/Resources-And-Publications/Guidelines-for-Womens-Health-Care. Retrieved December 20, 2015.

e. US Preventive Services Task Force. Final Recommendation Statement: Obesity in Adults: Screening and Management, June 2012. June 2012. Available at: www.uspreventiveservicestaskforce.org/Page/Document/RecommendationStatementFinal/obesity-in-adults-screening-and-management. Retrieved December 22, 2015.

References

1. Slawson, D., Fitzgerald, N., and Morgan, K. Position of the academy of nutrition and dietetics: The role of nutrition in health promotion and chronic disease prevention. *J Acad Nutr Diet.* 2013, **113**(7):972–9.

2. Todd, J.E. *Changes in Eating Patterns and Diet Quality among Working-Age Adults, 2005–2010*, ERR-161. US Department of Agriculture, Economic Research Service, January 2014.

3. Nield, L., Summerbell, C.D., Hooper, L., Whittaker, V., and Moore, H. Dietary advice for the prevention of type 2 diabetes mellitus in adults. Cochrane Metabolic and Endocrine Disorders Group. *Cochrane Database Syst Rev.* 2008, **3**: CD005102

4. Freeland-Graves, J.H. and Nitzke, S. Position of the academy of nutrition and dietetics: Total diet approach to healthy eating. *J Acad Nutr Diet.* 2013, **113**(2):307–17.

5. Finkelstein, E.A., Trogdon, J.G., Cohen, J.W., and Dietz, W. Annual medical spending attributable to obesity: Payer- and service-specific estimates. *Health Aff.* 2009, **28**:w822–31.

Fitness and Exercise

Maureen E. Farrell

Why Screen and Counsel?

In 2014, the World Health Organization (WHO) estimated that 25 percent of the world's adults and 80 percent of the adolescents were not active enough [1]. The Centers for Disease Control and Prevention (CDC) reports similar statistics with 21 percent of adults in the United States not getting the recommended amount of exercise weekly [2]. Fewer than 30 percent of high schoolers get at least 60 minutes of any form of physical activity daily. Getting enough physical activity is a tenet of the CDC's healthy lifestyle pentad [3]. Studies have shown that a regimen of cardiovascular, weight-bearing, and flexibility exercises is necessary to maintain a healthy body mass index (BMI) and combat obesity, to help prevent heart disease, to decrease the risk of osteoporosis, and to improve mental health and cognition [4,5,6]. For these reasons, the American College of Obstetricians and Gynecologists Well-Woman Task Force (WWTF) recommends screening and counseling adolescents and adult women regarding fitness and physical activity [a]. Other chapters in The Well Woman Visit address recommendations for Obesity, Cardiovascular Health, and Diet & Nutrition.

Rationale for Screening and Counseling

According to the CDC, physical fitness is "the ability to carry out daily tasks with vigor and alertness, without undue fatigue, and with ample energy to enjoy leisure-time pursuits and respond to emergencies" [4]. Fitness is linked to cardiorespiratory endurance, skeletal muscle performance, flexibility, balance, and

other components. Fitness and exercise combine to form a foundational pillar of women's preventive health care. A vast body of literature supports the importance of physical fitness and activity in the prevention and treatment of disease, particularly obesity and cardiovascular disease. Women have access to a tremendous amount of information regarding exercise and fitness on the internet, in popular magazines, on television, and from friends. However, studies have shown that information women receive from their physicians is taken more seriously and is more likely to lead to behavioral change [4,7]. Exercise not only helps to prevent morbid conditions such as cardiovascular disease, obesity, and osteoporosis but also is part of the recommended treatment for hypertension, hypercholesterolemia, and mental health diagnoses such as depression and anxiety [1–6].

Factors That Affect Screening and Counseling

Obesity: Obesity presents a particular challenge as it relates to physical activity. The less active a woman is, the more weight she is likely to gain, ultimately making physical activity more difficult. Unless interrupted, this vicious cycle continues. Physical activity benefits obese patients by increasing muscle mass, which makes it easier to burn calories and thus maintain or lose weight.

Eating disorders: Screening your patients' physical activity can also uncover related health issues or concerns. In younger women, excessive or "problematic exercise" can be a sign of an eating disorder or body dysmorphic issues [8].

Age: Addressing weight and fitness with adolescents should be handled delicately as many adolescents have a distorted body image. As women approach menopause, they may not focus as much on physical fitness as an

The views expressed herein are those of the author and do not necessarily reflect the official policy or position of the Department of the Navy, Department of Defense, or the United States Government.

important aspect of healthy living. Up to 75 percent of women over 65 do not exercise at the levels recommended. In addition to the health benefits already reviewed, osteoporosis, osteoarthritis, and neurocognitive function are improved with regular fitness [5]. Specifically, weight-bearing and muscle-strengthening exercises help to improve balance and prevent falls.

Recommended Guidelines and How to Find Them

The WWTF considered a variety of guidelines during the process of forming its recommendations. The WWTF recommends screening women during their appointments at all stages of their lives [a]. The US Preventive Services Task Force (USPSTF) further separates screening into specific groups including children, and adults with and without cardiovascular risk factors. It provides a summary of the evidence supporting behavioral counseling on the topic [b]. Given the prevalence of cardiovascular disease worldwide, the American Heart Association (AHA) remains the premier organization for physical activity recommendations. The guidelines are regularly reviewed based on available data; the current guidelines include revisions made in 2015 [c]. The CDC echoes the AHA recommendations [d] and cites the 2008 Physical Activity Guidelines for Americans published by the Department of Health and Human Services [e].

How to Screen and Counsel

Each well-woman visit provides an opportunity to screen patients for their current level of fitness and physical activity. Whether asked directly or on an intake questionnaire, it is necessary to determine what level and amount of exercise each patient is getting, specifically the number of days per week and the time she spends exercising. To assist in determining the intensity of her physical activities, the National Institutes of Health provides a list of common daily activities and athletic endeavors [9]. Accurate appraisal of physical activity is a requirement for effective counseling.

The AHA recommends 150 minutes of moderate exercise or 75 minutes of vigorous exercise per week in order to prevent heart disease and stroke. The AHA, in addition to its aerobic exercise

guidelines, recommends moderate- to high-intensity muscle-strengthening activity at least 2 days per week [c]. The AHA further recommends that if the goal is to lower blood pressure or cholesterol, then moderate to vigorous exercise should occur three–four times per week and be sustained for a minimum of 40 minutes [c].

If a change in behavior is required, it is of utmost importance to partner with the patient and provide focused counseling. First, determine what her health goals are if she has any. You also need to know what obstacles or concerns she perceives as barriers to participating in physical activity [4,5]. Setting graduated goals provides the patient a manageable plan and provides her supporters the opportunity to celebrate and reinforce the achievement of intermediate goals. The AHA provides an easy-to-read handout ideal for counseling patients on its current recommendations. It can be found at www.heart.org/HEARTO RG/HealthyLiving/PhysicalActivity/FitnessBasics/Am erican-Heart-Association-Recommendations-for-Phys ical-Activity-Infographic_UCM_450754_SubHomePa ge.jsp.

The Well-Woman Visit Book includes a chapter on Promoting Lifestyle Modification and Behavior with additional strategies for motivating patients.

New Developments Likely to Affect Future Guidelines

As new research emerges, the respective organizations and institutions will undoubtedly refine their recommendations. In 2016, the USPSTF is developing physical activity recommendations for adults without risk factors for cardiovascular disease, as well as an accompanying summary of evidence on behavioral counseling interventions [b].

Billing

The annual health assessment includes evaluation and counseling about maintaining a healthy lifestyle and minimizing health risks. This includes determining whether the patient is obtaining the recommended level of physical activity. The encounter for an established patient would be coded an established preventive medicine visit 9939X with the age-based "X" variable. The ICD-10 code is Z01.419, encounter for gynecological examination (general) (routine) without abnormal findings. If an abnormality exists, the code is modified to Z01.411 with the relevant additional code, obesity for example E66.9.

Illustrative Cases

A 15-year-old G0 presents for her first well-woman examination. Her BMI is 27. When asked about her physical activity, she reports that she is not involved in sports at school and hates her required physical education classes.

This young woman already meets the criteria for being overweight. With this age group, addressing concerns with weight and fitness has to be handled delicately as many adolescents have a distorted body image. By focusing on physical activity and its many health benefits, you redirect the conversation away from weight and on to fitness. This topic may have not been addressed with her before or if it has, your reiteration of its importance reinforces the point and lends an air of authority.

Screen and counsel now? Yes

Next screening and counseling: 6–12 months

A 20-year-old G0 collegiate athlete presents for her well-woman examination and needs a contraceptive refill. Her BMI is 17.5. She has no other medical complaints. You ask her about her weekly fitness regimen and she says she runs about 35–40 miles per week and is in the weight room lifting 2 days a week with her team.

Asking this patient specifically about her weekly fitness regimen can assist you in determining if her thin stature is an expected normal variant or if there is a pathologic component. In this situation, you may recognize that this level of training is normal for a collegiate-level runner. If instead you are concerned that based on her physical activity, she may suffer from body dysmorphic disorder or anorexia nervosa, you can tailor further evaluation and management.

Screen and counsel now? Yes

Next screening and counseling: (assuming there is no disorder) 12 months

A 28-year-old G0 with a BMI of 30 comes to see you for her well-woman examination. As part of the visit, she talks to you about her desire to have a baby in the next year or 2. When you question her about her physical activity, she says that she walks when she has time.

This is a golden opportunity to address physical activity and fitness. You can educate this patient about the increase in pregnancy complications in women with obesity. Complications include increases in spontaneous abortions, fetal anomalies, gestational diabetes, preeclampsia, cesarean delivery, and fetal death [10]. She will also tolerate the physical changes of pregnancy better with a baseline level of cardiovascular fitness.

Screen and counsel now? Yes

Next screening and counseling: 6–12 months

A 33-year-old G2P2 comes to your office for her annual examination. She has 1- and 4-year-old children at home and she works full time. Since the birth of her last child, she has not been able to lose her "baby weight." On review, you note that she has progressively gained weight over the course of her childbearing years and currently weighs 165 lbs (75 kg) at a height of 65 inches (165 cm). Her BMI is 27.5. When asked about her physical activity, she says that she gets exercise daily running after her kids, but that she doesn't have time to work out.

Addressing physical activity and fitness with this patient highlights its importance. By exercising at this point in her life, she can help to mitigate medical diseases such as heart disease, hypertension, diabetes, and osteoporosis. Additionally, it can set the tone for her family and healthy lifelong habits can be established. Your emphasis of her need to incorporate fitness into her life reminds her that she needs to care for herself as well as her family.

Screen and counsel now? Yes

Next screening and counseling: 12 months

A 57-year-old postmenopausal woman presents for her well-woman visit. She is thin, Asian, and has a BMI of 20. Upon questioning regarding physical activity, she says that she does not do much of anything except go to the grocery store once a week and watch television.

It is important to address exercise and fitness with women in all age groups. By asking about it, you can gauge the level of activity as well as the patient's understanding of its importance. It is an excellent opportunity to review the myriad of benefits that the different types of exercise offer. You can emphasize that joint flexibility and muscle strengthening are necessary components to her overall fitness and quality of life. You can also talk to her about concerns she may have regarding her other medical conditions and the safety of exercise with respect to these.

Screen and counsel now? Yes

Next screening and counseling: 12 months

Guidelines

a. American Congress of Obstetricians and Gynecologists. Well-Woman Recommendations. Available at: www.acog.org/About-ACOG/ACOG-Departments/Annual-Womens-Health-Care/Well-Woman-Recommendations, www.acog.org/-/media/Departments/Annual-Womens-Health-Care/Primary-and-Preventive-Care-ONLINE.pdf?dmc=1&ts=20160124T1159463170. Retrieved January 05, 2017.

b. US Preventive Services Task Force. Available at: www.uspreventiveservicestaskforce.org/BrowseRec/Search?s=physicalactivity. Retrieved January 05, 2017.

c. American Heart Association. Available at: www.heart.org/HEARTORG/HealthyLiving/PhysicalActivity/FitnessBasics/American-Heart-Association-Recommendations-for-Physical-Activity-in-Adults_UCM_307976_Article.jsp#.VqUCm2bSli4. Retrieved January 05, 2017.

d. Centers for Disease Control and Prevention. Available at: www.cdc.gov/physicalactivity/index.html. Retrieved January 05, 2017.

e. Department of Health and Human Services. Available at: http://health.gov/paguidelines/pdf/paguide.pdf. Retrieved January 05, 2017.

References

1. World Health Organization. Physical Activity Fact Sheet. January 2015. Available at: www.who.int/mediacentre/factsheets/en/

2. Centers for Disease Control and Prevention. Facts about Physical Activity. May 2014. Available at: www.cdc.gov/DiseasesConditions/.

3. Centers for Disease Control and Prevention. Tips for a Safe and Healthy Live. Available at: www.cdc.gov/family/tips/.

4. Fletcher, G.F. et al. Statement on exercise: Benefits and recommendations for physical activity programs for all Americans. *Circulation*. 1996, **94**(4):857–62.

5. Nied, R.J. and Franklin, B. Promoting and prescribing exercise for the elderly. *Am Fam Physician*. 2002, **65**(3):419–27.

6. Carek, P.J., Laibstain, S.E., and Carek, S.M. Exercise for the treatment of depression and anxiety. *Int J Psychiatry Med*. 2011, **41**(1):15–28.

7. Kreuter, M.W., Chheda, S.G., and Bull, F.C. How does physician advice influence patient behavior? Evidence for a priming effect. *Arch Fam Med*. 2000, **9**(5):426–33.

8. Rizk, M., Lalanne, C., Berthoz, S., and Kern, L. Problematic exercise in Anorexia Nervosa: Testing potential risk factors against different definition. *PLoS One*. 2015, **10**(11): 26618359.

9. National Institutes of Health. Available at: www.nhlbi.nih.gov/health/educational/lose_wt/phy_act.htm.

10. American College of Obstetricians and Gynecologists. Practice Bulletin 156: Obesity in Pregnancy. December 2015. Available at: www.acog.org/Resources-And-Publications/Practice-Bulletins/Committee-on-Practice-Bulletins-Obstetrics/Obesity-in-Pregnancy. Retrieved January 05, 2017.

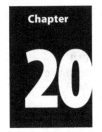

Obesity

Christopher M. Morosky

Chapter 20

Why Screen?

In 2011–2012, approximately 34.9 percent of American adults aged 20 or older, and 16.9 percent of adolescents aged 2–19 were obese [1]. While the prevalence of obesity has remained stable in the United States since 2003–2004, it has essentially doubled since the 1980s. Obesity places adolescent girls and adult women at risk for medical, reproductive, and psychological morbidity and is associated with an increased risk of all-cause mortality [2,3].

Overweight and obese adolescent girls suffer from low self-esteem and depression at greater rates than their normal-weight peers. Obese adolescents also have an increased prevalence of moderate to severe asthma, sleep apnea, hypertension, dyslipidemia, increasing fasting insulin levels, polycystic ovarian syndrome (PCOS), nonalcoholic fatty liver disease (NAFLD), and sudden death. Slipped capital femoral epiphysis and Blount disease, which is a growth disorder of the shin, have an increased prevalence among obese adolescents [4].

With increasing levels of obesity adult women are at increased risk of developing health-related conditions such as insulin resistance, type 2 diabetes, PCOS, hypertension, dyslipidemia, coronary vascular disease, and endometrial cancer [2]. Obesity also carries an increased risk of poor prenatal outcomes such as infertility, gestational diabetes, preeclampsia, cesarean delivery, wound infection, congenital anomalies, fetal macrosomia, and stillbirth [5].

Rationale for Screening and Counseling

Overweight and obese girls and women may not be aware of the definitions of normal and abnormal weight and body mass index (BMI) and may feel that their weight is normal relative to others in their peer group or community [6]. Annual calculation of

a BMI allows clinicians to explain the meaning of BMI to patients, and counsel patients regarding the impact of their weight on their current and future health and fertility.

BMI has been shown to correlate with body fat, and is also correlated with increasing health risks including cardiovascular risks. More precise measurements of body fat such as dual-energy x-ray absorptiometry are not feasible in the clinical setting. Other assessments of body fat such as waist circumference or skin-fold thickness are difficult to perform accurately and reference data are not easily available. BMI calculation is reliable, efficient, has acceptable clinical validity, and is a much better predictor of obesity than subjective assessment by the clinician.

Recent evidence suggests that following screening of BMI, referral of obese adolescents and adults to comprehensive moderate- to high-intensity multicomponent behavioral interventions is successful in producing weight loss and improvements of cardiovascular risk factors, such as glucose intolerance, lipid levels, blood pressure, and waist circumference [7]. These programs take a staged approach and focus on healthy eating, increased physical activity, and behavioral management techniques. Some patients benefit from the addition of pharmacologic agents such as sibutramine, orlistat, or metformin [2,3,7]. Finally, surgical intervention is a viable option for the treatment of obesity in some patients as well [2,8].

Factors That Affect Screening and Counseling

Age: In children and adolescents, BMI is reported as a percentile-for-age, and there is a large differential in the cutoff values used for girls compared to boys. Also, there is good evidence to suggest that as women age, the impact of obesity on health risk may be attenuated [9]. Due to age-related changes in metabolism, decreased muscle mass, and increased visceral obesity, BMI may not serve as an adequate measure of total body fat as women reach and surpass the sixth decade of life [9]. Lifestyle modifications designed to lower BMI may also reduce lean muscle mass and bone mineral density in elderly women.

Body composition: Bone and muscle are denser than fat, and people with elevated bone and muscle mass can have misleadingly high BMI measurements. These healthy individuals can be grouped with a similarly unhealthy cohort if BMI alone is used to screen for overall health.

Fat distribution: Central adiposity places an individual at an increased cardiovascular risk, whereas peripheral adiposity is less associated with such health consequences. Unlike waist circumference measurements, BMI does not take into consideration the location of body fat.

Recommended Guidelines and How to Find Them

The Well-Woman Task Force considered guidelines from the US Preventive Services Task Force (USPSTF), the American Academy of Pediatrics (AAP), the American Academy of Family Physicians (AAFP), and the American College of Obstetricians and Gynecologists (ACOG) as it developed its recommendations for obesity screening. The overall summary of these recommendations is that BMI should be calculated from height and weight measurements at all health maintenance visits for adolescents and adults, and that patients identified as being obese should be offered or referred to intensive counseling and multicomponent behavior interventions.

For obesity screening among children and adolescents, the USPSTF recommendations can be found on its website at www.uspreventiveservicestaskforce.org [a]. The AAP Committee on Nutrition conducted a formal review of the literature related to childhood obesity screening and prevention with results that are similar to those of the USPSTF and are available at www.aap.org [b]. The USPSTF also has recommendations for the screening and management of obesity for adults available on its website [c]. The AAFP supports these recommendations [d] and the ACOG expresses in a Committee Opinion the various aspects of ethical issues related to the screening and care of obese women [e].

Table 20.1 Recommended Weight Terminologies and Categories

Terminology	Adult (BMI)	Adolescent (BMI Percentile-for-Age)
Under weight	<18.5	<5th percentile
Normal weight	18.5–24.9	5th–84th percentile
Over weight	25.0–29.9	85th–94th percentile
Obesity	30 or greater	95th percentile or greater
Category I	30–34.9	
Category II	35–39.9	
Category III	40.0 or greater	

BMI: body mass index

How to Screen and Counsel

BMI is calculated from the measured weight and height of an individual and is calculated through the following formula:

$$\frac{\text{Weight in kilograms}}{(\text{Height in meters})^2}$$

Previously, BMI was calculated through the use of tables and charts; however, there are now several web-based and mobile application software programs available to assist with calculating BMI, for example, www.nhlbi.nih.gov/health/educational/lose_wt/BMI/bmicalc.htm.

The original 1998 BMI classification system proposed by the National Heart, Lung, and Blood Institute has been endorsed by the American College of Cardiology, the American Heart Association, and the Obesity Society. The classification system can be seen in Table 20.1. Obesity is defined as a BMI of 30.0 or greater and is divided into Class I Obesity (BMI 30.0–34.9), Class II Obesity (BMI 35.0–39.9), and Class III Obesity (BMI 40.0 or greater). As adolescent girls are continuing to grow and develop, BMI is therefore calculated as a percentile-for-age. A useful online BMI percentile calculator for children and teens is available from the Center for Disease Control and Prevention at https://nccd.cdc.gov/dnpabmi/calculator.aspx. The pediatric cutoffs and terminology were revised by an expert committee in 2007 and can be seen in Table 20.1. Overweight is defined as the 85th–94th BMI percentile-for-age, and obesity is defined as the 95th BMI percentile-for-age or higher.

The calculation of BMI is relatively straightforward for most adolescent girls and adult women. Height should be measured after removal of shoes with the feet flat against the floor. The person should stand comfortably with most of the back touching the wall and the head looking comfortably forward. A flat headpiece should be brought down to form a right angle with the wall and rest firmly on the crown of the head. Height should be measured to the nearest 1/8 of an inch or centimeter.

Weight should ideally be measured on a calibrated mechanical or an electronic scale. Shoes and heavy clothing should be removed. Bags and items such as cells phones, books, and parcels should be placed aside. As mentioned earlier, BMI for adults and BMI percentile-for-age for children and adolescents should be calculated using an online calculator. It is important to keep in mind that in certain subgroups of the population including the elderly, those with an increased peripheral distribution of adiposity and those fit individuals with high bone and muscle mass, waist circumference or waist-to-hip ratio may be better predictors of future health outcomes than BMI [7,9].

For both obese adolescents [a, b] and adults [c, e], the recommendation is for referral to moderate- to high-intensity multicomponent behavioral interventions. For children, this begins with a focus on the following parameters: increasing the amount of fruits, vegetables, and lean meats while decreasing the number of high-calorie food items eaten throughout the day, increasing moderate to vigorous activity to 60 minutes per day while limiting total television and screen time to 2 hours per day, and eliminating sugar-sweetened beverages altogether from the diet [b]. Evidence-based interventions that are successful for adults include: weight-loss goal setting, improving nutrition, increasing physical activity, addressing barriers to change, self-monitoring, and focusing on long-term maintenance of health [c]. These patients often require a multidisciplinary approach with assistance from dieticians, behavioralists, physical therapists, family counselors, psychologists, and psychiatrists.

The chapters on Fitness & Exercise, Diet & Nutrition, Metabolic Syndrome, and Promoting Lifestyle Modification & Behavior Change provide additional information relevant to obese patients.

New Developments Likely to Affect Future Guidelines

The USPSTF has planned updates for obesity screening and weight-loss management in children and adolescents as well as adults. These updates can be found on their website at www.uspreventiveservicestaskforce .org. The recommendation topic "Obesity in Children and Adolescents: Screening and Interventions" will be released in 2016. The key questions that are being addressed focus on whether obesity screening and weight management programs for children and adolescents lead to a reduction in age-related excess weight gain, improve health outcomes, and reduce adult obesity. This topic also plans to address if these screenings and interventions have adverse side effects. Similar key questions are being addressed for adults in the recommendation topic "Weight Loss to Prevent Obesity-Related Morbidity and Mortality in Adults: Behavioral and Pharmacotherapy Interventions," which will be released in 2018. Recommendation updates from the AAP, AAFP, and ACOG can be expected to follow the release of these updates from the USPSTF.

Billing

Overweight and obesity codes are listed in ICD-10 under the category E66. The correct coding within this category requires further attention to proper documentation of Severity (Overweight, E66.3; Obesity, E66.8; or Morbid Obesity, E66.01), Contributing Factors (Obesity due to excess calories, E66.09 or Drug-induced obesity, E66.1), Associations (Obesity complicating pregnancy, O99.21), and Manifestations (Morbid obesity with alveolar hypoventilation, E66.2). If documentation of BMI by the clinician is performed in the medical record, a table under the ICD-10 category Z68 can be used for correct coding of the BMI category (from BMI 19 or less, Z68.1, up to BMI 40 or greater, Z68.4, for adults and age-related BMI percentile for children and adolescents, Z68.5).

Illustrative Cases

A 15-year-old adolescent girl presents with her mother for a well-woman visit. Her height is 5 feet 1–1/8 inches and her weight is 170 pounds.

BMI: 32.0 BMI-for-age (girls): 97th percentile, Obese

This patient is at risk for lifelong obesity and health-related problems due to her weight. Screening should focus on her parents' obesity and her mother's obesity, weight gain, and presence of gestational diabetes in the patient's pregnancy. The patient should then be asked about her current dietary habits and daily physical activity. Initial interventions would include reducing or eliminating all sugar-sweetened drinks. The patient and her family should focus on increasing the amount of fruits, vegetables, and lean meats in her diet while reducing the number of high-calorie foods eaten. The patient should strive to increase her daily vigorous activity to 60 minutes per day, while limiting her television and screen time to less than 2 hours per day.

Screen now? Yes

Next screen: With the diagnosis of obesity, follow-up would be arranged to monitor the progress of recommended interventions, and not to screen.

A 22-year-old woman presents for a well-woman visit. She is interested in initiating contraception. Her height is 5 feet 4–3/4 inches and her weight is 220 pounds. She is otherwise healthy.

BMI: 36.9 BMI Category: Class II Obesity

This visit in an important opportunity for the physician to discuss the patient's obesity in the context of her current and future health risks. Screening should include a family history of obesity-related illnesses such as diabetes, hypertension, hyperlipidemia, and cardiac disease. Lifestyle modifications resulting in weight loss could greatly reduce her risks of these conditions in the future. The patient should be counseled that systemic forms of hormonal contraception may have diminished efficacy in the setting of increasing obesity. While the patient should not be discouraged from any particular form of contraception, this visit does allow the physician to recommend or refer the patient to intensive, multicomponent behavioral modifications to encourage weight loss and likely improve the efficacy of her chosen form of contraception.

Screen now? Yes

Next screen: With the diagnosis of obesity, follow-up would be arranged to monitor the progress of recommended interventions, and not to screen.

A 26-year-old woman presents for a well-woman visit. She is considering becoming pregnant in the next year.

Her height is 5 feet 6–1/4 inches and her weight is 255 pounds.

BMI: 40.8 BMI Category: Class III Obesity

The patient is at risk for current obesity-related health conditions. She should undergo testing for hypertension, dyslipidemia, insulin resistance, type 2 diabetes, and NAFLD. The diagnosis and management of these medical conditions are an important component of her preconception counseling. The patient's obesity puts her at risk for several adverse pregnancy outcomes including infertility, miscarriage, gestational diabetes, pregnancy-related hypertension, respiratory compromise, thromboembolic disease, cesarean delivery, wound infection, endometritis, and anesthesia complications. Initiating prenatal vitamins along with increased amounts of folic acid, this patient should be referred to services that can provide specific behavioral strategies to decrease her caloric intake and increase her vigorous physical activity. Enrollment in a structured weight-loss program and setting a weight-loss goal prior to conception should be encouraged.

Screen now? Yes

Next screen: With the diagnosis of obesity, follow-up would be arranged to monitor the progress of recommended interventions, and not to screen.

A 47-year-old woman presents for a well-woman visit. She complains of heavy and irregular menstrual bleeding. Her height is 5 feet 4–3/4 inches and her weight is 315 pounds. She has type 2 diabetes.

BMI: 52.8 BMI Category: Class III Obesity

This patient already has manifestations of obesity-related medical illness. She is at risk for future morbidity and mortality. A multidisciplinary team should be in place for this patient, including a primary care physician and endocrinologist. She should be encouraged to enroll in a high-intensity program that focuses on diet, physical activity, and behavioral counseling. Consultation with a bariatric surgeon would also be appropriate. There is now sufficient evidence to suggest that due to her obesity this patient is at increased risk for most all women's health cancers, including breast, endometrial, cervical, and ovarian cancers. A family history of these cancers should be recorded. She should undergo screening mammography and Pap smear screening according to current breast and cervical cancer screening guidelines. Endometrial sampling should be performed to rule out endometrial hyperplasia or carcinoma, and sonographic imaging of the pelvic organs is appropriate for this patient.

Screen now? Yes

Next screen: With the diagnosis of obesity, follow-up would be arranged to monitor the progress of recommended interventions, and not to screen.

A 68-year-old woman presents for a well-woman visit. Her height is 5 feet 7-1/2 inches and her weight is 195 pounds. She has hypertension that is well controlled with a single agent.

BMI: 30.1 BMI Category: Class I Obesity

This patient's obesity and hypertension put her at an increased risk of cardiovascular morbidity and mortality. The patient is also at increased risk of cancer due to her obesity. After a thorough medical and family history is conducted, appropriate cancer screening recommendations should be made according to current screening guidelines. The recommendation for weight loss in this patient should keep in mind the potential harms for screening and behavioral interventions in the elderly population. These harms include loss of lean muscle mass and bone mineral density, resulting in an increased risk of fracture. There is also a small risk of serious injury resulting from increased physical activity. Dietary modifications should focus on increased lean protein and sufficient levels of vitamins and minerals such as calcium, vitamin D, and iron. Recommended physical activities would include moderate weight-bearing exercises and resistance training. A focus on overall health is likely to be more beneficial for quality of life compared to specific weight-loss goals in the elderly population.

Screen now? Yes

Next screen: With the diagnosis of obesity, follow-up would be arranged to monitor the progress of recommended interventions, and not to screen.

Guidelines

Children and Adolescents

a. US Preventive Services Task Force. Final Update Summary: Obesity in Children and Adolescents: Screening. July 2015. Available at: www.uspreventiveservicestaskforce.org.

b. Daniels, S., Hassink, S.; Committee on Nutrition. The role of the pediatrician in prevention of obesity. *Pediatrics.* 2015, **136**(1):e275–92.

Available at: http://pediatrics.aappublications.org/content/136/1/e275.

Adults

c. Moyer, V. Screening for and management of obesity in adults: US Preventive Services Task Force recommendation statement. *Ann Intern Med.* 2012, **157**:373–8. Available at: www.uspreventiveservicestaskforce.org.

d. US Preventive Services Task Force. Screening for and management of obesity in adults: Recommendation statement. *Am Fam Physician.* 2012, **86**(10):1–3. Available at: www.aafp.org/afp/2012/1115/od3.html.

e. American College of Obstetricians and Gynecologists. Ethical issues in the care of the obese woman. Committee Opinion No. 600. *Obstet Gynecol.* 2014, **123**:1388–93.

References

1. Ogden, C., Carroll, M., Kit, B., and Flegal, K. Prevalence of childhood and adult obesity in the United States, 2011–2012. *JAMA.* 2014, **311**(8):806–14.

2. Fitness. *Guidelines for Women's Health Care: A Resource Manual,* 4th edition. Washington, DC: American College of Obstetricians and Gynecologists, 2014, pp. 245–63.

3. Obesity in Adolescents *Guidelines for Adolescent Health Care,* 2nd edition. Washington, DC: American College of Obstetricians and Gynecologists, 2011, pp. 148–63.

4. Gurnani, M., Birken, C., and Hamilton, J. Childhood obesity. Causes consequences, and management. *Pediatr Clin N Am.* 2015, **62**:821–40.

5. Liat, S., Cabero, L., Hod, M., and Yogev, Y. Obesity in obstetrics. *Best Pract Res Clin Obstet Gyneacol.* 2015, **29**:79–90.

6. Mueller, A. The role of school context in adolescents' weight-loss behaviors and self-perceptions of overweight. *Sociol Inq.* 2015, **85**(4):532–55.

7. Leblanc, E., O'Connor, E., Whitlock, E., Patnode, C., and Kapka, T. Effectiveness of primary care-relevant treatment for obesity in adults: A systematic evidence review for the US Preventive Services Task Force. *Ann Intern Med.* 2011, **155**:434–47.

8. Bour, E. Evidence supporting the need for bariatric surgery to address the obesity epidemic in the United States. *Curr Sports Med Rep.* 2015, **14**(2):100–3.

9. Woo, J. Obesity in older persons. *Curr Opin Clin Nutr Metab Care.* 2015, **18**:5–10.

The Metabolic Syndrome

Nguyet Anh Nguyen

Why Screen?

Metabolic syndrome (MetS) affects one in five Americans. MetS increases the risk of diabetes mellitus (DM), cardiovascular disease (CVD), and death. Although MetS is closely related to obesity, it also affects lean and normal-weight women. The dangers of obesity alone are well defined, but it is the additional risk factors (insulin resistance, dyslipidemia, and hypertension) that markedly elevate disease risk [1]. According to the World Health Organization (WHO), CVD and DM are among the top four leading noncommunicable causes of death globally with CVD responsible for 48 percent of these deaths. The profound rise in child and adolescent obesity underscores the importance of accurate diagnosis and timely, intensive behavior modifications to prevent the occurrence of irreversible health consequences [1].

Rationale for Screening

MetS screening allows physicians to identify early warning signs to prevent the development of DM or CVD. The components of MetS, such as insulin resistance, hypertension, and dyslipidemia, do not act independently to increase disease risk. The pathophysiology of MetS is not yet fully characterized but insulin resistance is thought to be a primary factor. Excess insulin elicits a variety of changes which lead to hypertension and a proinflammatory state that is characteristic of CVD [1–2]. In MetS, the excess adipose tissue leads to increased hepatic production of glucose and triglycerides and secretion of very low-density lipoprotein (VLDL), in turn stimulating insulin production, reducing high-density lipoproteins (HDL), increasing low-density lipoproteins (LDL), and further worsening atherosclerosis and CVD [1–4]. The lifetime risk of developing DM in patients with MetS increases five-fold and the risk of developing CVD over the first 5–10 years of disease increases

two-fold compared to individuals without MetS [a]. The interplay of dyslipidemia, hypertension, and insulin resistance justifies screening for MetS in addition to individual risk factors. Diet and lifestyle modifications can slow or prevent such sequelae, and there are other effective treatments that prevent disease progression [5].

Factors That Affect Screening

Age: Risk of MetS increases with age, but as the obesity epidemic spreads to children and adolescents, MetS is occurring more often in young women and girls. The interplay between childhood obesity, growth, puberty, and MetS is poorly defined. Even adolescents without risk factors may have dyslipidemia, which increases their risk of developing MetS later in life [1].

Ethnicity and race: Waist circumference (WC) is the most frequently applied diagnostic criteria for the diagnosis of MetS. A relative increase in visceral, more so than subcutaneous, adipose tissue has been associated with increased risk of MetS [3]. Subtle differences in the location of fat deposition may explain why the prevalence of MetS fails to correlate with WC measurements in some races and populations, and why different race-specific thresholds for WC have been recommended [2,3].

Recommended Guidelines and How to Find Them

The Well-Woman Task Force (WWTF) reviewed major organizational guidelines to develop final screening recommendations to assist clinicians in diagnosing MetS [1–5]. A joint Interim Statement was released in 2009 by multiple organizations including the American Heart Association (AHA), International Diabetes Federation (IDF), and the

Table 21.1 Criteria for Clinical Diagnosis of Metabolic Syndrome

Measure	Categorical Cut Points
Elevated waist circumference*	Population- and country-specific definitions
Elevated triglycerides (drug treatment for elevated triglycerides is an alternate indicator†)	≥150 mg/dL (1.7 mmol/L)
Reduced HDL-C (drug treatment for reduced HDL-C is an alternate indicator†)	<40 mg/dL (1.0 mmol/L) in males; <50 mg/dL (1.3 mmol/L) in females
Elevated blood pressure (antihypertensive drug treatment in a patient with a history of hypertension is an alternate indicator)	Systolic ≥130 and/or diastolic ≥85 mm Hg
Elevated fasting glucose‡ (drug treatment of elevated glucose is an alternate indicator)	≥100 mg/dL

HDL-C: high-density lipoprotein cholesterol

* It is recommended that the IDF cut points be used for non-Europeans and either the IDF or AHA/NHLBI cut points used for people of European origin until more data are available.

† The most commonly used drugs for elevated triglycerides and reduced HDL-C are fibrates and nicotinic acid. A patient taking one of these drugs can be presumed to have high triglycerides and low HDL-C. High-dose ω-3 fatty acids presumes high triglycerides.

‡ Most patients with type 2 diabetes mellitus will have the metabolic syndrome by the proposed criteria.

Source: Courtesy of Alberti, K.G. et al. Harmonizing the metabolic syndrome: A joint interim statement of the International Diabetes Federation Task Force on Epidemiology and Prevention; National Heart, Lung, and Blood Institute; American Heart Association; World Heart Federation; International Atherosclerosis Society; and International Association for the Study of Obesity. *Circulation*. 2009, 120(16):1640–5.

National Heart, Lung, and Blood Institute (NHLBI) that aimed to unify the MetS definition (available at http://circ.ahajournals.org/content/120/16/1640.full) [a]. They agreed that the presence of three out of five criteria would be sufficient for diagnosis (Table 21.1). One of the criteria – WC – uses different thresholds based on gender and ethnicity (Table 21.2) [a]. The major guidelines listed in this chapter were used to develop the WWTF final recommendations, which unify all the criterion variations between organizations and simplify screening. The WWTF recommends screening all patients for dyslipidemia once in late adolescence regardless of risk factors, screening adolescents and women with elevated BMI for dyslipidemia and hyperglycemia, and providing or referring screen positive patients for counseling about lifestyle modification and/or medication treatment. The WWTF makes separate screening recommendations for obesity and hypertension.

How to Screen

In the United States, MetS is diagnosed if (not using) three out of five criteria from the National Cholesterol Education Program Adult Treatment Panel III are present (NCEP ATP III): elevated WC, blood pressure (BP), triglycerides, and fasting glucose, as well as reduced HDL-C (Table 21.1) [1]. The benefit of this definition lies in clinicians' ability to screen patients using simple in-office measurements without the need for laboratory assessments [a, b].

Waist circumference: WC should be measured in all women with elevated BMI. WC should also be measured in patients who are at increased risk of DM or CVD even in those with normal weight. To measure a patient's waist, the clinician should palpate the hip to identify the top of the iliac crest. A line is then drawn at this level at the midpoint between the patient's abdomen and back. A tape measure is then wrapped around the waist and should be snug without indenting the skin. The clinician should then ask the patient to take two–three normal breaths and the final measurement should be taken at the end of normal expiration and measured to the nearest millimeter.

Dyslipidemia: For patients with elevated BMI or other CVD risk factors, a fasting lipid profile including TG and HDL levels is warranted [c]. For adolescents, the WWTF recommends one-time screening late in adolescence (no later than age 18) due to existing data that shows MetS in patients of normal BMI and absence of risk factors. Patients should be counseled on any abnormal findings and treated according to the USPSTF recommendations

Table 21.2 Current Recommended Waist Circumference Thresholds for Abdominal Obesity by Organization

Population	Organization (Reference)	Recommended Waist Circumference Threshold for Abdominal Obesity	
		Men	Women
Europid	IDF [4]	≥94 cm	≥80 cm
Caucasian	WHO [7]	≥94 cm (increased risk)	≥80 cm (increased risk)
		≥120 cm (still higher risk)	≥88 cm (still higher risk)
United States	AHA/NHLBI (ATP III)* [5]	≥102 cm	≥88 cm
Canada	Health Canada [8,9]	≥102 cm	≥88 cm
European	European Cardiovascular Societies [10]	≥102 cm	≥88 cm
Asian (including Japanese)	IDF [4]	≥90 cm	≥80 cm
Asian	WHO [11]	≥90 cm	≥80 cm
Japanese	Japanese Obesity Society [12]	≥85 cm	≥90 cm
China	Cooperative Task Force [13]	≥85 cm	≥80 cm
Middle East, Mediterranean	IDF [4]	≥94 cm	≥80 cm
Sub-Saharan African	IDF [4]	≥94 cm	≥80 cm
Ethnic Central and South American	IDF [4]	≥90 cm	≥80 cm

IDF: American Heart Association; WHO: World Health Organization; AHA: International Diabetes Federation; NHLBI: National Heart, Lung, and Blood Institute; ATP III: Adult Treatment Panel III

*Recent AHA/NHLBI guidelines for metabolic syndrome recognize an increased risk for CVD and diabetes at waist circumference thresholds of ≥94 cm in men and ≥80 cm in women and identify these as optional cut points for individuals or populations with increased insulin resistance.

Source: Courtesy of Alberti, K.G. et al. Harmonizing the metabolic syndrome: A joint interim statement of the International Diabetes Federation Task Force on Epidemiology and Prevention; National Heart, Lung, and Blood Institute; American Heart Association; World Heart Federation; International Atherosclerosis Society; and International Association for the Study of Obesity. Circulation. 2009, 120(16):1640–5.

with dietary and behavioral modifications and medications when indicated [d].

Blood pressure: The WWTF recommends BP screening for all groups starting in adolescence (age 13 and above). The goal is to maintain BP <140/90 mm Hg (or <130/80 mm Hg in diabetic patients). Dietary and lifestyle modifications are recommended for BP ≥120/80 mm Hg and BP medication initiated if BP >140/90 (or >130/80 mm Hg in diabetic or renal disease patients) according to the Eighth Joint National Committee (available at http://jama.jamanetwork.com/article.aspx?articleid=1791497) [e].

Hyperglycemia: In patients less than age 45, fasting blood glucose (FBS) testing is recommended in patients with elevated WC, obesity, or elevated BP >135/80 to assist in MetS diagnosis. Lifestyle modifications should be initiated when patients have abnormal FBS; however, if a patient is diagnosed with frank DM, then drug therapy should be initiated according to ADA guidelines (available at http://professional.diabetes.org/content/clinical-practice-recommendations).

Each component of MetS should be treated according to standard care guidelines to correct abnormalities of weight, BP, and glycemic control [3,5]. Normalization in these conditions may also ameliorate lipid abnormalities. Women diagnosed with MetS should be referred to a primary care physician for frequent monitoring of progress and continuity of care. Additional information on Obesity, Cardiovascular Disease, and Diabetes, Diet & Nutrition, Fitness & Exercise, and Promoting Lifestyle Modification and Behavior Change appears in other chapters.

New Developments Likely to Affect Future Recommendations

In 1998, the WHO defined MetS to provide clinicians a guide for treatment and prevention of DM and CVD [b]. Since that time, many organizations have developed definitions of MetS. A lack of a unified clinical definition makes interpretation of research and clinical strategies inconsistent [5]. Efforts to create a single international standard could affect future screening recommendations; however, WWTF guidelines align with current AHA recommendations (Table 21.1).

Some have challenged the idea that MetS is a true "syndrome" citing the lack of conclusive evidence regarding a true unifying pathophysiology [6]. Empiric tools, such as the NHLBI risk calculator (http://cvdrisk.nhlbi.nih.gov), perform better in predicting cardiovascular events. A WHO expert consultation report published in 2010 questioned the utility of MetS [7]. The ongoing debate may affect future guidelines regarding MetS screening and treatment.

Billing

The well-woman exam visit is typically covered under the International Classification of Diseases, Tenth Revision (ICD-10) code Z01.419, the encounter for the gynecological examination (general) (routine) without abnormal findings. If a woman meets the criteria for screening, then the appropriate Current Procedural Terminology (CPT) code for the test is used under the preventive service visit codes 99394–99397 (age dependent) with ICD-10 codes (cholesterol screening is Z13.220 and diabetes screening is Z13.1) for diagnoses. If a patient has CVD risk factors or meets criteria for obesity, the code E66.x should be used; in patients with diabetes, the code E11.xxx should be used with the appropriate specifications for the laboratory test performed. Hypercholesterolemia and its variations are coded under E78.x code.

The Center for Medicare and Medicaid Services (CMS) requires a unique set of Healthcare Common Procedures Coding System (HCPCS) codes. Dyslipidemia screening is covered annually during ages 11–17 and once during ages 18–21 under code 80061 with diagnosis code Z13.220. For routine cholesterol screening, CMS covers screening for women greater than 45 years and older (also for women ages 20–45 who are at risk for CVD) performed every 5 years using codes 82465 or 83718 with routine diagnosis. DM screening is covered under code 82947 – glucose; quantitative blood, 82950 – glucose post glucose dose (includes glucose); or 82951 – glucose tolerance test, three specimens (includes glucose) with ICD-10 code Z13.1. CMS states DM testing is covered for at-risk patients or those diagnosed with "prediabetes" with two screening test per year; or one screening per year if previously tested but not diagnosed with prediabetes or if never tested.

Illustrative Cases

A 15-year-old female presents for her first well-woman visit. She is accompanied by her mother. During your evaluation you note significant acne and a dark velvety rash behind her neck. Her BMI is 31. Her mother denies any history of CVD in their family.

The patient's elevated BMI alone warrants screening for MetS; therefore, a lipid profile, FBS, and WC should be measured, even in the absence of the other findings such as acanthosis nigricans. In the adolescent group (13–18 years), BP screening is recommended at every visit. Obese children and adolescents should receive close follow-up by a pediatrician and a multidisciplinary team to assist with healthy diet, weight loss, and physical activity.

Screen now? Yes

Next screen: Annually for BMI and BP. If obesity not corrected by age 18, rescreen for dyslipidemia and hyperglycemia.

A 19-year-old female presents for her well-woman exam. She is sexually active and in a monogamous relationship. She has been on the same birth control pill for 2 years with no complaints. Her mother denies any history of CVD in their family.

MetS screening should be done once in late adolescence or early adulthood (18–21 years) to detect patients with normal BMIs who may be affected. If screening is negative, no additional screening until indicated until the patient develops risk factors such as obesity.

Screen now? Yes

Next screen: As clinically indicated

A 47-year-old woman with a history of polycystic ovarian syndrome (PCOS) presents for a well-woman visit. Her family history is notable for a maternal history of a myocardial infarction at age 59.

The patient has CVD risk factors (family history of early-onset CVD) and should be offered MetS screening starting with BP and BMI. If either is elevated, a WC, fasting lipid profile, and FBS should be performed.

Screen now? Yes

Next screen: BP and BMI annually if all other testing is normal

A 67-year-old woman who had a hysterectomy due to fibroids years ago presents for her well-woman exam. She is up to date with her mammogram, dual-energy x-ray absorptiometry (DXA) scan, and colonoscopy. She reports doing well and denies any significant past medical history.

MetS and CVD risk increases with age; therefore, screening with BP, fasting lipid profile, weight and WC, and FBS should be performed even if the patient has a normal BMI.

Screen now? Yes

Next screen: BP at every visit or at least annually, WC in overweight patients or those with CVD risk factors, FBS in 3 years, and lipid profile in 5 years

Guidelines

a. American Heart Association and National Heart, Lung and Blood Institute, Alberti, K.G. et al. Harmonizing the metabolic syndrome: A joint interim statement of the International Diabetes Federation Task Force on Epidemiology and Prevention; National Heart, Lung, and Blood Institute; American Heart Association; World Heart Federation; International Atherosclerosis Society; and International Association for the Study of Obesity. *Circulation.* 2009, **120**(16): 1640–5. Available at: www.nhlbi.nih.gov/health/health-topics/topics/ms. Retrieved January 18, 2016.

b. World Health Organization, Alberti, K.G., and Zimmet, P.Z. Definition, diagnosis and classification of diabetes mellitus and its complications. Part 1: Diagnosis and classification of diabetes mellitus provisional report of a WHO consultation. *Diabet Med.* 1998, **15**(7):539–53.

c. National Cholesterol Education Program and Adult Treatment Panel III. Treatment of High Blood Cholesterol in, Third Report of the National Cholesterol Education Program (NCEP) Expert Panel on Detection, Evaluation, and Treatment of High Blood Cholesterol in Adults (Adult Treatment Panel III) final report. *Circulation.* 2002, **106**(25):3143–421. Available at: http://circ.ahajournals.org/content/106/25/3143.full.pdf±html?sid=e0896a5d-0e3d-4c66-afc0-2e64f7a199d4. Retrieved January 18, 2016.

d. US Preventive Services Task Force. Final Update Summary: Lipid Disorders in Adults (Cholesterol, Dyslipidemia): Screening. July 2015. Available at: www.uspreventiveservicestaskforce.org/Page/Document/UpdateSummaryFinal/lipid-disorders-in-adults-cholesterol-dyslipidemia-screening?ds=1&s=lipidscreening.

e. Eighth Joint National Committee, James, P.A., Oparil, S., Carter, B.L. et al. 2014. Evidence-based guideline for the management of high blood pressure in adults: Report from the panel members appointed to the Eighth Joint National Committee (JNC 8). *JAMA.* 2014, **311** (5):507–20.

References

1. Miranda, P.J., DeFronzo, R.A., Califf, R.M., and Guyton, J.R. Metabolic syndrome: Definition, pathophysiology, and mechanisms. *Am Heart J.* 2005, **149**(1):33–45.

2. Grundy, S.M., Brewer, H.B. Jr, Cleeman, J.I., Smith, S.C. Jr, and Lenfant C. Definition of metabolic syndrome: Report of the National Heart, Lung, and Blood Institute/American Heart Association conference on scientific issues related to definition. *Arterioscler Thromb Vasc Biol.* 2004, **24**(2):e13–8.

3. Eckel, R.H., Grundy, S.M., and Zimmet, P.Z. The metabolic syndrome. *Lancet.* 2005, **365** (9468):1415–28.

4. Grundy, S.M. Metabolic syndrome: Connecting and reconciling cardiovascular and diabetes worlds. *J Am Coll Cardiol.* 2006, **47**(6):1093–100.

5. American Heart Association, et al. Diagnosis and management of the metabolic syndrome. An American Heart Association/National Heart, Lung, and Blood Institute Scientific Statement. Executive summary. *Cardiol Rev.* 2005, **13**(6):322–7.

6. D'Agostino, R.B., Sr., Vasan, R.S., Pencina, M.J., Wolf, P.A., Cobain, M., Massaro, J.M., Kannel, W.B. General cardiovascular risk profile for use in primary care: The Framingham Heart Study. *Circulation.* 2008, **117** (6):743–53.

7. Simmons, R.K., Alberti, K.G., Gale, E.A., Colagiuri, S., Tuomilehto, J., Qiao, Q., Ramachandran, A., Tajima, N., Brajkovich Mirchov, I., Ben-Nakhi, A., Reaven, G., Hama Sambo, B., Mendis, S., Roglic, G. The metabolic syndrome: Useful concept or clinical tool? Report of a WHO Expert Consultation. *Diabetologia.* 2010, **53**(4):600–5.

Chapter 22

Iron Deficiency Anemia

Moune Jabre Raughley

Why Screen?

According to the World Health Organization's (WHO) *Global Database on Anaemia*, the prevalence of anemia in nonpregnant women in the United States from 1993 to 2005 was 6.9 percent [1]. However, the extent of clinically relevant disease is unclear.

Rationale for Not Screening

There are currently no established recommendations supporting routine screening for iron deficiency anemia in asymptomatic nonpregnant women and adolescents [1,2]. The American Congress of Obstetricians and Gynecologists Well-Woman Task Force (WWFT) specifically summarized that "routine screening for anemia is not recommended," although this is a qualified recommendation [1]. This is likely due to limited data on the clinical impact of iron deficiency anemia in nonpregnant women in the United States and lack of evidence of improved outcomes with screening and treatment. Symptomatic anemia does benefit from diagnosis and treatment.

Factors That Affect Screening

Signs and symptoms: Women presenting with signs or symptoms concerning for anemia should be screened. Symptoms may be nonspecific and include palpitations, dizziness, fatigue, shortness of breath, and pica. Evaluation for anemia may be reasonable if pallor or tachycardia is noted on physical examination.

Abnormal uterine bleeding: The WWTF does not address risk factor assessment in deciding whom to screen. However, abnormal uterine bleeding affects nearly 15 percent of women and is a frequent cause of iron deficiency anemia [2]. It may be reasonable to screen otherwise asymptomatic women with a history of significant abnormal uterine bleeding.

Additional risk factors to consider in the adolescent population include a prior history of iron deficiency anemia or a diet lacking iron-rich foods.

Recommended Guidelines and How to Find Them

At present in the United States, no major societies have guidelines recommending routine screening for iron deficiency anemia in asymptomatic nonpregnant women as there is no data to support the practice. The WWTF final recommendation addresses adolescents and adults of all ages and states that routine screening for anemia is not recommended [1]. This is a qualified statement because it is based on expert opinion alone given the relative paucity of data on this subject.

In general, the WWTF adopted the American Academy of Pediatrics (AAP) Bright Futures guidelines for adolescents. The WWTF recommendation differs from the Bright Futures guidelines for anemia, and it is not clear if this was deliberate. The AAP recommends that all adolescents have an anemia risk assessment at the annual visit, which should be followed by screening if risk factors are present [2–4].

In 1998, the Centers for Disease Control published guidelines recommending periodic screening of all nonpregnant women of childbearing age [5]. This recommendation was not carried forward in any subsequent revisions. The current US Preventive Services Task Force guidelines on iron deficiency anemia are limited to children and pregnant women and do not address nonpregnant women at all [6].

How to Screen/Test

Asymptomatic adult women should not be screened. The usual review of systems should encompass questions covering potential anemia symptoms and routine physical examination may detect pallor or tachycardia. If a woman presents with symptoms concerning for anemia, such as palpitations, dizziness, fatigue, shortness of breath, or signs such as tachycardia or pallor, then an anemia evaluation is reasonable.

For adolescent girls, the clinician should screen for presence of anemia risk factors at each annual well-adolescent visit. According to the AAP guidelines, these risk factors are a diet lacking in iron-rich foods, menses that are heavy or last ≥5 days, or a prior history of iron deficiency anemia. The presence of any of these risk factors should trigger screening [2–4].

A complete blood count is cost effective, provides much valuable information, and should be the initial test of choice. Once anemia is confirmed by a low hemoglobin (<12 g/dL), additional testing should be undertaken to assess iron stores and determine the etiology [1].

New Developments Likely to Affect Future Guidelines

Currently, the prevalence of iron deficiency anemia in nonpregnant women in the United States is relatively low, which in part drives the absence of recommendations for screening. Screening might be warranted if the prevalence were to increase significantly. Large population studies are needed to determine not only the prevalence of anemia in asymptomatic nonpregnant women but also the extent of clinically significant anemia in those women that screen positive. Studies would also have to answer the question of whether iron supplementation would then improve outcomes and justify the costs of routine screening.

Billing

Health maintenance billing codes are not applicable if the testing is being done for diagnostic rather than for screening purposes. For diagnostic testing in symptomatic women, the ICD-10 billing codes corresponding to the presenting signs and symptoms should be used. If true screening is being done, as in the case of adolescents with positive risk factors, the appropriate ICD-10 health maintenance code is Z13.0 – encounter for screening for diseases of the blood.

Illustrative Cases

A healthy 23-year-old female presents for her well-woman visit. She reports feeling well and has a negative review of systems.

Screen now? No. This patient is asymptomatic and should not be screened for anemia.

Next screen: Only if becomes symptomatic or develops signs.

A 42-year-old overweight female presents for her well-woman visit. She reports feeling well. On review of systems, she reports fatigue as well as dyspnea with climbing stairs.

Screen now? Yes. She has subtle symptoms that may be consistent with anemia. Testing would be better described as diagnostic testing rather than screening.

Next screen: If symptoms recur in future.

A 16-year-old female who plays competitive sports and is a vegetarian presents for routine evaluation. She has heavy menses. Review of systems is negative. Further history reveals that her vegetarian diet rarely includes eggs, beans, or iron-fortified cereals.

Screen now? Yes. This is an adolescent patient who, although asymptomatic, has two risk factors for anemia, heavy menses and a diet lacking iron-rich foods. She should be screened according to the AAP guidelines.

Next screen: Should have symptoms and risk factors reviewed at subsequent well-adolescent visits.

Guidelines

Nonpregnant Pre- and Postmenopausal Women

a. Conry, J.A. and Brown, H. Well-Woman Task Force: Components of the Well-Woman Visit. *Obstet Gynecol.* 2015, **126**(4):697–701.

Adolescent Girls

b. Hagan, J.F., Shaw, J.S., and Duncan, P.M., editors. *Bright Futures Guidelines for Health Supervision of Infants, Children and Adolescents*, 3rd edition. Elk Grove Village, IL: American Academy of Pediatrics, 2008.

References

1. DeBenoist, B., McLean, E., Egli, I. et al. *Worldwide Prevalence of Anemia 1993–2005: WHO Global Database on Anemia*. Geneva: World Health Organization, 2008. Available at: www.who.int/vmnis/anaemia/prevalence/en/. Retrieved January 3, 2015.

2. Short, M.W. and Domagalski, J.E. Iron deficiency anemia: Evaluation and management. *Am Fam Physician*. 2013, **87**:98–104.

3. Bright Futures Medical Screening Reference Table for Adolescent Visits. Available at: https://brightfutures.aap .org/Bright%20Futures%20Documents/MSRTable_Ad olVisits.pdf.

4. Simon, G.R., Baker, C., Barden, G.A. et al.; Committee on Practice and Ambulatory Medicine and Bright Futures Periodicity Schedule Workgroup. Recommendations for pediatric preventive health care. *Pediatrics*. 2016, **137**(1):1–3.

5. Centers for Disease Control and Prevention. Recommendations to prevent and control iron deficiency anemia in the United States. MMWR Morb Mortal Wkly Rep. 1998, 47:1–36.

6. United States Preventive Services Task Force. Iron Deficiency Anemia in Pregnant Women: Screening and Supplementation. Available at: www .uspreventiveservicestaskforce.org/Page/Document/ RecommendationStatementFinal/iron-deficiency-anemia-in-pregnant-women-screening-and-supplementation.

Osteoporosis

Anitra Beasley

Why Screen?

Osteoporosis is a common disease characterized by low bone mass, microarchitectural disruption and deterioration of bone tissue, and skeletal fragility that together result in an increased fracture risk, especially of the hip, spine, and wrist [a]. More than 8 million women in the United States older than 50 years have osteoporosis, and one half of all postmenopausal women will have an osteoporosis-related fracture during their lifetime [1,2 ['(b)']]. Osteoporotic fractures, particularly hip fractures, are associated with chronic pain and disability, loss of independence, decreased quality of life, and increased mortality [b]. Additionally, caring for these fractures is expensive. Direct care costs for osteoporotic fractures range from $12 to $18 billion annually, and indirect costs add greatly to this estimate [2].

Rationale for Screening

The goal of screening for osteoporosis is to identify women at increased risk of sustaining a fracture and who could benefit from intervention to minimize this risk. The World Health Organization (WHO) provides diagnostic thresholds for low bone mass and osteoporosis based upon bone mineral density (BMD) measurements in a young-adult female reference population (T-score). Normal bone density is defined as a value within 1 standard deviation (SD) of the reference population mean. A T-score 1–2.5 SD below the mean is termed low bone mass, formerly known as osteopenia, and a score that is 2.5 SD or more below the mean is osteoporosis [3]. Although women with T-scores of less than or equal to −2.5 have the highest risk of fracture, more fractures actually occur in patients with low bone mass as there are many more patients in this category [a]. The WHO diagnostic criteria for osteoporosis should not be applied to children or premenopausal women.

Bone mass in older adults is defined as the peak bone mass achieved by young adulthood minus the amount of bone subsequently lost. The process of bone remodeling maintains a healthy skeleton by continuously removing older bone and replacing it with new bone. Bone loss occurs when this balance is altered, resulting in greater bone removal than replacement. The substantial decline in estrogen levels at menopause causes a time-limited rapid bone loss in women. This bone loss leads to an increased risk of fracture that is magnified by other age-associated declines in functioning.

Bone measurement tests correlate with bone strength and predict short-term risk for osteoporotic fractures. Early diagnosis and quantification of bone loss and fracture risk are important because lifestyle modifications and available therapies can slow or reverse the progression of osteoporosis. A combination of fall prevention strategies, dietary and behavioral modifications, and pharmacologic therapy can treat osteoporosis and decrease the risk of fracture [a].

Factors That Affect Screening

Age: Age is one of the most important factors related to bone quality, and bone loss increases significantly with age [c]. The associated increased fracture risk is low in premenopausal and early menopausal women, and therefore major guidelines recommend against routine screening for osteoporosis in younger women without risk factors.

Other factors: Additional risk factors for low-trauma fracture include previous fragility fracture, medical causes of bone loss such as long-term glucocorticoid therapy or rheumatoid arthritis, low body weight, family history of hip fracture, current cigarette smoking, or excessive alcohol intake (Box 23.1).

Previous fragility fracture
Medical causes of bone loss
Low body weight
Family history of hip fracture
Current cigarette smoking
Excessive alcohol intake
Advanced age

Recommended Guidelines and How to Find Them

In the United States, there are no consensus guidelines governing screening for osteoporosis, and the WWTF did not include it in its review. However, major organizations and medical societies recommend screening for osteoporosis with BMD assessment in postmenopausal women starting at age 65 regardless of risk factors, and most, including the American College of Obstetrics and Gynecology (ACOG) and the US Preventive Services Task Force (USPSTF), recommend screening younger postmenopausal women with risk factors [a–c]. The USPSTF [c] specifically recommends "screening for osteoporosis in women aged 65 or older and in younger women whose fracture risk is equal to or greater than that of a 65-year-old white woman who has no additional risk factors." They note that there are a number of instruments to predict risk, and specifically used the Fracture Risk Assessment (FRAX) tool to make estimates. The 10-year risk of a 65-year-old white woman is 9.3 percent using this tool, and following USPSTF recommendations, screening should be done on postmenopausal women under age 65 with greater than 9.3 percent 10-year risk using this tool. The National Osteoporosis Foundation Guidelines [a] specifically recommend BMD measurements of the hip and spine with dual-energy x-ray absorptiometry (DXA) for screening, while the USPSTF and ACOG note that it is the generally used test.

How to Screen

Bone health should be addressed in all age groups, including puberty and adolescence, because of the effect of nutrition and lifestyle on bone health. Patients should be evaluated for reversible risk factors such as smoking, excessive alcohol consumption, and sedentary lifestyle, and appropriate counseling performed to attempt to modify these risks. Since the majority of osteoporosis-related fractures result from falls, it is also important to evaluate the risk of falling. Counseling should include fall prevention.

Major guidelines for women recommend BMD screening for osteoporosis in all women 65 years or older, and most recommend screening in younger postmenopausal women with an increased fracture risk [a–c]. Use of a formal tool to assess risk in menopausal women under age 65 should be incorporated into well-woman care. The WHO Fracture Risk Assessment (FRAX®) tool estimates the 10-year probability of a major osteoporotic fracture using easily obtainable clinical data and is one of the most widely used instruments to predict fracture risk (www.sheffield.ac.uk/FRAX). Women with greater than 9.3 percent 10-year fracture risk (the risk of a 65-year-old white woman without other risk factors) should be screened. Routine screening of a newly postmenopausal woman or a "baseline" screen is not recommended.

Multiple modalities are available and can be used for BMD screening. While DXA is the most commonly used bone measurement test in the United States, its high cost and lack of portability have led to the development of other techniques to measure peripheral sites. These include ultrasound, peripheral DXA (pDXA), radiograph absorptiometry, and peripheral quantitative computerized tomography (pQCT) of the heel, radius, or hand.

All available technologies measuring central and peripheral skeletal sites provide site-specific and global assessment of future fracture risk; however, DXA measurement at the hip is the best predictor of risk of future hip fracture [a]. Measurement of BMD using DXA has become the gold standard for the diagnosis of osteoporosis and for guiding decisions about which patients will benefit from therapy [b]. The WHO criteria for diagnosis of osteoporosis are based on BMD measured by DXA and, therefore, do not apply to the other technologies. Although peripheral sites such as the wrist and heel are predictive of osteoporosis and fractures, they cannot be used for monitoring treatment effects. Bone turnover markers have been used in clinical trials of osteoporosis therapies to demonstrate response to treatment; however, bone turnover markers cannot be used to diagnose osteoporosis, and the usefulness of markers as an incentive for adherence has been questioned [c].

Evidence is lacking about optimal timing of repeated screening and whether repeated screening is necessary in a woman with normal BMD. In the absence of an increased fracture risk, data from the Study of Osteoporotic Fractures suggests a screening interval of 15 years for a woman older than 65 years with normal BMD or mild bone loss (T-score greater than or equal to −1.5), a 5-year screening interval for a T-score from −1.5 to −1.99, and a 1 year screening interval for a T-score between −2.0 and −2.49 [4]. Because of limitations in the precision of testing, a minimum of 2 years may be necessary to improve fracture risk prediction [b].

New Developments Likely to Affect Future Recommendations

Further research that could inform clinical decisions about screening for osteoporosis is needed. Insufficient evidence exists with regard to treatment parameters for peripheral screening methods, the true incidence of major osteoporotic fractures in nonwhite ethnic groups in the United States, optimal screening intervals, and the effect of clinical and subclinical vertebral fractures on health-related quality of life [b]. An update to the USPSTF guidelines is in progress.

Billing

Screening for osteoporosis is covered under the ICD-10 code Z13.820. Several screening tests for osteoporosis are available. Medicare is the largest payer for osteoporosis; however, coverage guidelines vary by payer and plan type.

Illustrative Cases

A 49-year-old G2P2, recently menopausal woman presents for a scheduled well-woman visit and requests a "baseline scan" for her bones.

Major guidelines, including ACOG, recommend against screening women under 65 years of age without additional risk factors for osteoporosis. If her history, physical, or biochemical testing is concerning for a heightened risk of osteoporosis, FRAX® may be used to determine if she would benefit from BMD screening.

Screen now? No

Next screen: age 65 unless she develops additional risk factors for osteoporosis before then

A 23-year-old G0P0 presents for her well-woman visit. She read on the internet about risk to her bones from prolonged use of depot medroxyprogesterone acetate (DMPA). She has used DMPA for contraception since she was 19. She is satisfied with this method and is not interested in longer-acting methods, such as intrauterine devices (IUDs) or the implant.

While DMPA use is associated with loss of BMD, it is generally temporary and reversible. Increased fractures are not seen in current or former DMPA users. There is no indication for osteoporosis screening in long-term users of DMPA nor is there a reason to limit the duration of DMPA use.

Screen now? No

Guidelines

a. Cosman, F., de Beur, S.J., LeBoff, M.S. et al. Clinician's guide to prevention and treatment of osteoporosis. *Osteoporos Int.* 2014, 25(10):2359–81. Available at: http s://my.nof.org/bone-soruce/education/clinicians-guide-to-the-prevention-and-treatment-of-osteoporosis. Retrieved May 21, 2016.

b. American College of Obstetricians and Gynecologists. Osteoporosis. Practice Bulletin No. 129. *Obstet Gynecol.* 2012, 120:718–34. Available at: www.acog.org/Resourc es-And-Publications/ Practice-Bulletins-List (membership required). Retrieved May 21, 2016.

c. US Preventive Services Task Force. Screening for osteoporosis: US Preventive Services Task Force recommendation statement. *Ann Intern Med.* 2011, 154: 356–64. Available at: www .uspreventiveservicestaskforce.org/Page/Document/Up dateSummaryFinal/osteoporosis-screening. Retrieved May 21, 2016.

References

1. Wright, N.C., Looker, A.C., Saag, K.G. et al. The recent prevalence of osteoporosis and low bone mass in the United States based on bone mineral density at the femoral neck or lumbar spine. *J Bone Miner Res.* 2014, 29(11):2520–6

2. US Department of Health and Human Services. *Bone Health and Osteoporosis: A Report of the Surgeon General.* Rockville, MD: US Department of Health and Human Services, Office of the Surgeon General, 2004.

3. Kanis, J.A., McCloskey, E.V., Johansson, H., et al. A reference standard for the description of osteoporosis. Bone. 2008, 42(3):467–75.

4. Gourlay, M.L., Fine, J.P., Preisser, J.S. et al. Bone-density testing interval and transition to osteoporosis in older women. *N Engl J Med.* 2012, 366(3):225–33.

Diabetes

Janeen Arbuckle

Why Screen?

Diabetes affects 29.1 million people in the United States, 13.4 million of whom are women. The incidence of diabetes in the United States has more than tripled since the 1980s with 1.4 million new cases of diabetes diagnosed in 2014 alone [1]. Diabetes develops as a result of the body's inability to properly process glucose, resulting in hyperglycemia. Prolonged episodes of hyperglycemia cause microvascular complications such as retinopathy, nephropathy, and neuropathy, as well as macrovascular diseases such as stroke and coronary artery disease. In addition to the morbidity and mortality associated with diabetes, the direct and indirect cost of diabetes in the United States in 2012 was estimated to be $245 billion annually [2]. Individuals with diabetes incur annual medical expenses that are more than twice those without diabetes [2]. Because the progression of disease can be mitigated or halted by intervention, early diagnosis serves as an opportunity to educate the patient and enables them to take steps to alter the course of their disease.

Rationale for Screening

Diabetes is a metabolic derangement in the processing of blood glucose due to defective insulin secretion, impaired insulin action, or both. Type 1 diabetes accounts for 5–10 percent of cases of diabetes and is a consequence of the autoimmune destruction of the β cells of the pancreas and loss of endogenous insulin production. Diagnosis of type 1 diabetes requires the identification of one or more autoimmune markers such as islet cell antibodies [3].

Type 2 diabetes accounts for 90–95 percent of cases of diabetes and is due to insulin insensitivity at the tissue level. In diabetes, hyperglycemia exists along a continuum and progresses from normal blood glucose levels to diabetic range levels over a course of 10 or more years [4]. There is a curvilinear relationship between blood glucose levels and the development of diabetes, with a disproportionate increase in risk of diabetes with small increases in blood glucose levels [3]. Due to the fairly slow onset of diabetes, individuals are often asymptomatic in the early stages of the disease and therefore do not seek medical therapy. Unfortunately, the hyperglycemia present in the early, asymptomatic stages of diabetes is sufficient to cause pathologic changes at the tissue level [3].

Routine screening for type 2 diabetes allows for earlier detection of the disease, allowing for interventions that can possibly slow these destructive processes. A number of trials have demonstrated that improved glycemic control among individuals with diabetes reduces the microvascular complications associated with the disease [5]. Although the benefit of intensive glycemic control on cardiovascular disease is less clear, the greatest opportunity for cardiovascular disease reduction appears to be among those individuals with newly diagnosed diabetes [5], underscoring the benefit of early detection.

In addition to identifying individuals with diabetes, screening allows for the identification of individuals who are at an especially high risk of developing diabetes. Individuals with blood glucose levels that are too elevated to be deemed normal but not diagnostic for diabetes are considered to have prediabetes [3]. Individuals with prediabetes have values in an intermediate range (Table 24.1) and are at risk for the subsequent development of diabetes and cardiovascular disease [3,4]. Individuals with elevated but nondiagnostic values on a fasting blood glucose test or an oral glucose tolerance test (OGTT) are referred to as having impaired fasting glucose (IFG) and impaired glucose tolerance (IGT), respectively. These terms are considered synonymous with prediabetes and may be used interchangeably. A number of randomized controlled trials have demonstrated that intensive lifestyle modifications

Table 24.1 Test Results for Normal Glucose, Prediabetes, and Diabetes

Test	Normal Result	Prediabetes	Diabetes
Hemoglobin A1C (%)‡	<5.7	5.7–6.4	≥6.5
Fasting plasma glucose*			
mmol/L	<5.6	5.6–6.9	≥7.0
mg/dL	<100	100–125	≥126
2-hour glucose tolerance test (75 g load)			
mmol/L	< 7.8	7.8–11.0	≥11.1
mg/dL	<140	140–199	≥200
Random blood glucose†			
mmol/L			≥11.1
mg/dL			>200

* Fasting is defined as no caloric intake for ≥8 hours.

† Only applicable in patients with symptoms of hyperglycemia or in hyperglycemic crisis. Individuals with positive test results should have repeat testing on a different day to confirm the diagnosis.

‡ AACE supports similar testing modalities but uses a hemoglobin A1C ≥5.5 percent to identify individuals with prediabetes.
Source: Adapted from the ADA and USPSTF guidelines [3,4].

among patients with prediabetes can result in sustained reduction in the rate of development of diabetes [6]. Pharmaceutical interventions such as metformin have also been shown to reduce the rate of progression to diabetes among women with prediabetes and should be considered in women with a BMI >35 or those with worsening blood glucose levels despite lifestyle modification [6].

Factors That Affect Screening

Age: The prevalence of diabetes and IGT increases with age [7].

Race: Individuals of African American, Latino, Native American, Asian American, or Pacific Islander descent are at increased risk of type 2 diabetes.

Body mass index: Being overweight (BMI >25) is a risk factor for type 2 diabetes. Asian American populations are at risk for diabetes at lower body mass indices (BMI >23) [3].

History of gestational diabetes: Women with a history of gestational diabetes are seven times more likely to develop diabetes than women without this history [8]. Approximately 35–60 percent of women with a history of gestational diabetes will develop diabetes within 10 years of their pregnancy [9]. (Women with a history of gestational diabetes are discussed in detail in the chapter on *Postpartum Screening of Gestational Diabetics*.)

Prediabetes: Individuals with impaired fasting blood glucose, IGT, or a hemoglobin A1C in the prediabetes range are at especially high risk for development of diabetes, with 15–30 percent of individuals with prediabetes progressing to diabetes within 5 years [4].

Comorbid conditions: Women with hypertension or hyperlipidemia are at increased risk for cardiovascular disease.

Polycystic ovarian syndrome (PCOS): Women with PCOS have a two- to five-fold increased risk of developing diabetes [10].

Family history: There is a familial component to type 2 diabetes, although the genetics and inheritance patterns are poorly understood. Those women with first-degree relatives with type 2 diabetes are at increased risk. Although there appears to be a genetic component to type 1 diabetes, it is not well characterized and does not appear to be associated with a significant increased risk in family members.

Recommended Guidelines and How to Find Them

The Well-Woman Task Force (WWTF) recommends screening for diabetes every 3 years beginning at age 45 or earlier for those with risk factors for diabetes. Screening for adolescents aged 13–18 is not recommended except for those who are obese, defined as a BMI of 30 or higher.

The WWTF recommendations are largely derived from the American Diabetes Association (ADA) recommendations. The ADA recommends:

- Testing to assess risk for future diabetes in asymptomatic people should be considered in adults of any age who are overweight or obese (BMI ≥25 kg/m^2 or ≥23 kg/m^2 in Asian Americans) and who have one or more additional risk factors for diabetes.
- For all patients, testing should begin at age 45.
- If tests are normal, repeat testing carried out at a minimum of 3-year intervals is reasonable.
- To test for prediabetes, fasting plasma glucose, 2-hour plasma glucose after 75-g OGTT, and A1C are equally appropriate.
- In patients with prediabetes, identify and, if appropriate, treat other cardiovascular disease risk factors.
- Testing to detect prediabetes should be considered in children and adolescents who are overweight or obese and who have two or more additional risk factors for diabetes.

The ADA recommends with prediabetes should be screened annually [a]. The ADA has developed a mobile application, ADA Standards of Care, available as a free electronic download (http://professional.diabetes.org/content/standards-care-app).

The American Association of Clinical Endocrinologists (AACE) and American College of Endocrinology (ACE) revised their recommendations after the Task Force convened, and now endorse screening by age 45 or earlier if one or more risk factors are present. The AACE/ACE support screening every 3 years with a consideration for screening annually in those with two or more risk factors [b].

The US Preventive Services Task Force (USPSTF) also updated their guidelines, which are more restrictive. They recommend "screening for abnormal blood glucose as part of cardiovascular risk assessment in adults aged 40 to 70 years who are overweight or obese. Clinicians should offer or refer patients with abnormal blood glucose to intensive behavioral counseling interventions to promote a healthful diet and physical activity." They noted that while there was limited evidence for the appropriate screening interval, rescreening every 3 years was reasonable, and that clinicians could consider earlier screening in persons with one or more risk factor [c].

The Centers for Disease Control and Prevention helps maintain the National Diabetes Prevention Program and the National Diabetes Education Program. A number of resources can be accessed through their website: www.cdc.gov/diabetes/prevention/.

How to Screen

Screening of individuals at average risk for diabetes should begin at age 45. Screening for diabetes risk factors and measurement of BMI should be routine parts of well-woman care. For women with additional risk factors, screening should begin earlier and be repeated every 3 years. Both the USPSTF (Box 24.1) and the ADA (Box 24.2) have recommendations for risk factor criteria for early screening. Screening in children and adolescents aged 13–18 should be performed in those individuals who are obese (BMI >30).

The WWTF recommendations do not specify which diagnostic tools and thresholds should be used for screening for diabetes. The ADA, USPSTF, and AACE/ACE support the use of any one of the four tests for screening (Table 24.1). Options include a fasting plasma glucose level, a 2-hour OGTT, or a hemoglobin A1C level. The 2-hour OGTT involves a fasting plasma glucose level followed by a repeat measurement, 2 hours after a 75-g oral glucose challenge. A random blood glucose level can also be used to identify diabetes among women with classic symptoms of hyperglycemia (e.g., polydipsia and polyuria) or those with hyperglycemic crisis (e.g., diabetic ketoacidosis). In asymptomatic women, an abnormal result should be confirmed on repeat testing, ideally using the same test, on a subsequent date. The decision with regards to which screening test should be individualized and consider cost, feasibility, and convenience [a, c].

Rescreening of women with normal tests who remain at risk should be done at 3-year intervals. The ADA supports annual screening for diabetes in those individuals with prediabetes [a].

BOX 24.1 Potential Indications for Early Screening – USPSTF

- Family history of type 2 diabetes
- History of gestational diabetes
- History of PCOS
- High-risk racial/ethnic group (African American, American Indian or Alaskan Native, Hispanics or Latinos, or Native Hawaiians or Pacific Islanders)

Source: Siu, A.L. Screening for abnormal blood glucose and type 2 diabetes mellitus: US Preventive Services Task Force recommendation statement. *Ann Intern Med.* 2015, 163:861–8.

BOX 24.2 Additional Risk Factors for Testing in Asymptomatic Overweight* Adults – ADA

- Physical inactivity
- First-degree relative with diabetes
- High-risk race/ethnicity (e.g., African American, Latino, Native American, Asian American, Pacific Islander)
- Delivered a baby weighing >9 lb or were diagnosed with gestational diabetes
- Hypertension (≥140/90 or on therapy for hypertension)
- HDL cholesterol level <35 mg/dL and/or triglyceride level >250 mg/dL
- PCOS
- Hemoglobin A1C ≥5.7% or IFG or GT on prior testing
- Other conditions associated with insulin resistance (e.g., severe obesity, acanthosis nigricans)
- HDL: high-density lipoprotein
  *BMI >=25 kg/m^2 or >= 23 kg/m^2 in Asian Americans

Source: Adapted from Table 24.2 in reference [3]

New Developments Likely to Affect Future Guidelines

Although a number of studies have shown the benefits of lifestyle modification and pharmacotherapy on preventing or delaying the progression of prediabetes to diabetes, to date, there have been no studies showing screening impacts on mortality rates or cardiovascular disease-related morbidity [4]. Trials conducted to date have been limited to 10-year follow-up. Additional studies with longer follow-up periods will provide further insight into the potential benefits and harms of screening and may lead to changes in recommendations for screening or intervals for repeat testing.

Billing

Diabetes screening is typically covered under CPT codes 82947 or 83036 with diagnosis code Z13.1, encounter for screening for diabetes mellitus.

Illustrative Cases

An 18-year-old African American female presents for a well-adolescent visit. She reports menarche at age 13 and infrequent periods occurring every 3–6 months. Her BMI is 34.

This patient's clinical history is worrisome for PCOS. In addition to the diagnostic evaluation of her abnormal uterine bleeding, screening for diabetes is recommended given her obesity. This patient's race is also a risk factor for diabetes, further supporting screening.

Screen now? Yes

Next screening: If the patient has a normal result and her risk factors are still present, she should have repeat testing in 3 years. If she is diagnosed with prediabetes, she should have repeat testing in 1 year.

A healthy 46-year-old Caucasian female presents for her annual well-woman visit. She is of normal weight and her vital signs are normal. She has no symptoms, but has not seen a health care provider since her last child was born 8 years ago.

In addition to her other health care needs, this patient is due for screening for diabetes. Diabetes is commonly asymptomatic and screening should begin at age 45, regardless of risk factors.

Screen now? Yes

Next screen: If her screen is normal, it should be repeated in 3 years. If she is diagnosed with prediabetes, she should have repeat testing in 1 year.

A healthy 25-year-old Caucasian female G0 presents for her annual well-woman visit. She is considering pursuing pregnancy in the coming year and wants to be assured that she is healthy enough to do so. She has regular, predictable cycles and denies any significant medical problems. Her family history is notable for hypertension in her grandmother but is otherwise negative. Her BMI is 22.

Screening asymptomatic women without risk factors for diabetes is not indicated until age 45. This patient's overall health, race, current BMI, and negative family history make her risk of diabetes low.

Screen now? No

Next screen: Age 45 or with the onset of risk factors for diabetes

A 33-year-old healthy Caucasian female presents for her annual well-woman visit. She notes a recent diagnosis of type 1 diabetes in her 9-year-old daughter and questions whether she and her other children should be screened. She is asymptomatic, has normal vital signs and a BMI of 19. No other family members have diabetes.

Routine screening for type 1 diabetes is not recommended outside of participation in a research trial. Given her current health and age, screening for type 2 diabetes is not recommended.

Screen now? No

Next screen: Age 45 or with the onset of risk factors for diabetes

A 38-year-old African American female presents for her annual well-woman visit. She has a history of hypertension which is currently well controlled on a calcium-channel blocker. She is asymptomatic, but is concerned about her weight which has increased by 15 pounds since her annual examination last year. Her BMI is 27.

This patient has multiple risk factors for diabetes including her race, history of hypertension, and being overweight.

Screen now? Yes

Next screen: If her test is normal, it should be repeated in 3 years. If she is diagnosed with prediabetes, she should have repeat testing in 1 year.

A 31-year-old Native American female presents for her well-woman visit. She has been followed in your practice for a personal history of PCOS and had an elevated hemoglobin A1C of 5.9 at her examination last year. She was referred to a nutritionist and has since begun exercising three times weekly.

Women with a history of PCOS are at increased risk of diabetes and warrant screening at an earlier age. This patient has previously diagnosed prediabetes. Women with prediabetes should be screened annually for the development of diabetes. This woman has implemented lifestyle changes which have been shown to prevent or delay progression of prediabetes to diabetes. If her testing remains consistent with prediabetes, then the addition of metformin should be considered.

Screen now? Yes

Next screen: 1 year

A 39-year-old obese Caucasian female presents for her annual well-woman visit. She reports increased thirst and hunger. Despite her increased appetite, she has noticed an unintentional 5-pound weight loss.

Screening for diabetes is recommended for symptomatic individuals. This patient reports polydipsia and polyphagia, common complaints among individuals with diabetes. This patient may be screened with a fasting blood glucose, a glucose tolerance test, a hemoglobin A1C, or a random blood glucose value. A random blood glucose of >200 mg/dL is sufficient to confirm the diagnosis of diabetes in symptomatic individuals.

Screen now? Yes

Guidelines

a. American Diabetes Association. Classification and diagnosis of diabetes. *Diabetes Care*. 2016, 39:S13–S22.

b. Handelsman, Y. et al. American Association of Clinical Endocrinologists and American College of Endocrinology – Clinical practice guidelines for developing a diabetes mellitus comprehensive care plan – 2015. *Endocr Pract*. 2015, 21(Suppl 1):1–87.

c. Siu, A.L. Screening for abnormal blood glucose and type 2 diabetes mellitus: US Preventive Services Task Force recommendation statement. *Ann Intern Med*. 2015, **163**:861–8.

References

1. Centers for Disease Control and Prevention. *National Diabetes Statistics Report: Estimates of Diabetes and Its Burden in the United States, 2014.* Atlanta, GA: US Department of Health and Human Services, 2014.

2. American Diabetes Association. Economic costs of diabetes in the US in 2012. *Diabetes Care.* 2013, **36:** 1033–46.

3. American Diabetes Association. 2. Classification and diagnosis of diabetes. *Diabetes Care.* 2016, **39:**S13–22.

4. Siu A.L. Screening for abnormal blood glucose and type 2 diabetes mellitus: US Preventive Services Task Force recommendation statement. *Ann Intern Med.* 2015, **163:**861–8.

5. American Diabetes Association. 5. Glycemic targets. *Diabetes Care.* 2016, **39:**S39–46.

6. American Diabetes Association. 4. Prevention or delay of type 2 diabetes. *Diabetes Care.* 2016, **39:**S36–8.

7. The DECODE Study Group. Age- and sex-specific prevalences of diabetes and impaired glucose regulation in 13 European cohorts. *Diabetes Care.* 2003, **26:**61–9.

8. American College of Obstetricians and Gynecologists. Gestational diabetes mellitus. ACOG Practice Bulletin No. 137. *Obstet Gynecol.* 2013, **122:**406–16.

9. Metzger, B.E., Buchanan, T.A., Coustan, D.R. et al. Summary and recommendations of the Fifth International Workshop-Conference on Gestational Diabetes Mellitus. *Diabetes Care.* 2007, **30:** S251–60.

10. American College of Obstetricians and Gynecologists. Polycystic ovary syndrome. ACOG Practice Bulletin No. 108. *Obstet Gynecol.* 2009, **114:**936–49.

Hypothyroidism Screening

Bryan K. Rone

Why Screen?

Hypothyroidism, defined by an elevation of serum thyroid-stimulating hormone (TSH) with a decrease in serum-free thyroxine (T4), and subclinical hypothyroidism, defined by an elevation of serum TSH with a normal serum T4, are well-known medical conditions. According to the US National Health and Nutrition Examination Survey (NHANES III) [1], 5.8 percent of women had either overt or subclinical hypothyroidism. Hypothyroidism has a wide range of clinical manifestations affecting almost every body system (Table 25.1), and can cause significant morbidity. Reproductive effects include infertility, miscarriage, and poor pregnancy outcomes [a].

Rationale for Screening

Hypothyroidism is common and easy to diagnose with safe and inexpensive serum laboratory tests. It is relatively easy to treat with oral thyroid replacement and clinical manifestations resolve with treatment. Given these characteristics, hypothyroidism seems very amenable to screening. However, for population screening to be effective, early diagnosis and treatment should have measurable positive impact to the patient or society. Unfortunately, there are no studies showing early detection and treatment of hypothyroidism fulfills this requirement [b]. A decision analysis showed that while hypothyroid screening had similar cost-effectiveness to other diseases where screening is generally accepted, there was no impact on the primary outcome, measurement of quality-adjusted life years [2].

Observational studies have suggested that untreated subclinical hypothyroidism in pregnancy is associated with impaired cognitive development. Screening women in their reproductive years or prior to pregnancy seems reasonable; however, two randomized trials [3,4] did not show improvement in cognitive outcomes with early pregnancy thyroid

screening and initiation of thyroid replacement, arguing against routine screening during or prior to pregnancy.

Screening women at higher than average risk is an alternative screening methodology. The well-woman visit is an opportunity to assess clinical symptoms and diagnoses associated with hypothyroidism and screen if present.

Factors That Affect Screening

Signs and symptoms: Hypothyroidism is associated with many clinical signs and symptoms such as constipation, fatigue, weight gain, and menstrual irregularities. Table 25.2 lists common signs and symptoms that should prompt consideration of screening.

Conditions with high association with hypothyroidism: Hypothyroidism is associated with a number of other medical problems, prior treatments, and medications (Table 25.3).

Recommended Guidelines and How to Find Them

In 2012, the American Association of Clinical Endocrinologists (AACE) and the American Thyroid Association (ATA) [a] published joint clinical practice guidelines for hypothyroidism in adults. They acknowledged a lack of consensus regarding universal population screening among medical societies. They advocate screening when a woman's medical diagnoses, surgical history, or medication history (Table 25.3) include conditions that place her at a higher risk of hypothyroidism. In 2015, the US Preventive Services Task Force (USPSTF) [b] published a clinical guideline stating that the current evidence is insufficient to assess the balance of benefits and harms of screening for thyroid dysfunction in nonpregnant, asymptomatic adults. The American Academy of Family Physicians adopted these guidelines. The Well-Woman Task Force (WWTF) [c]

Table 25.1 Clinical Manifestations of Hypothyroidism by Body System

Body System	Clinical Manifestations of Hypothyroidism
General	Fatigue Weight gain Depressed mood
Skin	Dry skin Edema Cold sensitivity Alopecia
Cardiovascular	Reduced exercise capacity Hypertension Hypercholesterolemia
Respiratory	Shortness of breath on exertion Sleep apnea
Gastrointestinal	Decreased taste sensation Constipation
Neurologic	Carpal tunnel syndrome Slowed autonomic reflexes
Musculoskeletal	Joint pain Muscle pain
Renal	Hyponatremia Renal insufficiency Hyperhomocysteinemia
Reproductive	Menstrual irregularities Infertility Decreased libido
Hematologic	Hypocoagulable state Anemia

Source: References [a, 5]

Table 25.2 Common Manifestations of Hypothyroidism

	ICD-10 Code
Menstrual irregularities	N92.6
Infertility	N97.9
Decreased libido	R68.82
Fatigue	R53.83
Weight gain	R63.5
Depressed mood	F32.9
Dry skin	L85.3
Edema	R60.1
Cold sensitivity	R68.89*
Alopecia	L65.9
Reduced exercise capacity	R68.89*
Shortness of breath on exertion	R06.02
Decreased taste sensation	R43.2
Constipation	K59.00

* R68.89 is a code for other general symptoms when no other unique code exists
Source: References [a, 5]

also reveal clinical symptoms or examination findings that are associated with hypothyroidism (Tables 25.1–25.3). Women with signs or symptoms or conditions with high association should have screening performed with measurement of serum TSH.

combined these guidelines in their final recommendations. The WWTF does not recommend universal screening for women at low risk for hypothyroidism or women who are pregnant or currently planning a pregnancy. They do support screening for hypothyroidism based on the signs, symptoms, and disease processes that are associated with hypothyroidism (Tables 25.2 and 25.3).

How to Screen

Risk assessment should be performed during the well-woman visit. Providers should review the patient's medical and surgical history for diagnoses that place her at risk of hypothyroidism (Table 25.3). A complete review of systems and physical examination may

New Developments Likely to Affect Future Guidelines

Subclinical hypothyroidism is more common than overt hypothyroidism, and there are a number of important gaps in knowledge. Treatment studies comparing the natural course of untreated subclinical hypothyroidism with treatment of asymptomatic patients could find important health outcome differences within the groups. Improvements in outcomes such as cardiovascular health, cognitive function, bone health, cancer risk, quality of life, and reproductive outcomes could provide evidence that population screening provides benefit [b].

Leveraging electronic health records is a novel approach to population screening. The ICD-10 codes associated with a high risk of hypothyroidism (Tables 25.2 and 25.3) could be used to identify women who might benefit from screening.

Table 25.3 Conditions, Diagnoses, and Symptoms That Should Prompt Screening for Hypothyroidism

Hypothyroidism screening is suggested for women with the following conditions that have a high association with hypothyroidism.	ICD-10 Codes
Type 1 diabetes	E10.9
Pernicious anemia	D51.0
Autoimmune thyroid disease in a first-degree relative	Z83.49
History of radiation to the thyroid gland, head, or neck; radioactive iodine therapy	Z51.0
History of thyroid surgery or thyroid dysfunction	E07.9
Abnormal thyroid examination	E04.9
Psychiatric disorders	
Use of amiodarone or lithium	
Hypothyroidism screening is also suggested for women with the following diagnoses or symptoms that may have an association with hypothyroidism.	
Adrenal insufficiency	E27.40
Alopecia	L63.0
Anemia	D64.9
Cardiac dysrhythmia	I49.9
Changes in skin texture	R23.4
Congestive heart failure	I50.9
Constipation	K59.00
Dementia	F03.90
Dysmenorrhea	N94.6
Hypercholesterolemia and/or mixed hyperlipidemia	E78.5
Hypertension	I10
Fatigue and malaise	R53.81
Prolonged QT interval	I45.81
Vitiligo	L80
Weight gain	R63.5

Source: References [a, c].

Billing

Hypothyroid screening may be performed as part of a preventive health encounter or during a problem-based visit. As screening is based on symptom or risk factor, providers should use the appropriate evaluation and management CPT code and ICD-10 code corresponding to the risk factor or symptom (Tables 25.1–25.3).

Illustrative Cases

A 21–year-old female presents for a well-woman visit. She is sexually active. She denies any medical problems, *previous surgeries, or significant family history. Her body mass index (BMI) is 23. Her review of systems is negative and her physical examination is normal.*

She does not have any symptoms or any history that would make her high risk. Screening is not recommended for asymptomatic low-risk women.

Screen now: No

Next screen: No routine screening for hypothyroidism is recommended. She should have regular medical history updates and review of systems at her well-woman visits, with screening if she becomes symptomatic or high risk.

A 60-year-old female presents for a well-woman visit. During the review of systems, she reports fatigue, pain with movement, and feeling cold. Her BMI is 32. Her blood pressure is 148/96. On examination, her skin is very dry and she has new lower extremity edema.

Her symptoms are consistent with hypothyroidism. Women over 50 have higher prevalence of hypothyroidism than other patient populations. Screening is recommended in symptomatic women.

Screen now: Yes

Next screen: Disease management if hypothyroidism is confirmed. If symptoms are not from hypothyroidism, she should have routine symptom and risk assessment at future well-woman visits.

A 45-year-old female presents for a well-woman visit. She is currently using an intrauterine device for contraception. When she was 35 years old, she was treated for Hodgkin's lymphoma with chemotherapy and chest/neck radiation. She denies any surgeries. Her review of systems is negative. Her BMI is 28. Her physical examination is normal.

Her medical history is significant for Hodgkin's lymphoma that was treated with chemotherapy and chest/neck radiation. The thyroid gland is very sensitive to radiation exposure. Prior head/neck radiation exposure makes her high risk (Table 25.2).

Screen now: Yes

Next screen: The patient's high risk factor for hypothyroidism will not change over time. She will need periodic rescreening.

Guidelines

a. Garber, J.R., Cobin, R.H., Gharib, H. et al. Clinical practice guidelines for hypothyroidism in adults: Cosponsored by the American Association of Clinical Endocrinologists and the American Thyroid Association. *Endocr Pract.* 2012, **18**(6):988–1028.

b. LeFevre, M.L. and US Preventive Services Task Force. Screening for thyroid dysfunction: US Preventive Services Task Force recommendation statement. *Ann Intern Med.* 2015, **162**(9):641–50.

c. Conry, J.A. and Brown, H. Well-Woman Task Force: Components of the Well-Woman Visit. *Obstet Gynecol.* 2015, **126**(4):697–701.

References

1. Hollowell, J.G., Staehling, N.W., Flanders, W.D. et al. Serum TSH, T(4), and thyroid antibodies in the United States population (1988 to 1994): National Health and Nutrition Examination Survey (NHANES III). *J Clin Endocrinol Metab.* 2002, **87**(2):489–99.

2. Danese, M.D., Powe, N.R., Sawin, C.T., and Ladenson, P.W. Screening for mild thyroid failure at the periodic health examination: A decision and cost-effectiveness analysis. *JAMA.* 1996, **276**(4):285–92.

3. Negro R., Schwartz A., Gismondi R., et al. Universal screening versus case finding for detection and treatment of thyroid hormonal dysfunction during pregnancy. *J Clin Endocrinol Metab.* 2010, **95**(4):1699–707.

4. Lazarus, J.H., Bestwick, J.P., Channon, S. et al. Antenatal thyroid screening and childhood cognitive function. *N Engl J Med.* 2012, **366**(6):493–501.

5. El-Shafie, K.T. Clinical presentation of hypothyroidism. *J Fam Community Med.* 2003, **10**(1):55–8.

Chapter

26

Kidney Disease

Julie Zemaitis DeCesare

Why Screen?

Chronic kidney disease (CKD) affects 1 in 10 adults in the United States. In 2010, the United States spent approximately 33 billion dollars annually, 6.3 percent of the Medicare budget, on the treatment of chronic and end-stage renal disease [1]. The two most common risk factors for CKD are diabetes and hypertension. These diseases are present in two-thirds of women with CKD. Early detection of CKD and control of comorbidities can potentially prevent and decrease end-stage renal disease and dialysis [2].

Rationale for Screening

CKD causes serious morbidity and mortality. It is typically asymptomatic until very advanced. If early intervention improved long-term outcome, screening to detect early disease would be very important. Unfortunately, studies supporting universal screening for CKD do not exist. Two systematic reviews [3,4] found no randomized controlled trials of screening. CKD is rare in patients without hypertension and diabetes [a], so screening asymptomatic patients without risk factors would likely be very low yield. There is the possibility of false positives in screening low-risk populations, so there is the potential for harm. Potential CKD treatments may be started for other CKD-related conditions [3] further diluting potential benefits from screening.

Factors That Affect Screening

Nonmodifiable Risk Factors

Age: CKD progresses and accelerates with age.

Race: African Americans are 3.5 times and Hispanics are 1.5 times more likely to develop end-stage kidney disease compared to Caucasians.

Gender: Female sex appears to be protective, as women are 50 percent less likely than men to develop end-stage kidney disease.

Modifiable Risk Factors

Obesity: According to the National Health and Nutrition Examination Survey (NHANES) 2011–2012 data, 65.8% of all women are overweight, 36.1% are obese, and 8.3% are morbidly obese. Obesity is a known risk factor for CKD. It is unclear if the obesity causes CKD or is just associated with other risk factors such as hypertension, diabetes, and proteinuria.

Glycemic control: Optimization of glycemic control can minimize the progression of CKD in diabetic patients.

Hypertension: Strict control of hypertension can prevent progression of CKD. If initiated early, two antihypertensive drug classes, angiotensin-converting enzyme inhibitors and angiotensin receptor blockers, appear to slow progression of renal disease [5].

Caffeine: Excessive caffeine consumption may be harmful to the kidneys and may promote progression of CKD.

Alcohol: Excessive consumption of alcohol is a risk factor. However, a moderate amount of alcohol consumption may be protective (1–2 glasses of wine per day) [6].

Proteinuria: Higher amounts of proteinuria (>3 g per 24-hour urine) are a known prognostic indicator for rapid progression of CKD.

NSAID exposure: Chronic nonsteroidal antiinflammatory drug (NSAID) users have a 1.18-fold increased risk of CKD. This effect is even more pronounced in patients who have baseline hypertension, and these two factors combined are associated with a 1.32-fold increased risk of CKD [7].

Smoking: Tobacco consumption increases the risk of progression from CKD to end-stage renal disease.

Hyperlipidemia: Elevated lipid profile is associated with higher rates of CKD.

Lupus: Almost half of all patients with lupus develop lupus nephritis, which in turn develops CKD [8].

Recommended Guidelines and How to Find Them

The American College for Obstetrics and Gynecologists (ACOG) Well-Woman Task Force guidelines support the recommendations of the US Preventive Services Task Force (USPSTF) [a], who found that there was insufficient evidence for routine screening in asymptomatic adults. The American College of Physicians (ACP) and the National Kidney Foundation (NKF) [b, c] recommendations are slightly different in that they separate out adults with risk factors. The ACP [c] recommends against screening asymptomatic adults without risk factors and the NKF [b] recommends screening at-risk individuals aged 18 and older, where risks include diabetes, hypertension, and family history of kidney disease. The American Society of Nephrology disagrees and recommends screening in the absence of risk factors [d]. Further useful information can be found at the CDC provider online surveillance project for CKD, which outlines latest recommendations and options for providers and patents. This resource can be accessed at https://nccd.cdc.gov/ckd/. Useful patient education can be accessed at www.cdc.gov/diabetes/pubs/pdf/kidney_factsheet.pdf.

How to Screen

Routine screening for CKD in not recommended in asymptomatic adults by the Well-Woman Task Force (WWTF) or USPSTF. Some providers may choose to follow the ACP or NKF guidelines, which include screening adults with risk factors for CKD such as diabetes, hypertension, and family history of kidney disease. Monitoring for CKD is part of chronic disease management of diabetes and hypertension. In these patients, testing involves assessment of creatinine derived estimates of glomerular filtration rate (GFR) and urine testing for albumin. CKD is typically a progressive disease. When impaired renal function is diagnosed or suspected, referral to an appropriate specialist is indicated.

New Developments Likely to Affect Future Recommendations

Current USPSTF recommendations are based on "insufficient evidence to balance benefits and harms." Obtaining evidence on benefits of early detection and management of CKD in asymptomatic adults could lead to guideline changes. As new treatments like targeted biologicals or bone marrow or stem cell transplantation to repair injured renal tubules becomes clinically available, early screening may be indicated to allow early intervention to slow or reverse the damage in CKD [2,8].

Billing

Screening for CKD is not billable separate from the well-women visit. Specific ICD-10 codes for CKD include N18.1 Chronic kidney disease, stage 1, N18.2 Chronic kidney disease, stage 2 (mild), N18.3 Chronic kidney disease, stage 3 (moderate), N18.4 Chronic kidney disease, stage 4 (severe), N18.5 Chronic kidney disease, stage 5, N18.6 End stage renal disease, N18.9 Chronic kidney disease, unspecified.

Illustrative Cases

A 50-year-old woman presents for a well-woman visit. She is without complaints. She has no other significant medical problems and no significant family history.

Screen now: No

Next screen: Screening not indicated in absence of symptoms. Screening may become relevant as part of chronic medical conditions that she may acquire over time.

A 33-year-old Caucasian G3P0303 woman presents for an annual well-women visit. She has a history of type 1 diabetes diagnosed at age 11 and chronic hypertension. Her blood pressure (BP) in the office today was 150/100. She is currently taking nifedipine for BP control. She had proteinuria during her last pregnancy 3 years ago.

Monitoring as part of chronic disease management of diabetes and chronic hypertension includes screening for CKD. Appropriate labs include HgbA1C, estimated glomerular filtration rate (eGFR), and a spot urine albumin-to-creatinine ratio (UACR). The UACR confirms the earlier history of proteinuria, so she needs to be counseled about the presence of CKD and referred to a renal specialist. She should also receive counseling about strict glycemic control, with a target HgbA1C <6.5. As her BP is not optimally controlled, further intervention is warranted after referral to a nephrologist.

Screen now? Yes

Next screen: Screening is no longer appropriate. She needs monitoring of renal function and management by an appropriate specialist.

Guidelines

a. Moyer, V.A. Screening for chronic kidney disease: US Preventive Services Task Force recommendation statement. US Preventive Services Task Force. *Ann Intern Med.* 2012, **157**:567–70.

b. National Kidney Foundation. K/DOQI clinical practice guidelines for chronic kidney disease: Evaluation, classification, and stratification. *Am J Kidney Dis.* 2002, **39**:S1–266.

c. Qaseem, A., Hopkins, R.H., Sweet, D.E., Starkey, M., and Shekelle, P. Screening, monitoring, and treatment of stage 1 to 3 chronic kidney disease: A clinical practice guideline from the American College of Physicians. Clinical Guidelines Committee of the American College of Physicians. *Ann Intern Med.* 2013, **159**:835–47.

d. ASN disagrees with new guidelines, says adults should be screened for kidney disease [press release]. *Nephrol News Issues* [electronic], 2013. Available at: www.nephrologynews.com/articles/109817-asn-disagrees-with-new-guidelines-says-adults-should-be-screened-for-kidney-disease. Retrieved December 23, 2015.

References

1. United States Renal Data System. *Annual Data Report: Epidemiology of Kidney Disease in the United States.* Bethesda, MD: National Institutes of Health, National Institute of Diabetes and Digestive and Kidney Diseases, 2014.

2. Meguid, A., El Nahas, B., and Aminu, K. Chronic kidney disease: The global challenge. *Lancet.* 2005, **365**(9456): 331–40.

3. Fink, H.A., Ishani, A., Taylor, B.C. et al. *Chronic Kidney Disease Stages 1–3: Screening, Monitoring, and Treatment.* Comparative Effectiveness Review 37. AHRQ Publication 11(12)-EHC075-EF. Rockville, MD: Agency for Healthcare Research and Quality, 2012.

4. Fink, H.A., Ishani, A., Taylor, B.C. et al. Screening for, monitoring, and treatment of chronic kidney disease stages 1 to 3: A systematic review for the US Preventive Services Task Force and for an American College of Physicians Clinical Practice Guideline. *Ann Intern Med.* 2012, **156**:570–81.

5. Ward, F., Holian, J., and Murray, P. Drug therapies to delay the progression of chronic kidney disease. *Clin Med.* 2015, **15**(6):550–7.

6. Sato, K., Hayashi, T., Uehara, S. et al. Drinking pattern and risk of chronic kidney disease: The Kansai Healthcare Study. *Am J Nephrol.* 2014, **40**(6):516–22.

7. Wang, H., Hsu, Y.H., Chuang, S.Y. et al. Use of nonsteroidal anti-inflammatory drugs and risk of chronic kidney disease in subjects with hypertension: Nationwide Longitudinal Cohort Study. *Hypertension.* 2015, **66**(3):524–33.

8. Rovin, B. and Parikh, S. Lupus nephritis: The evolving role of novel therapeutics. *Am J Kidney Dis.* 2014, **63**(4):677–90.

Chapter 27

Bacteriuria

Lauren E. Nelson

Why Screen?

Asymptomatic bacteriuria is the presence of bacteria in the urine of a woman not complaining of symptoms concerning for a urinary tract infection (UTI). The Well-Woman Task Force (WWTF) recommends against screening for asymptomatic bacteriuria in the nonpregnant population [a]. Bacteriuria is a common finding in healthy female patients and increases with age, sexual activity, and genitourinary abnormalities [b]. Bacteriuria is present in about 1 percent of girls less than 14 years of age and increases to approximately 20 percent in women greater than 80 years of age [1]. Screening for bacteria in the urine of asymptomatic patients has not shown improvement in the outcomes. Some evidence for harm resulting from the treatment of asymptomatic bacteriuria has been demonstrated [b].

Rationale for Screening

Despite the relatively common finding of asymptomatic bacteriuria, studies have not shown any related long-term adverse outcomes and treatment has not been shown to decrease rates of UTI [c]. A Swedish study followed 1,462 women aged 38–60 with asymptomatic bacteriuria for 24 years. No difference in mortality or progression to chronic kidney disease was found when compared with a nonbacteriuric population [2]. Additionally, a randomized controlled trial (RCT) demonstrated that women who were treated with an antibiotic course for bacteriuria had a higher rate of *Escherichia coli* with resistance to amoxicillin-clavulanic acid, trimethoprim-sulfamethoxazole, and ciprofloxacin [3]. A Cochrane Review in 2015 of nine RCTs comparing antibiotic treatment versus placebo or no treatment of asymptomatic bacteriuria showed that while antibiotic treatment was superior in achieving bacteriological cure, there was no difference in the rate of developing

a symptomatic UTI. However, the antibiotic treatment groups showed a significantly higher rate of adverse events, leading the authors to conclude that there is no clinical benefit to treating asymptomatic bacteriuria [4].

Factors That May Affect Screening

Pregnancy: Many professional organizations including the American College of Obstetricians and Gynecologists (ACOG) recommend screening for asymptomatic bacteriuria in the first trimester [d]. Unlike asymptomatic nonpregnant patients, treatment of bacteriuria in the pregnant population has been shown to decrease the incidence of pyelonephritis, preterm delivery, and low-birth-weight infants [b].

Patients with diabetes: Both the American Academy of Family Physicians (AAFP) and the IDSA recommend against screening for or treating asymptomatic bacteriuria in women with diabetes [b, c]. Studies of women with diabetes have not shown a difference in incidence of UTI, mortality, or progression to diabetic complications in patients with asymptomatic bacteriuria when compared to nonbacteriuric patients [5].

Older patients: The IDSA does not recommend screening for asymptomatic bacteruria in older adults [c]. Studies have shown similar outcomes regardless of age when evaluating the sequelae of treating asymptomatic bacteriuria [b].

Patients with spinal cord injuries: Patients with spinal cord injuries have a higher rate of both asymptomatic bacteriuria and UTI [b]. Limited data are available on treating asymptomatic bacteriuria in this population. However, the IDSA recommends against screening and treatment of asymptomatic bacteriuria, as bacteriuria is common in patients with spinal cord injuries and treatment did not confer long-term cure [c]. A study evaluating the treatment of asymptomatic bacteriuria in this population for 7–14 days showed that 93 percent of patients had recurrence of bacteriuria when retested in 30 days [6].

Patients with indwelling urethral catheters: Patients with chronic indwelling catheters should not be screened or treated for asymptomatic bacteriuria [b, c]. Cloudy or foul-smelling urine is not an indication for screening or treatment [b]. In patients with chronic indwelling catheters, who were positive for bacteriuria, treatment with cephalexin versus no treatment showed no difference in fever or reinfection [7].

Recommended Guidelines and How to Find Them

The three major organizations that discuss asymptomatic bacteriuria and publish recommendations for screening and treatment are the US Preventive Services Task Force (USPSTF), AAFP, and IDSA. These organizations agree in their recommendation against screening for asymptomatic bacteriuria in nonpregnant female patients [b, c, e]. These recommendations and a discussion of the available data in relevant populations can be found on the respective websites for each professional organization.

How to Screen

Screening for asymptomatic bacteriuria is only recommended in the pregnant population [4,5]. The quantitative criteria for diagnosing asymptomatic bacteria are at least 100,000 colony-forming units (CFUs) per mL of urine in a culture obtained from voided midstream clean-catch specimen or at least 100 CFUs per mL of urine from a catheterized specimen [3]. Additionally, the IDSA states that the diagnosis of asymptomatic bacteriuria can be made only after two consecutive voided specimens show at least 100,000 CFUs of the same bacteria [3].

New Developments Likely to Affect Future Recommendations

The IDSA statement on asymptomatic bacteriuria is currently in the process of being updated with a projected publication date of Spring 2017.

Billing

No special billing considerations that apply to this recommendation as screening is not recommended.

Illustrative Cases

A 47-year-old patient presents for a well-woman visit. She was recently diagnosed with diabetes. She remembers being told that diabetes can make her more susceptible to infections and asks if she should be checked for UTI. She denies urinary symptoms including incontinence.

Screening for asymptomatic bacteriuria is not recommended in nonpregnant female patients, including in the setting of diabetes. You advise the patient against screening, unless she experiences symptoms concerning UTI.

Screen: No

Next screen: No screening ever if remains asymptomatic

A home-health nurse notifies you that a 50-year-old patient of yours with neurogenic bladder and chronic indwelling urethral catheter had foul-smelling urine on home-health rounds. The nurse was concerned for UTI, but the patient denied all urinary symptoms. She asks if you would like to order a urine culture or prescribe an antibiotic.

The AAFP and IDSA recommend against screening for bacteriuria in the setting of an indwelling catheter or for cloudy or foul-smelling urine. The patient should be screened only if she develops symptoms of a UTI.

Screen: No

Next screen: No screening ever if remains asymptomatic

A 24-year-old patient presents to the office with symptoms of frequency and dysuria. Office urinalysis demonstrates no leukocytes and no nitrites. She asks if any other urine testing could be performed to better evaluate for UTI.

This patient should be screened for bacteriuria with urine culture given her symptoms, regardless of her urinalysis result.

Screen: Yes

Next screen: No further testing as long as her symptoms resolve

A 38-year-old patient presents to your office for a well-woman visit. She recently attended a health fair sponsored by her workplace. She brings the results of several screening tests for you to review. Included in her results is a urine culture positive for greater than 100,000 CFUs of E. coli. She denies symptoms of UTI. She is concerned that her urine tested positive for bacteria and asks if any treatment is necessary.

Treatment of asymptomatic bacteriuria has not been shown to decrease the incidence of symptomatic UTI. Additionally, the use of antibiotics in this situation may lead to increased antibiotic resistance or increased risk of adverse medication side effects.

Treatment: No

Next screen: No screening ever if remains asymptomatic

Guidelines

a. Conry, J.A. and Brown, H. Well-Woman Task Force: Components of the Well-Woman Visit. *Obstet Gynecol.* 2015, **126**(4):697–701.

b. Colgan, R., Nicolle, L.E., McGlone, A., and Hooton, T.M. Asymptomatic bacteriuria in adults. *Am Fam Physician.* September 15, 2006, 74(6):985–90. Available online at: www.aafp.org/afp/2006/0915/p985.html.

c. Nicolle, L.E., Bradley, S., Colgan, R. et al. Infectious diseases society of America guidelines for the diagnosis and treatment of asymptomatic bacteriuria in adults. *Clin Infec Dis.* 2005, **40**(5):643–54. Available at: http://cid.oxfordjournals.org/content/40/5/643.full#ref-50.

d. Guidelines for Perinatal Care. American Academy of Pediatrics [and] the American College of Obstetricians and Gynecologists. 7th ed. Perinatal care. March 2013. Available at: www.acog.org/Resources-And-Publications/Guidelines-for-Perinatal-Care.

e. Clinical Summary: Asymptomatic Bacteriuria in Adults: Screening. US Preventive Services Task Force. October 2014. Available at: www.uspreventiveservicestaskforce.org/Page/Document/ClinicalSummaryFinal/asymptomatic-bacteriuria-in-adults-screening.

References

1. Nicolle, L.E. Asymptomatic bacteriuria: When to screen and when to treat. *Infect Dis Clin North Am.* 2003, **17**: 367–94.

2. Bengtsson, C., Bengtsson, U., Bjorkelund, C., Lincoln, K.M., and Sigurdson, J.A. Bacteriuria in a population sample of women: 24-year follow-up study. Results from the prospective population-based study of women in Gottenburg, Sweden. Scand J Urol Nephrol. 1998, **32**: 284–9.

3. Cai, T., Nesi, G., Mazzoli, S. et al. Asymptomatic bacteriuria treatment is associated with a higher prevalence of antibiotic resistant strains in women with urinary tract infections. *Clin Infect Dis.* December 1, 2015, **61**(11):1655–61. Epub August 12, 2015.

4. Zalmanovici Trestioreanu, A., Lador, A., Sauerbrun-Cutler, M.T., and Leibovici, L. Antibiotics for asymptomatic bacteriuria. *Cochrane Database Syst Rev.* April 8, 2015.

5. Geerlings, S.E., Stolk, R.P., Camps, M.J. et al. Consequences of asymptomatic bacteriuria in women with diabetes mellitus. *Arch Intern Med.* 2001, **161**: 1421–7.

6. Waites, K.B., Canupp, K.C., and DeVivo, M.J. Eradication of urinary tract infection following spinal cord injury. *Paraplegia.* 1993, **31**:645–52.

7. Warren, J.W., Anthony, W.C., Hoopes, J.M., and Muncie, H.L. Jr. Cephalexin for susceptible bacteriuria in afebrile, long-term catheterized patients. *JAMA.* 1982, **248**:454–8.

Pelvic Floor Disorders

Erica Nelson

Why Screen?

Pelvic floor disorders affect 20–40 percent of women and have the potential to profoundly impact the quality of life [1]. Screening is simple and focused on symptoms. Symptoms include leakage of urine with activity, urgency to void, nocturia, leakage of stool or flatus, or sensation of a vaginal bulge. Once identified, treatments range from simple outpatient therapy to complex surgery to improve a woman's overall health and decrease the risk of serious illness.

Rationale for Screening

Women can expect to live on average to 86 years. Symptoms of incontinence and prolapse most commonly develop in the sixth decade. These conditions affect a large percentage of older women, with prevalence of up to 50 percent of all women [1]. In addition to urinary, bowel, and vaginal symptoms, these conditions are associated with depression, anxiety, poor work performance, social isolation, and sexual dysfunction. Women with incontinence or prolapse tend to be less active, reclusive, depressed, and withdrawn. Correction of these disorders has the potential for significant impact on their overall health and well-being [1,2]. Pelvic prolapse also increases the risk of serious illness. For example, incontinence can be a symptom of lower urinary tract infection (UTI), which untreated in an older woman can lead to sepsis or chronic renal disease. Identifying and treating women with urinary or fecal incontinence or pelvic prolapse has the potential to improve the quality of life and decrease the costs of health care including female hygiene products, surgical treatments, and nursing home admissions.

There are effective treatments for women with pelvic floor disorders. Identification of the type of urinary incontinence (Box 28.1) guides treatment [2]. Overactive bladder symptoms can be controlled with dietary modifications, pelvic floor rehabilitation,

and medications. Stress incontinence can be controlled with pelvic floor rehabilitation or surgical management with either a mid-urethral sling or urethral bulking procedures. Pelvic organ prolapse can be treated with a pessary or surgical management for the specific vaginal defect.

Factors That Affect Screening

Age: The risk of pelvic organ prolapse increases with age.

Obesity: Overweight and obese women have a higher prevalence of pelvic organ prolapse.

Obstetrical history: Increasing parity is associated with greater risk of prolapse.

Other: Conditions that increase mechanical forces and decrease tissue integrity such as chronic constipation, smoking, and chronic lung disease may also predispose to pelvic organ prolapse. Hysterectomy may contribute to compromise of the vaginal apex. Pelvic radiation may also increase the risk of prolapse. These procedures change the normal pelvic support structure, muscle tone, and neurologic input, which may weaken vaginal tissue.

Recommended Guidelines

While pelvic floor disorders span both incontinence and prolapse, guidelines focus on incontinence. The American College of Obstetrics and Gynecology (ACOG) recommends all women over the age of 18 be routinely screened for symptoms of urinary or fecal incontinence [a]. The World Health Organization (WHO) recommends screening women over the age of 50 for urinary incontinence [b]. The Centers for Disease Control and Prevention (CDC) recommends health care providers should routinely ask patients aged 65 and older about urinary incontinence [c]. The Centers for Medicare and Medicaid Services (CMS) includes screening all

---

BOX 28.1 Types of Urinary Incontinence

Stress incontinence – Loss of urine with cough, sneeze, or other physical activity usually related to anatomic displacement of the bladder neck

Overactive bladder – Involuntary contraction of the bladder which leads to symptoms of urinary urgency and can lead to loss of urine

Mixed incontinence – Combination of stress incontinence and overactive bladder that can lead to a sense of urgency and leakage with physical activity.

BOX 28.2 Essential Components of the Basic Office Evaluation for Urinary Incontinence [2]
1. History
2. Physical examination with assessment for pelvic organ prolapse
3. Cough stress test and assessment of urethral hypermobility for women with urinary symptoms
4. Postvoid residual of urine volume
5. Urinalysis/urine culture

---

women over the age of 65 for urinary incontinence as one of its Physician Quality Reporting System (PQRS) measures [d]. Based on uniform expert agreement, the Well-Woman Task Force (WWTF) recommends routine screening of all adult women aged 50 and older.

How to Screen

While the recommendations are not specific about how to screen, several validated screening questionnaires for urinary incontinence and pelvic floor disorders have been developed. A short questionnaire focusing on leakage of urine related to physical activity or urge can help evaluate symptoms in a 3-month interval [3]. The guidelines focus on screening for incontinence, and related questions should ask about urination, loss of urine, bowel habits, and leakage of stool or flatus. While not specifically part of the screening guidelines, prolapse is also common, and additional questions about sexual history, pelvic pressure, and vaginal bulge may lead to detection of symptomatic prolapse without incontinence.

The most common symptoms involve leakage of urine. Some women might feel reluctant to discuss these issues due to embarrassment or a perception that leakage is a "normal" consequence of aging. Women should be reassured, put at ease, and encouraged to discuss their symptoms and pursue evaluation and treatment.

Positive responses about urine leakage should be followed by evaluation including obtaining a clean-catch urinalysis, urine culture, physical examination, and postvoid residual to identify stress incontinence, urethral hypermobility, or defects in vaginal support (Box 28.2). Physical examination should begin with examination of any obvious lesions or prolapse, followed by provocative testing with valsalva and cough, noting any leakage of urine, passage of stool, or further worsening of prolapse. Inspection should also note any excoriations or bleeding from prolonged prolapse. A rectal examination assesses the integrity of the anal sphincter and the posterior vaginal wall. Women with abnormal findings might benefit from further diagnostic evaluation and testing [2]. Depending on the practitioner's scope of practice, some aspects of the evaluation may require referral to a specialist.

Future Developments

Development of simplified tools to efficiently and effectively screen women for pelvic floor disorders would improve the opportunity for providers and patients to address these disorders in a comfortable and routine manner. Treatments including behavioral changes, pessary devices, pharmaceutical agents, pelvic floor rehabilitation, and surgical procedures continue to evolve and expand to provide safe and effective options for women.

Billing

Pelvic floor disorders screening is typically covered under the ICD-10 code for annual examination –

BOX 28.3 Common ICD-10 Codes for Pelvic Floor Disorders

Diagnosis	Code
Urinary tract infection	N39.0
Urinary incontinence	R32
Urinary frequency	R35.0
Stress incontinence	N39.3
Overactive bladder	N32.81
Cystocele, midline	N81.11
Rectocele	N81.6
Uterine prolapse	N81.4

Procedure	Code
Urinalysis	81005
Postvoid residual (catherization)	51701

preventive health care. If a urinalysis (81005) is obtained, then the diagnosis specific to the patient's symptom should be used, for example, stress incontinence (N39.3), overactive bladder (32.81), or cystocele (N81.11). Postvoid residual (51701) should be billed as a procedure paired with the appropriate diagnosis. Follow-up visits would be billed as separate evaluation and management (E/M) codes. Common codes for pelvic floor disorders are listed in Box 28.3.

Illustrative Cases

An active 51-year-old G1P1001 presents for her well-woman visit. She denies any problems.

The WWTF recommends all adult women aged 50 or older be screened for symptoms of urinary and fecal incontinence.

Screen now? Yes

Next screen: Next well-woman visit unless symptoms develop in interim

A healthy 55-year-old G3P3003 presents for her well-woman visit and complains of feeling "a bulge like an egg" in her vaginal area.

She reports symptoms consistent with pelvic organ prolapse and should undergo further evaluation. This should include history and examination and measurements of the descent of the vaginal wall during valsalva. A cystocele, rectocele, or enterocele may be found, and treatment with pessary or surgery

may improve the patient's symptoms and quality of life.

Screen now? Yes

Next screen: Interval based on findings

A 52–year-old G4P4004 presents for well-woman visit. She states she does not exercise due to urine leakage.

She is reporting urinary incontinence and needs further evaluation. This evaluation can include physical examination including assessment for pelvic organ prolapse with and without valsalva, cough stress test, measurement of postvoid residual, and urinalysis/urine culture [2]. Providers may choose to refer for further evaluation and management depending on their scope of practice. Correction of her incontinence will likely improve her overall well-being and health.

Screen now? No – screening is not necessary. The patient reports urinary incontinence and should be offered further evaluation to determine the etiology.

Next screen: No – future questions about urinary incontinence will track her treatment response and not be for screening.

A 67-year-old G3P2012 with a history of a forceps delivery and chronic constipation complains of a bulge in her vaginal area especially before she has a bowel movement. She frequently feels she is unable to completely move her bowels and sometimes has to splint to complete a bowel movement.

The patient is reporting symptoms consistent with a rectocele. The symptoms should be further evaluated with detailed history and physical examination for pelvic organ prolapse with and without valsalva. Providers may choose to refer for further evaluation and management depending on their scope of practice. Identification of a posterior wall defect and treatment might improve her bowel function.

Screen now? Yes

Next screen: Interval based on findings

An 82-year-old G2P2002 woman presents for a well-woman visit. She is accompanied by her daughter who is concerned that her mother no longer wants to participate in activities.

CDC, CMS, WHO, ACOG, and the WWTF all recommend screening women in this age group for urinary incontinence. The WWTF also recommends screening for fecal incontinence. Screening should include history, with focused questions on incontinence of stool and urine. Screening questions for prolapse are also reasonable. Examination should include assessment for pelvic organ prolapse with and without valsalva. This patient could be avoiding social interactions and becoming withdrawn because of incontinence of urine or stool. Identification and treatment might improve her overall quality of life.

Screen now? Yes

Next screen: Interval based on findings

Guidelines

a. American College of Obstetricians and Gynecologists. *Well-woman Recommendations*. Washington, DC: American College of Obstetricians and Gynecologists, 2015. Available at: //www.acog.org/About-ACOG/A COG-Departments/Annual-Womens-Health-Care/W ell-Woman-Recommendations. Retrieved March 12, 2015.

b. World Health Organization. *Age-Friendly Primary Health Care Centres Toolkit*. Geneva: WHO, 2008. Available at: www.who.int/ageing/publications/upco ming_publications/en/. Retrieved May 17, 2016.

c. Centers for Disease Control and Prevention. Knowledge, attitudes, and practices of physicians regarding urinary incontinence in persons aged > or

= 65 years – Massachusetts and Oklahoma, 1993. *MMWR Morb Mortal Wkly Rep.* 1995, **44**(747):753–4.

d. Centers for Medicare and Medicaid Services. *Physician Quality Reporting System (PQRS): Measures List.* Baltimore, MD: CMS, 2016. Available at: www.cms.gov/ Medicare/Quality-Initiatives-Patient-Assessment-Inst ruments/PQRS/MeasuresCodes.html. Retrieved May 17, 2016.

References

1. Wu, J., Vaugh, C., Goode, P. et al. Prevalence and trends of symptomatic pelvic floor disorders in US women. *Obstet Gynecol.* 2014, **123**:141–8.

2. American College of Obstetricians and Gynecologists. Urinary Incontinence in Women. Practice Bulletin No. 155. *Obstet Gynecol.* 2015, **126**:e66–81.

3. Brown, J., Bradley, C., Subak, L. et al. The sensitivity and specificity of a simple test to distinguish between urge and stress urinary incontinence. *Ann Intern Med.* 2006, **144**:715–23.

4. Grarely, A. and Noor, N. Diagnosis and surgical treatment of stress urinary incontinence. *Obstet Gynecol.* 2014, **124**:1011–27.

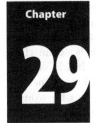

Chapter

29

Contraception

Rebecca Cohen

Why Counsel?

Approximately half (51 percent) of the 6.6 million pregnancies that occur annually in the United States are unintended [1]. Unintended pregnancies can impact individuals' social and economic well-being. From a public health perspective, unintended pregnancies lead to adverse maternal and child health outcomes [1]. In the United States, many women faced with an unintended pregnancy seek abortion care; in 2011, there were 1.06 million abortions, and the abortion rate was 16.9 per 1,000 women aged 15–44 [2].

Rationale for Counseling

Contraception is key to preventing unintended pregnancies. At an individual level, contraception reduces the probability of having an abortion by 85 percent [3]. At a program level, publicly subsidized US family planning services in the United States have helped women prevent 20 million pregnancies over the last 20 years [3]. Methods that are nondaily and not coital dependent are much more effective [4]. Thus, it is imperative that providers caring for women provide detailed counseling about and access to highly effective methods.

Improving the quality of contraceptive counseling, thus potentially improving satisfaction and with adherence to a contraceptive plan, is one strategy to prevent unintended pregnancy [5]. Women's selection of a new contraceptive method is influenced by whether providers mention or recommend specific methods. In addition, development of a close, trusting patient–provider relationship and a shared decision-making approach that focuses on patient preferences has resulted in improved contraceptive continuation [5]. Providing counseling about side effects and using strategies to promote contraceptive continuation and adherence can also help optimize women's use of contraception [5].

Factors That Affect Counseling

Desire for future childbearing: For women who are certain that they do not desire more children, permanent contraception in the form of male or female sterilization should be discussed. Women who desire future childbearing should be provided information on time to return to fertility after contraceptive discontinuation.

Medical conditions: For women interested in hormonal methods, providers must first distinguish whether or not the woman is a candidate for combined hormonal methods that incorporate both estrogen and progestin (e.g., oral contraceptive pill, patch, ring). The primary concern with estrogen therapy is the increased risk of arterial and venous thromboembolism. Certain genetic or medical conditions such as Factor V Leiden or ischemic heart disease have an unacceptable risk of thromboembolism with the addition of estrogen. Other conditions such as hormonally sensitive breast cancers and certain liver diseases can also worsen with the addition of estrogen.

Age: Adolescents should be assured of confidentiality and providers should be aware of local laws regarding contraceptive provision to minors. Adolescents can receive contraceptive services without parental consent in some, but not all, states. Perimenopausal women may have vasomotor symptoms that respond well to an estrogen-containing method and perimenopausal bleeding patterns that may be regulated with estrogen-containing methods or lightened with progestin-only methods.

Concurrent gynecologic problems: Some contraceptive methods are also effective treatments for some of the underlying etiologies of abnormal uterine bleeding and pelvic pain. The Mirena levonorgestrel intrauterine device (IUD) is Food and Drug Administration (FDA)–approved to treat idiopathic heavy menstrual bleeding. Levonorgestrel IUDs can also decrease bleeding among women with fibroids. Pain from endometriosis or primary dysmenorrhea may respond to combined oral and implantable progestin contraception.

Recommended Guidelines and How to Find Them

Evidence-based contraception guidelines from the Institute of Medicine (IOM) and Centers for Disease Control and Prevention (CDC) formed the basis of the Well-Woman Task Force recommendations. In 2010, the CDC released the contraceptive US Medical Eligibility Criteria (US MEC). The US MEC was adapted from the World Health Organization recommendations to reflect current scientific evidence, the US patient population, and local contraceptive service provision, and to include methods available in the United States [a]. The majority of US recommendations are consistent with global recommendations; when necessary, changes were made through systematic review by a panel of family planning experts. Most major organizations, including the American College of Obstetricians and Gynecologists (ACOG) [b] have adopted these guidelines.

In 2013, the CDC published *US Selected Practice Recommendations for Contraceptive Use* (US SPR), to address common concerns and eliminate barriers to contraceptive use. The US SPR is supported by ACOG [c]. Both ACOG [d] and the American Academy of Pediatrics (AAP) [e] recommend long-acting reversible contraceptive (LARC) methods as first-line contraception for adolescents, including those who have never given birth.

The Affordable Care Act (ACA), passed in 2010, specified that preventive health services were to be covered without a patient co-pay. An IOM committee reviewed effective women's health preventive services and concluded that adult women with reproductive capacity should have access to the full range of FDA-approved methods, including sterilization procedures, as part of the preventive health services covered by the ACA [f].

In 2016, the CDC released updates of both the US MEC and US SPR [6–7]. These documents are available on the CDC website (www.cdc.gov/repro ductivehealth/contraception/contraception_gui dance.htm). The website includes access to down-loadable resources: summary tables, counseling tools, and applications for handheld devices. The 2016 US MEC includes eligibility recommendations not included in previous versions for women with cystic fibrosis, multiple sclerosis, or exposure to specific psychotropic drugs. The revised recommendations for emergency contraception now include ulipristal acetate. Recommendations for postpartum and breast-feeding women are also updated, as well as eligibility for women with chronic medical conditions, such as dyslipidemia, migraine headaches, superficial venous disease, and with sexually transmitted diseases including human immunodeficiency virus. The 2016 US SPR provides revised recommendations for starting regular contraception after the use of emergency contraceptive pills and new recommendations for the use of medications to ease insertion of IUDs.

How to Counsel

Before focusing on the choice of a contraceptive method, providers should obtain a full history to assess for contraindications to specific methods. If the patient is currently using contraception at the time of the well-woman visit, the provider should briefly assess her satisfaction with the method and whether it continues to meet her contraceptive needs. If the patient is not using contraception, but does not desire pregnancy, the provider should review all options available to the patient and help her select a method. A short-acting reversible method such as pills, patch, ring, or injectable may be appropriate for a woman who desires conception in the near future. LARC methods such as implants or IUDs are effective for at least 3 years (dependent on the method) but can be removed sooner to attempt conception. As summarized above, there are multiple factors other than desire/timing of future childbearing that may affect counseling for specific subgroups of patients.

The discussion between provider and patient should build trust, provide unbiased information, and allow the patient to express concerns [5]. Providers should share a realistic picture of anticipated side effects and address barriers to adherence. It is important to remember that no single method is right for all women; some may prioritize method characteristics other than efficacy and it is important to avoid coercive or overly directive counseling [8]. For women at risk for sexually transmitted infections (STIs), providers should encourage dual method contraception, which is the use of condoms with a highly effective contraceptive method [5]. Use of visual aids such as physical models of contraceptive methods and a handout with methods grouped by effectiveness level may help women select the best contraceptive method for them [4].

The CDC recommends use of a Reproductive Life Plan to guide contraceptive counseling [6]. With this plan, the provider asks each reproductive-aged, nonsterile woman if she wants to have any (more) children, and if so, how many. For women who desire future pregnancy, the provider asks when the woman would like to become pregnant, and what contraceptive method she would like to use until that time. Women who do not desire future childbearing are also asked about contraceptive methods. The provider then guides discussion and method selection in partnership with the patient and addresses relevant factors described above.

While most women can safely use any form of contraception, women with medical comorbidities or other risk factors have fewer options. In the US MEC, a specific category of medical eligibility (ranging from no restrictions on use to unacceptable health risk) is applied to each contraceptive method for each condition. The full text of the US MEC, arranged by contraceptive method class, is available along with updates and summary charts on the CDC website (www.cdc.gov/reproductivehealth/contraception/usmec.htm).

New Developments Likely to Affect Future Recommendations

Political and legal forces may influence access to recommended methods of contraception. ACA mandated that women be covered for preventive health services, including FDA-approved contraceptive methods, without a co-pay or deductible. However, both the ACA itself and the religious exemptions have been subject to ongoing legal challenges that may limit access (if contraceptive coverage is reduced or eliminated) or expand access (if faith-based exemptions are removed).

Evidence on optimal methods of contraceptive counseling may inform future recommendations. The Contraceptive CHOICE Project, a cohort study

of almost 10,000 women who desired to delay pregnancy at least 12 months, used a structured counseling method that prioritized highly effective LARC methods (IUDs and contraceptive implants) [7]. Counselors engaged in personalized counseling to review all available contraceptive methods and help each participant select a method that best fits her needs. When this technique was used and financial barriers to LARC were removed, 73 percent of women chose a LARC method.

Billing

Contraceptive encounters are covered under the ICD-10 code group Z30, encounter for contraceptive management. Z30.01X codes are for initiation of contraception (where the "X" varies by method initiated), while Z30.4X codes are for management of a currently used method. These encounter codes do not include the insertion procedure or removal procedure for LARC methods, nor do they include the LARC device itself. IUD insertion is coded with CPT 58300, and removal is 58301. The devices are billed with J3700 (Paragard® brand copper IUD), J3701 (Skyla® brand 13.5 mg levonorgestrel IUD), or J3702 (Mirena® or Liletta® brand 52 mg levonorgestrel IUD). Implant insertion is coded as 11981, removal as 11982, and the Nexplanon® device (the only FDA–approved contraceptive implant in the United States) is J7307. Women who desire sterilization and are covered by publicly funded insurance must sign a "Consent for sterilization" form between 30 and 180 days prior to the sterilization procedure.

Illustrative Cases

A 16-year-old G0 presents for a well-adolescent visit. She has been sexually active for 3 months with one partner, uses condoms "most of the time," and desires to avoid pregnancy "at least until I'm done with college."

If her pregnancy test is negative and the provider is reasonably sure she is not pregnant (she has not had unprotected sex within 2 weeks or since last menses), she should be counseled on all methods. LARC methods align with her goal to delay pregnancy for several years, are recommended by ACOG and AAP, and should be prioritized. She should be encouraged to use condoms consistently to protect against STIs. Providers should know their state's laws about providing contraception to a minor without parental consent.

Contraception counseling? Yes

Next counseling: Annually

A 37-year-old G2P2 presents for a well-woman exam. She has smoked 1 pack of cigarettes per day since age 17. She is currently using combined oral contraceptive pills and is happy with this method.

Due to this patient's age and smoking status, use of estrogen-containing methods (such as combined oral contraceptives) is contraindicated. The provider should work with the patient to find an alternate method of contraception that does not contain estrogen; this discussion can focus on the patient's reproductive goals and characteristics of methods that are safe for her. The patient should be encouraged to quit smoking and could resume use of combined oral contraceptives if she is able to quit.

Contraception counseling: Yes

Next counseling: Annually

A 47-year-old healthy G3P1Ab2 presents for her well-woman exam. She is currently using condoms for contraception. She reports that her periods have become less frequent and lighter over the past year and that she has started to experience hot flushes.

This patient has likely started the perimenopausal transition. Although the risk of unintended pregnancy is low at her age, she may benefit from an estrogen-containing contraceptive method that is both more effective than condoms and could help with her vasomotor symptoms.

Contraception counseling: Yes

Next counseling: Annually (if menopause has not occurred)

A 14-year-old presents for a well-adolescent exam. She has no concerns today. She currently has regular periods and is not, and has never been, sexually active.

After confirming in a confidential manner (without the parent or guardian present) that the patient is not sexually active, she should be offered brief counseling on all methods (including delaying sexual activity). Her visit is an opportunity to build trust and provide information. A pelvic examination should not be performed unless it is part of contraceptive fitting or placement.

Contraception counseling: Yes

Next counseling: When she desires to initiate contraception

Guidelines

Women with Medical Risk Factors

a. US Medical Eligibility Criteria for Contraceptive Use. MMWR recommendations and reports: Morbidity and mortality weekly report recommendations and reports/Centers for Disease Control. June 18, 2010, 59(RR-4):1–86.

b. Committee Opinion No. 505. Understanding and using the US medical eligibility criteria for contraceptive use, 2010. *Obstet Gynecol.* September 2011, **118**(3):754–60.

US Select Practice Recommendations

c. ACOG Committee Opinion No. 577. Understanding and using the US selected practice recommendations for contraceptive use, 2013. *Obstet Gynecol.* November 2013, **122**(5):1132–3.

Adolescent Women

d. Committee Opinion No. 539. Adolescents and long-acting reversible contraception: Implants and intrauterine devices. *Obstet Gynecol.* October 2012, **120**(4):983–8.

e. Ott, M.A. and Sucato, G.S. Contraception for adolescents. *Pediatrics.* October 2014, **134**(4): e1257–81.

Affordable Care Act

f. Committee on Preventive Services for Women. *Clinical Preventive Services for Women: Closing the Gaps.* Washington, DC: Institute of Medicine, 2011. Available at: www.nap.edu/download.php?record_id=13181. Retrieved February 25, 2016.

Guideline Updates Published after the Well-Woman Task Force Report

g. Curtis, K.M., Tepper, N.K., Jatlaoui, T.C. et al. US medical eligibility criteria for contraceptive use, 2016. *MMWR Recomm Rep.* 2016, 65(RR-3):1–104.

h. Curtis, K.M., Jatlaoui, T.C., Tepper, N.K. et al. US selected practice recommendations for contraceptive use, 2016. *MMWR Recomm Rep.* 2016, 65 (RR-4):1–66.

References

1. Unintended pregnancy in the United States. Available at: www.guttmacher.org/pubs/FB-Unintended-Pregnancy-US.html. Retrieved January 22, 2016.

2. Jones, R.K. and Jerman, J. Abortion incidence and service availability in the United States, 2011. *Perspect Sex Reprod Health*. March 2014, **46**(1):3–14.

3. Contraceptive use is key to reducing abortion worldwide. Available at: www.guttmacher.org/pubs/tgr/06/4/gr060407.html. Retrieved January 23, 2016.

4. Contraception: How effective are birth control methods? Available at: www.cdc.gov/reproductive health/unintendedpregnancy/contraception.htm. Retrieved January 22, 2016.

5. Dehlendorf, C., Krajewski, C., and Borrero, S. Contraceptive counseling: Best practices to ensure quality communication and enable effective contraceptive use. *Clin Obstet Gynecol*. December 2014, **57**(4):659–73.

6. Reproductive Life Plan Tool for Health Professionals. Available at: www.cdc.gov/preconception/rlptool.html. Retrieved January 22, 2016.

7. Madden, T., Mullersman, J.L., Omvig, K.J., Secura, G.M. , and Peipert, J.F. Structured contraceptive counseling provided by the contraceptive CHOICE project. *Contraception*. August 2013, **88**(2):243–9.

8. Madden, T., Secura, G.M., Nease, R.F., Politi, M.C., and Peipert, J.F. The role of contraceptive attributes in women's contraceptive decision making. *Am J Obstet Gynecol*. July 2015, **213**(1):46 e1–6.

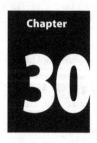

Sexual Health

Brett Worly

Why Screen?

Sexual problems are common, burdensome, and underreported. While 12–40 percent of women will experience female sexual dysfunction at some point in their lives, 68 percent of women with sexual dysfunction say they would not volunteer this information at a health care visit for fear of embarrassing their provider [a, b, c, d]. Addressing a woman's sexual health status can provide young women with correct terminology and factual understanding of their bodies and sexual response while helping to prepare them for safe and healthy relationships with future partners. Women at other life stages may encounter problems with sexual desire, lubrication, and arousal/orgasm; may not have a sexual partner; or may have a partner with sexual problems [1–3]. Furthermore, healthy sexuality enriches a woman's overall well-being and quality of life, and enhances the quality of her relationships with intimate partners.

Screening for sexual violence and other aspects of sexual health are covered in the chapters on Mental Health and Psychosocial Issues, Suicide and Behavioral Assessment, Domestic and Intimate Partner Violence, and Sexually Transmitted Infections.

Rationale for Screening

Screening women for sexual health problems is a part of a well-woman visit, as sexual health has important components of physical, mental, and relationship health. Sexual health can improve a woman's sexual satisfaction and general overall sense of wellness. Untreated sexual dysfunction may lead to interpersonal relationship problems and even cause problems in the workplace [1]. Women with healthy sexual function will have an improved quality of life and improved relationships with intimate partners.

Factors That Affect Screening

Age and culture: Adolescents, young women, and older women, as well as women from specific religious or ethnic communities, may be embarrassed to discuss sexuality with physicians particularly when there are age or gender differences. A common misperception is that extremes of age preclude interest in sexuality. In fact, women develop an age- and situation-appropriate interest in sexuality throughout their lives [1]. Women raised in particular families or cultures may lack the appropriate vocabulary or language skills to have an open, healthy discussion about sexuality and sexual health.

Lesbian, gay, bisexual, and transgender (LGBT) patients: Health care providers may lack experience discussing sexuality with women from the LGBT community, as these women are estimated to comprise less than 5 percent of US women. Lesbian and bisexual women may have had health care experiences that make them less likely to disclose their sexual orientation and discuss sexual problems. Transgender patients may come for a screening visit and encounter intake forms and questions forcing them to choose a male or female gender identity. Using inclusive intake procedures and an LBGT-friendly sticker or lapel pin can identify a welcoming place for all patients and facilitate disclosure of sexual health issues [4].

Cancer status: Around 20–40 percent of women with breast cancer experience sexual problems, but many hesitate to discuss these problems with providers due to alterations in physical appearance and body image, comorbid depression, or other difficulties coping with cancer. Cancer survivors may be complacent with sexual problems as an acceptable trade-off for extended life. Many doctors fail to discuss sexual health with cancer survivors, and many patients are afraid to bring up their sexual concerns without being asked.

Patients without sexual partners: Patients without partners often have strong sexually healthy lives with fantasy, toys, and masturbation. These patients may encounter new sexual problems, or may have had such severe sexual problems in the past that their relationships were destroyed.

Recommended Guidelines and How to Find Them

The ACOG Well-Woman Task Force (WWTF) relied on evidence-informed recommendations summarized in a 2011 ACOG Practice Bulletin [a] and a report from the World Health Organization [4], as well as multiple sources of expert opinion summarized in the WWTF Report [e].

How to Screen

Adolescents: The WWTF recommends that providers offer the opportunity for respectful and open dialogue about sexual health and sexuality for women and girls aged 13–18, including topics of sexual orientation, gender identity, and sexual dysfunction. Screening, guidance, and education on issues including sexual development, menses, human papillomavirus (HPV) vaccine, and pregnancy/sexually transmitted infection (STI) prevention, may occur. Start with a normalizing statement and open-ended question, such as "Many people in your age group are having sexual experiences, by themselves or with a partner. How is that going for you?" Additional prompts include, "Tell me about your sexual partner or partners." This question can be a relatively safe gauge of a woman's interest in discussing this issue, and is asked in a gender-neutral manner. As the conversation continues, the healthcare provider could say, "Sexual problems can happen to people at any age. Is this a particular challenge for you?" [a, c].

Adult women: The annual visit provides the opportunity to screen for sexual health issues, but a follow-up visit is more appropriate to fully evaluate and treat sexual problems. The WWTF recommends screening with just one or two questions such as "Are you satisfied with your sex life?" or "Do you have any questions or concerns about sex?" [a, e] Other screening options include objective questionnaires,

such as the FSFI, Brief Sexual Symptom Checklist for Women, and the Decreased Sexual Desire Screener (www.obgynalliance.com/files/fsd/DSDS_Pocketcard.pdf) [1].

Specific subgroups may benefit from framing statements and questions tailored to their situations. These can be posed after the two questions recommended by the WWTF. For older women, "Many women have sexual problems in the years after menopause, specifically when it comes to dryness and pain. Is this an issue for you?" A similar approach can be used to invite dialogue in women with cancer [2]. For women who are not in a sexual relationship, one can ask about previous partners, reasons for ending relationships, and reasons the patient is not currently in a sexual relationship.

New Developments Likely to Affect Future Guidelines

The current WWTF recommendations rely primarily on evidence-informed positions published by ACOG and the WHO. The emergence of systematic reviews and evidence summaries on sexual health screening could spur changes in the guidelines. In the coming years, some professional organizations, including the American Academy of Pediatrics (AAP), may develop new guidelines. The *Diagnostic and Statistical Manual of Mental Disorders-5* published in 2013 included changes in the definitions and classification of some forms of female sexual dysfunction [4]. Sexual interest and arousal disorders were combined to replace hypoactive sexual desire disorder. Genito-pelvic sexual pain/penetration disorder replaced sexual pain disorder. Future changes in the diagnostic criteria for sexual problems could influence future guidelines.

Billing

The ICD-10 billing codes for common sexual health issues are included in the following:

Female Sexual Interest/Arousal Disorder: F52.22
Genito-pelvic Sexual Pain/Penetration Disorder: F52.6
Female Orgasmic Disorder: F52.31

These problems may be included in the well-woman visit and may be separately reimbursed. Local variations regarding health insurance may apply, and it is best to check with common insurance companies used by patients in your area. Often, full evaluation of sexual dysfunction takes longer than the allotted time for the well-woman visit, and it may be more appropriate to bill based on the time spent with the patient, or have the patient return for further evaluation and management with an appointment on another day.

Illustrative Cases

A 23-year-old G0 is seen for a well-woman visit. She is sexually active with one partner regularly for 2 years. Screening reveals that she is satisfied with her sex life but is concerned that she has never had an orgasm.

Additional questions indicate there are no other sexual symptoms or relationship problems. The patient can experience orgasm during masturbation but not with this partner. A follow-up visit is scheduled for further discussion and counseling.

Screen now? Yes

Next screening: N/A – the problem will be addressed at a follow-up visit and monitored at subsequent visits

A 52-year-old G3P3 is seen for a well-woman visit and discloses vaginal dryness over the past year. Screening indicates that she is not satisfied with her sex life due to decreased interest and arousal.

Additional questions indicate she is having entry and deep dyspareunia, which further decreases her interest and arousal. She is also having bothersome vasomotor symptoms and difficulty sleeping. She is satisfied with her relationship – the only problems are sexual ones. A follow-up visit is scheduled for further evaluation.

Screen now? Yes

Next screening: N/A – the problem will be addressed at a follow-up visit and monitored at subsequent visits

A 16-year-old G0 is seen for her first well-woman visit. She is accompanied by her mother and discloses no questions or concerns. After the majority of the history is completed, the patient's mother is asked to leave the room so the remainder of the history can be completed confidentially. When asked about her sexual experiences, the patient says that her friends have started experimenting with sex, alcohol, and marijuana. She has questions about her reproductive and sexual anatomy, gender identity, and sexuality.

In discussing sexuality with young women, confidentiality should be established before the patient encounter begins. Local, state, and federal laws may dictate what information needs to be disclosed to parents of minor children. This should be clearly explained to the patient. Once the appropriate confidentiality parameters have been agreed upon, the provider should answer the patient's questions about her anatomy, gender identity, and sexuality. More information may be shared over subsequent visits. Counseling should also occur on prevention of pregnancy, STIs, and non-consensual sex.

Invite discussion now? Yes

Next opportunity: Next comprehensive health visit

A 67-year-old G3P3 with diabetes, chronic hypertension, obesity, and depression presents for a well-woman visit. Screening indicates that she is happy with her sex life, but notes that for the past 2 years it takes more stimulation to have an orgasm.

Screening for sexual dysfunction should continue throughout adulthood. Additional questioning should focus on the health of her partner, satisfaction with their relationship, the presence of sexual pain, and problems with sexual interest. A discussion about female anatomy, normal sexual experiences with aging, and the use of sex toys to assist with stimulation, may also be helpful.

Screen now? Yes

Next screening: 1 year

Guidelines

a. American College of Obstetricians and Gynecologists committee on practice bulletins – Gynecology. Female sexual dysfunction. *Obstet Gynecol.* 2011, **117** (4):996–1007. This comes from the American College of Obstetrics and Gynecology and is an evidence-based review of the literature.

b. Lamont, J. Female sexual health consensus clinical guidelines. *J Obstet Gynaecol Can.* 2012, **34**(8):S1–56. This is an evidence-based review of the literature from the Society of Obstetricians and Gynecologists of Canada.

c. Brook, G., Bacon, L., Evans, C. et al. 2013 UK national guideline for consultations requiring sexual history taking. Clinical Effectiveness Group. British Association for Sexual Health and HIV.

d. World Health Organization Sexual Health Guidelines. Available at: www.who.int/topics/sexual_health/en/. Retrieved February 25, 2016.

e. American College of Obstetrics and Gynecology 2013–2014 Well-Woman Task Force. *Obstet Gynecol.* October 2016. [Epub ahead of print]

References

1. Kingsberg, S.A. and Woodard, T. Female sexual dysfunction: Focus on low desire. *Obstet Gynecol.* 2015, **125**(2):477–86.

2. Huffman, L.B., Hartenbach, E.M., Carter, J., Rash, J.K., and Kushner, D.M. Maintaining sexual health throughout gynecologic cancer survivorship: A comprehensive review and clinical guide. *Gynecol Oncol.* November 7, 2015. [Epub ahead of print]

3. Carpenter, K.M., Williams, K., and Worly, B. (forthcoming). Treating women's orgasmic difficulties.

In Peterson, Z.D., editor. *Handbook of Sex Therapy*, Hoboken, NJ: Wiley-Blackwell.

4. American Psychiatric Association. *Diagnostic and Statistical Manual of Mental Disorders*, 5th edition. Washington, DC: American Psychiatric Association, 2013.

5. Nastri, C.O., Lara, L.A., Ferriani, R.A. et al. Hormone therapy for sexual function in perimenopausal and postmenopausal women. Cochrane Database Syst Rev. 2013, (**6**):CD009672.

6. American College of Obstetrics and Gynecology. Healthcare for lesbians and bisexual women. Committee Opinion No. 525. *Obstet Gynecol.* 2012, **119** (5):1077–80.

Chapter 31

Hepatitis B and C Screening

Kimberly S. Gecsi

Why Screen?

There are an estimated 3.2 million people in the United States living with chronic hepatitis C virus (HCV) infection [1,2]. Incidence rates of acute hepatitis C decreased among females from 2000 to 2003 and remained fairly constant from 2004 to 2010. From 2010 to 2013, the rates of acute hepatitis C increased among females with a rate of 0.7 cases per 100,000 population. Chronic liver disease develops in 60–70 percent of infected patients, with close to 20 percent developing cirrhosis. More than 30 percent of liver transplant cases and the recent three-fold increase in hepatocellular carcinoma are attributed to HCV infection [a]. Hepatitis B virus (HBV) is less common, with 1.2 million persons in the United States living with chronic infection. Incidence rates of acute hepatitis B decreased for females from 2000 to 2012, but slightly increased from 2012 to 2013. In 2013, the rate for females was 0.73 cases per 100,000 population. The natural history of the infection is varied, with 15–25 percent of patients developing chronic infection that can progress to cirrhosis, liver failure, and liver cancer [3].

Rationale for Screening

Most people with viral hepatitis B or C do not know they are infected. Chronic disease is associated with cirrhosis, liver cancer, and liver failure. Screening with serologic testing is the primary means for identifying persons with viral hepatitis. Each year in the United States 17,000 people die from HCV-related liver disease and 1,800 die from HBV-related liver disease [2]. Early identification and treatment of chronic infection with the use of antiviral therapy improves clinical outcomes, including decreasing hepatocellular carcinoma. Current antiviral regimens for HCV have been shown to result in a sustained virologic response (SVR) with low side effects, demonstrating the benefit of screening for early detection. SVR is associated with a reduced risk of all-cause mortality, including

decreasing need for liver transplants [4]. For hepatitis B, chronic disease is much more likely to develop in infected infants, with 30–40 percent of all chronic HBV infections resulting from vertical transmission [b]. For this reason, identification of infected pregnant patients is important [a]. Prophylaxis of infants born to infected mothers with hepatitis B vaccine and immune globulin within 12 hours of birth can significantly reduce transmission of the virus. Harms of screening for both HBV and HCV are limited but potentially include anxiety, patient labeling, and feelings of stigmatization. Harms of antiviral therapy are small, and adverse events are limited.

Factors That Affect Screening

HCV is primarily acquired through the sharing of contaminated needles or syringes and less commonly through sexual contact, vertical transmission at birth, or needle stick injuries. There are a number of well-established risk factors (Box 31.1).

Peak prevalence of HCV was 4.3 percent in individuals that were between the ages of 40–49 during 1999–2002 [5].

BOX 31.1 Risk Factors for Hepatitis C Virus Infection

Current or former injection drug users

Incarcerated women

Recipients of blood transfusions or donated organs before 1992

Long-term hemodialysis patients

HIV-positive women

Intranasal drug use

Getting an unregulated tattoo

Infants born to infected mothers

Individuals born between 1945 and 1965

Infants born to infected mothers

Sex partners of infected persons

Women with multiple sexual partners

Women who have a sexually transmitted disease

Injection drug users

Household contacts of infected persons

Health care and public safety workers exposed to blood on the job

Hemodialysis patients

Residents and staff of facilities for developmentally disabled persons

Travelers to regions with intermediate or high rates of hepatitis B (>2%)

Women born in countries with a high prevalence of HBV infection (>2%)

US-born persons not vaccinated as infants whose parents were born in regions of very high prevalence of HBV infection (>8%)

Hepatitis B

HBV is primarily transmitted through contact with infectious blood, semen, or other bodily fluids at the time of birth, sexual contact, or needle sharing with an infected individual. Needle sticks or other sharp instrument injuries are another route for transmission. There are a number of well-established risk factors (Box 31.2).

Recommended Guidelines and How to Find Them

Screening guidelines for HCV and HBV are published by the US Preventive Services Task Force (USPSTF) and are updated on a regular basis [a, c, d]. Input from the Agency for Healthcare Research and Quality (AHRQ) and the Centers for Disease Control and Prevention (CDC) is used to help develop the guidelines. The USPSTF publishes full guidelines statements as well as consumer guides that give helpful patient information about screening. The CDC website offers useful tables and flow sheets for guidance with screening recommendations and risk stratification. The American Academy of Family

Medicine website also offers helpful case studies on screening recommendations [6]. The Well-Woman Task Force recommendation is in line with the USPTF recommendations for both HBV and HCV.

How to Screen HCV

History should be assessed for potential risk factors (Table 31.1), and women at high risk of infection should be screened. Women born between 1945 and 1965 should undergo one-time screening. Patients in the birth cohort (1945–1965) without the presence of other risk factors only need to be screened once. Patients who continue to be at increased risk of new infection (intravenous [IV] drug users) should be screened periodically. Women at high risk include IV drug users, having a history of blood transfusion before 1992, those born to an HCV-infected mother, current or former incarceration, intranasal drug use, and those with other percutaneous exposures.

Hepatitis C screening should start with anti-HCV antibody serum testing. A nonreactive test in patients that are not immunocompromised and have no recent known exposure to HCV is satisfactory in ruling out the presence of disease. Patients with a positive HCV antibody screen should undergo HCV RNA polymerase chain reaction (PCR) testing to identify the presence of viremia. A negative HCV RNA test confirms absence of current HCV infection. A positive test confirms presence of current infection, and follow-up tests to determine the presence of liver fibrosis or cirrhosis are recommended (Figure 31.1).

Hepatitis B Virus

History should be assessed for potential risk factors (Table 31.2), and women at high risk of infection should be screened. History should include questions related to IV drugs use and should ascertain whether use ever occurred, even just once or many years in the past. While individuals at high risk of HBV infection should be screened, the general asymptomatic nonpregnant population should not undergo screening [c]. Women that should undergo screening include persons born in countries and regions with a high prevalence of HBV infection (>2 percent) (Table 31.1), US-born persons not vaccinated as infants whose parents were born in regions with a very high prevalence of HBV infection (>8 percent) [7], HIV-

Table 31.1 Geographic Regions with a Prevalence of Hepatitis B Surface Antigen ≥2%

Region	Country
Africa	All (sub-Saharan Africa >5%)
Asia	All (Southeast Asia >5%)
Australia and South Pacific	All except Australia and New Zealand
Middle East	All except Cyprus and Israel
Eastern Europe	All except Hungary
Western Europe	Malta, Spain, and indigenous populations of Greenland
North America	Alaskan Natives and indigenous populations of northern Canada
Mexico and Central America	Guatemala and Honduras
South America	Ecuador, Guyana, Suriname, Venezuela, and Amazonian areas of Bolivia, Brazil, Colombia, and Peru
Caribbean	Antigua and Barbuda, Dominica, Grenada, Haiti, Jamaica, St. Kitts and Nevis, St. Lucia, and Turks and Caicos Islands

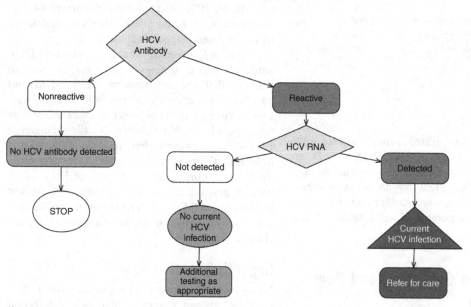

Figure 31.1 Recommended Testing Sequence for Identifying Current Hepatitis C Virus (HCV) Infection.

positive persons, IV drug users, and household contracts or sexual partners of persons with HBV infection. Pregnant women should undergo screening at their first prenatal visit [b].

Hepatitis B screening differs based on the risk category that prompts testing. Most patients at high risk, as well as all pregnant women, should be screened using a serum test for antibodies to HBsAg, which has a reported sensitivity and specificity greater than 98 percent [8]. A positive test indicates acute or chronic infection. IV drug users, immunocompromised patients, hemodialysis patients, and patients whose sex partners are HBsAg positive should have additional screening tests for anti-HBs and anti-HBc. Patients with negative tests should be assessed for ongoing risk factors and vaccinated against HBV if indicated.

New Developments Likely to Affect Future Guidelines

Screening individuals born between 1945 and 1965 for HCV was prompted by the recognition of the

Table 31.2 ICD-10 Diagnosis Codes for HBV and HCV Screening

ICD-10 Code	Description	When to Use
F19.1	Other psychoactive substance abuse	HBV or HCV screening
F11.10	Intravenous nondependent opioid abuse	HBV or HCV screening
Z72.51	High-risk heterosexual behavior	HBV screening
Z72.89	Other problems related to lifestyle	HBV screening
Z00.00	Encounter for general medical examination without abnormal findings	HCV screening in birth cohort

HBV: hepatitis B virus; HCV: hepatitis C virus

increased incidence of infection and the development of effective new medications. Outside this birth cohort, screening recommendations for both HBV and HCV are limited to testing patients at high risk. Limited screening programs miss patients with infection, and these patients will not benefit from early identification and treatment. Screening guidelines may change if additional treatments for HCV or HBV become available or if the prevalence of disease in the US population increases. Furthermore, the development of an HCV vaccine, currently being tested in human subjects, may change screening recommendations to identify candidates for vaccination.

Billing

Effective June 2, 2014, the Center for Medicare and Medicaid Services (CMS) began covering HCV screening for the following conditions: current or past history of illicit injection drug use, transfusion prior to 1992, and individuals born between 1945 and 1965 who have not had prior screening. Repeat screening will only be approved by CMS in patients with continued IV drug use. Most private insurance plans, including plans on the Health Insurance Marketplace, will cover these screening recommendations.

Hepatitis B screening in pregnant women at the time of their first prenatal visit and again at delivery if there are new or ongoing risk factors is covered by all insurance plans including Medicare and Medicaid. Screening for HBV will also be covered by CMS for individuals with the following risk factors: multiple sex partners, using barrier protection inconsistently, having sex under the influence of alcohol or drugs, having sex in exchange for money or drugs, having a sexually transmitted infection (STI) within the past year, and IV drug use. Private insurance coverage of screening for HBV in high-risk individuals depends on individual plan specifications. See Table 31.2 for ICD-10 codes that can be used for HCV and HBV screening.

Illustrative Cases

A 27-year-old woman presents as a new patient for her well-woman visit. She recently moved to the United States from Canada and has an unremarkable medical history. She reports that she used IV heroin a few times in her early 20s but is no longer using any drugs or alcohol. She is currently sexually active with one partner and has had more than ten lifetime partners.

Screening for HCV is recommended in the presence of risk factors. Her most important risk factor is a history of IV drug use. She will only need rescreening if there is continued possible exposure. Since her IV drug use has stopped, she will not need to be rescreened. A history of multiple sexual partners and IV drug use are both risk factors for HBV. Canada is not a country with high prevalence (>2 percent) of disease, so screening is not recommended based on her prior country of residence.

Screen now for HCV? Yes

Screen now for HBV? Yes

Next screening for HCV: Only if new risk factors present

Next screening for HBV: Only if new risk factors present or with pregnancy

A 50-year-old woman born in 1964 presents for her well-woman visit. She has a negative medical and surgical history. She has worked at the local hospital as a labor and delivery nurse for 25 years and is recently divorced. She denies any history of illicit drug use but does drink alcohol on a nightly basis. She is not sexually active.

One-time HCV screening is recommended for persons born between 1945 and 1965. Moderate alcohol intake is not a risk factor for HCV infection. Persons who are at high risk of HBV infection include those who are infected with HIV, injection drug users, household contacts or sex partners of persons with HBV infection, and men who have sex with men. Her work as a labor and delivery nurse does not alone put her at enough risk to recommend screening.

Screen now for HCV? Yes

Screen now for HBV? No

Next screening for HCV: Only if new risk factors present

Next screening for HBV: Only if new risk factors present

A 28-year-old woman who was born in China and works as a lab technician at the local university presents for well-woman visit. She denies any history of blood transfusion, IV drug use, alcohol use, or tattoos. She is married and has only been sexually active with one partner. She uses a copper IUD for contraception.

Women at high risk of HCV include IV drug users, having a history of blood transfusion before 1992, those born to an HCV-infected mother, current or former incarceration, intranasal drug use, and those with other percutaneous exposures. The highest incidence rate of HCV infection is found among American Indians and Alaska Natives, and the lowest incidence among persons of Asian or Pacific Islander descent. In the United States, persons at high risk of HBV infection include those born in countries and regions with a high prevalence of HBV infection (2 percent or greater) and US-born persons who were not vaccinated as infants and whose parents are from a country or region with a very high prevalence of HBV infection (8 percent or greater), such as sub-Saharan Africa, central and southeast Asia, and China.

Screen now for HCV? No

Screen now for HBV? Yes

Next screening for HCV: Only if new risk factors present

Next screening for HBV: Only if new risk factors present or with pregnancy

Guidelines

a. Moyer, V.A. Screening for hepatitis C virus infection in adults: US Preventive Services Task Force Recommendation Statement. *Ann Intern Med.* 2013, 159:349–35.

b. US Preventive Services Task Force. Screening for hepatitis B virus infection in pregnancy: US Preventive Services Task Force reaffirmation recommendation statement. *Ann Intern Med.* 2009, 150:869–73.

c. LeFevre, M.L. Screening for hepatitis B virus infection in nonpregnant adolescents and adults: US Preventive Services Task Force recommendation statement. *Ann Intern Med.* 2014, 161:58–66.

d. Conry, J.A. and Brown, H. Well-Woman Task Force: Components of the Well-Woman Visit. *Obstet Gynecol.* 2015, 126:697–701.

References

1. Smith, B.D., Patel, N., Beckett, G.A., Jewett, A., and Ward, J.W. Hepatitis C virus antibody prevalence, correlates and predictors among persons born from 1945 through 1965, United States, 199–2008. *Hepatology.* 2011, 544(suppl 1):554A–5A.

2. Chou, R., Cottrell, E.B., Wasson, N., Rahman, B., and Guise, J.M. *Screening for Hepatitis C Virus Infection in Adults.* Comparative Effectiveness Review No. 69. AHRQ Publication No. 12-EHC090-EF. Rockville, MD: Agency for Healthcare Research and Quality; 2012. Available at: www.effectivehealthcare.ahrq.gov/search-for-guides-reviews-and-reports/?pageaction=displayproduct&productid=1284.

3. Kowdley, K.V., Wang, C.C., Welch, S., Roberts, H., and Brosgart, C.L. Prevalence of chronic hepatitis B among foreign-born persons living in the United States by country of origin. *Hepatology.* 2012, 56:422–33.

4. Van der Meer, A.J., Veldt, B.J., Feld, J.J. et al. Association between sustained virological response and all-cause mortality among patients with chronic hepatitis C and advanced hepatic fibrosis. *JAMA.* 2012, 308:2584–93.

5. Chou, R., Cottrell, E.B., Wasson, N., Rahman, B., and Guise, J.M. A systematic review to update the 2004 US Preventive Services Task Force recommendation. *Ann Intern Med.* 2013, 158:101–8.

6. Mabry-Hernandez, I. and Blackmer, S. Screening for hepatitis C virus infection in adults. *Am Fam Physician.* 2014, 90(6):405–6.

7. Geographic prevalence of Hepatitis B. CDC Yellowbook. 2016; chapter 3. Available at: wwwnc.cdc.gov/travel/yellowbook/2016/infectious-diseases-related-to-travel/hepatitis-b.

8. Weinbaum, C.M., Williams, I., Mast, E.E. et al.; Centers for Disease Control and Prevention. Recommendations for identification and public health management of persons with chronic hepatitis B virus infection. *MMWR Recom Rep.* 2008, 57(RR-8):1–20.

Chapter 32

HIV Screening

Sarah Milton

Why Screen?

Human immunodeficiency virus (HIV) is a single-stranded RNA virus that is transmitted by exposure to infected bodily fluids. While the incidence of HIV infection in the United States has been stable over the last 20 years, the overall burden of the disease has increased substantially. The Centers for Disease Control and Prevention (CDC) estimates there were 47,500 new cases of HIV in 2010 and that over 1.2 million people in the United States are currently living with HIV or AIDS. Women represent one-quarter of HIV-infected individuals in the United States. African American women are disproportionately affected, comprising over 60 percent of the female HIV-infected population. Despite efforts to increase HIV screening, one in five people infected with HIV are unaware of their diagnosis [a]. In contrast to other at-risk populations, the majority of new HIV infections in women are contracted via heterosexual contact. The risk of acquiring HIV during unprotected heterosexual intercourse is much greater for women than it is for men [a]. Medical professionals providing preventive care to women are uniquely positioned to screen for HIV infection and counsel regarding effective prevention strategies.

Screening for HIV infection is critical, as early HIV diagnosis improves overall survival [1]. Awareness of HIV infection provides infected individuals with insight regarding risk-taking behavior and allows for education and intervention to decrease transmission of the virus. Prompt identification of persons infected with HIV allows for early initiation of treatment [2].

Rationale for Screening

Providing appropriate screening for HIV infection and counseling regarding disease status requires a basic understanding of the pathophysiology of HIV infection. Approximately 10 days after HIV infection, HIV-1 RNA is detectable in plasma. Four to ten days later, the HIV-1 p24 antigen is transiently detectable. This time period represents "acute" HIV infection. Ten to thirteen days after HIV RNA is first detected in plasma, HIV immunoglobulin M (IgM) antibodies are expressed at levels detectable by most immunoassays. Approximately 3 weeks following HIV infection, HIV immunoglobulin (IgG) antibodies are detectable and subsequently persist, indicative of established infection [2] (Figure 32.1).

From 1989 to 2014, HIV screening was performed with a repeatedly reactive immunoassay for HIV antibodies. Positive screening tests were then confirmed with either an HIV-1 Western blot or HIV-1 immunofluorescence assay. Comprehensive review of HIV screening practices led the CDC to identify several weaknesses in this screening strategy. Specifically:

- The algorithm failed to identify acute HIV-1 infections.
- Assays that detect HIV-1 infection earlier are now widely available.
- The risk of HIV-1 transmission from persons with acute and early infection is much higher than that from a person with established infection.
- Initiation of antiretroviral therapy during the early stage of HIV-1 infection can benefit the patient and reduce HIV transmission.
- The use of HIV-1 Western Blot in the previous algorithm misclassifies the majority of HIV-2 infections. HIV-2 is rare in the United States, but appropriate identification of HIV-2 infection is critical as effective retroviral therapy for HIV-2 differs from HIV-1 [2].

In light of these weaknesses, the CDC has recommended a new testing strategy [2]. The new screening recommendations increase the sensitivity of diagnosis of acute HIV infection compared to prior screening algorithms [3].

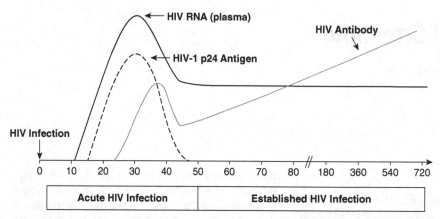

Figure 32.1 Immune Response to Human Immunodeficiency Virus (HIV) Infection (Adapted from CDC Laboratory Testing for the Diagnosis of HIV Infection)

Source: Centers for Disease Control and Prevention, Association of Public Health Laboratories. Laboratory Testing for the Diagnosis of HIV Infection Updated Recommendations. *Atlanta, GA: CDC; Silver Spring, MD: APHL; 2014. Available at: www.cdc.gov/hiv/pdf/hivtestingalgorithmrecommendation-final.pdf.*

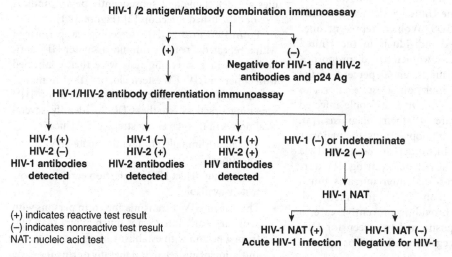

Figure 32.2 Human Immunodeficiency Virus (HIV) Screening Algorithm (adapted from CDC Laboratory Testing for the Diagnosis of HIV Infection)

Source: Centers for Disease Control and Prevention, Association of Public Health Laboratories. Laboratory Testing for the Diagnosis of HIV Infection Updated Recommendations. *Atlanta, GA: CDC; Silver Spring, MD: APHL; 2014. Available at: www.cdc.gov/hiv/pdf/hivtestingalgorithmrecommendation-final.pdf.*

The new screening test is a serum HIV-1/2 antigen/antibody immunoassay that detects antibodies to both HIV-1 and HIV-2 and the HIV-1 p24 antigen. This test identifies both acute and long-standing infections and distinguishes HIV-1 from HIV-2 infection (Figure 32.2).

The most important benefit of the new screening algorithm compared to prior screening methods is sensitivity in the detection of acute HIV infection [3]. Early diagnosis is associated with an overall decrease in morbidity. HIV screening has been proven to be cost-effective from a population health perspective [a].

Factors That Affect Screening

Age: HIV infection can occur at any age, including adolescents and women over age 65.

Risk factors for transmission:

- More than one sex partner since last HIV test
- Use of intravenous drugs
- Sex partners who use intravenous drugs
- Patients who exchange sex for money or drugs
- HIV-infected sex partner(s)
- Sex partner(s) including men who have sex with other men [a, b]

Blood and organ donors: HIV testing is mandatory in persons who donate blood or organs to prevent unintended infection of patients receiving the donated tissue.

Possible acute HIV infection: Around 40–90 percent of HIV-infected individuals will experience symptoms of viral illness (fever, chills, and myalgias) during the acute phase of the infection. These symptoms often come to clinical attention when patients seek care from primary care providers. In this setting, identification of risk factors for HIV infection should result in HIV screening and can lead to identification of early HIV infection [a].

Occupational exposure: Persons who have an occupational exposure to blood or bodily fluids should be screened for HIV unless the source patient's HIV status is immediately available [a].

Specimen source: The commercially available home HIV testing kits or rapid HIV tests only test for HIV-1 antibodies (evidence of established infection). HIV tests that use dried blood or saliva are also less sensitive and test only for HIV antibodies. A positive result with rapid and home HIV test kits requires confirmatory testing [2].

Recommended Guidelines and How to Find Them

While the Well-Women Task Force (WWTF) included sexually transmitted infections in their work plan, they did not review or make specific recommendations regarding HIV screening guidelines. The CDC is the primary source for HIV screening guidelines. Their 2006 "Recommendations for HIV Testing in Adults, Adolescents, and Pregnant Women in Health-Care Settings" serves as the source of the recommendations for most other professional societies and outlines screening parameters [a]. The CDC also makes recommendations on the specific laboratory tests to be used for screening. The most recent update to this document, in 2014, introduced a new screening algorithm [2]. The US Preventive

Services Task Force (USPSTF) recommendations are similar to those outlined by the CDC [b]. The American Medical Association also recommends routine HIV screening as recommend by the CDC [c]. The American College of Obstetrics and Gynecology (ACOG) endorses the CDC screening recommendations [d]. HIV screening is recommended in at-risk adolescent patients.

How to Screen

All women between the ages of 13 and 64 should be tested for HIV at least once in their lifetime.

Special considerations related to consent and privacy may be present for minors. Although providers should encourage open communication between adolescents and their parents or guardians, most states allow for adolescent sexually transmitted disease (STD) screening without parental consent or notification. Information regarding state laws and minor consent for care is maintained by the Guttmacher Institute [4]. Providers should be familiar with local laws to allow for safe and proactive care for at-risk adolescents in their practice.

Following initial screening, annual assessment of risk factors is recommended. Screening should continue in women aged 65 and older if they have risk factors for HIV infection. At least annual HIV testing should be performed in women with any of the following risk factors:

- More than one sex partner since their last HIV test
- Use of intravenous drugs
- Sex partners who use intravenous drugs
- Exchange sex for money or drugs
- HIV-infected sex partner
- Have sex with men who have sex with other men [a]

HIV screening is also indicated for:

- *Pregnancy*: HIV screening is routinely performed during initial prenatal visits. Identification of HIV-infected pregnant women is critical for the prevention of perinatal transmission [5].
- *Sexually transmitted infections*: Any woman with concern for or diagnosis of an STD should be screened for HIV [a].
- *New sexual relationship*: Providers should encourage women to be screened for all sexually transmitted infections, including HIV, prior to initiation of a new sexual relationship [a].

- *Occupational exposure*: Persons who have an occupational exposure to blood or bodily fluids should be screened unless the source patient's HIV status is immediately available [a].
- *Possible acute HIV infection*: Screening with plasma RNA for acute HIV infection is indicated in patients with symptoms of acute HIV infection (fever, chills, myalgias) and recent high-risk behavior [a].

No written consent is necessary to screen for HIV; however, patients should be informed that this test is being ordered based on clinical history, risk factors, occupational exposure, or other factors. Clear documentation should be outlined in the medical record if a patient declines HIV screening [a, d]

Based on the 2014 CDC recommendations, screening should be done with the HIV-1/2 antigen/antibody combination immunoassay. This test has increased sensitivity for detection of early, acute HIV infection [2]. Rapid HIV tests are available that yield results in less than 1 hour. If a rapid HIV test is positive, confirmatory testing is necessary before assigning definitive HIV diagnosis [6].

Communication of positive test results should be done in person by a provider with experience in counseling patients regarding HIV. Prompt referral to an infectious disease specialist to initiate care is prudent. Providers should encourage women to discuss HIV status with current and prior sexual partners so that they can also be tested. If women are reticent to disclose results personally, local health departments often provide anonymous partner notification systems that encourage screening without revealing the identity of the infected person [a][2]. It is mandatory that new HIV cases are reported to state health departments [a].

All women, but particularly women who are at risk for HIV infection, should be counseled regarding prevention strategies and screening expectations. While prevention counseling is not a mandatory part of HIV screening, it is an important component of well-woman care. Safe sex practices, condom use, and education on risk factors should be addressed as part of prevention counseling [a][2].

New Developments Likely to Affect Future Guidelines

Increasing compliance with the new HIV screening algorithm (HIV-1/2 antigen/antibody combination immunoassay) will result in more specific efficacy data. Identification of an increasing number of acute HIV infections may allow for more tailored treatment of early infection and changes in screening recommendations. There is insufficient data to determine if the new screening algorithm is sufficient to identify seroconversion in patients taking retroviral medications or pre- or postexposure prophylaxis prior to or following exposure to HIV infection. This remains an area of ongoing research [2].

Billing

HIV screening can be billed independent of other components of the well-woman visit with the following codes:

1. Z11.3 – Encounter for screening for infections with a predominantly sexual mode of transmission
2. Z11.4 – Encounter for screening for human immunodeficiency virus

Illustrative Cases

A 24-year-old female presents for annual well-woman examination. When she was seen last year, she was screened for HIV and the test was negative. She has had two sexual partners in the last year. She is in a monogamous relationship with her current partner and uses condoms.

HIV screening is recommended for all women with more than one sexual partner since their last HIV test. The patient should be counseled about the recommendation and offered screening.

Screen now? Yes

Next screen? Dependent upon risk assessment, which should be performed annually

A healthy 16-year-old presents for a well-adolescent care. She has been sexually active with one lifetime partner and reports using a condom with all acts of intercourse. She is accompanied by her mother who is aware of her sexual history and is supportive of her daughter receiving reproductive health care.

Screening for HIV is recommended in adolescents who are sexually active. Providers should encourage parental involvement. In most states, HIV screening can be performed without parental consent or notification. It is important that providers are aware of individual state laws related to consent for reproductive health care service in minors. Access to minor reproductive health laws is available via the Guttmacher Institute at www.guttmacher.org/state center/spibs/spib_OMCL.pdf.

Screen now? Yes

Next screen? Well-woman visits should include assessment for HIV risk factors and repeat testing if risk factors are identified

> *A 34-year-old gravida 0 woman presents for a well-woman visit. She is sexually active with her husband. She is in a monogamous committed relationship for the last 4 years. She has never had an HIV test.*

The CDC recommends all women aged 13–65 be screened at least once for HIV infection. HIV screening is best performed with HIV-1/2 antigen/antibody combination immunoassay.

Screen now? Yes

Next screen? Dependent upon risk assessment, which should be performed at each well-woman visit

Guidelines

a. Branson, B.M., Handsfield, H.H., Lampe, M.A., et al. *Revised Recommendations for HIV Testing of Adults, Adolescents, and Pregnant Women in Health-Care Settings.* MMWR 2006;**55**(RR14);1–17. Available at: www.cdc.gov/mmwr/preview/mmwrhtml/rr5514a1.htm. Retrieved January 28, 2017.

b. Screening for HIV: US Preventive Services Task Force: Recommendation Statement. VA Moyer, on behalf of the US Preventive Services Task Force. *Ann Intern Med.* 2013, **159**:51–6.

c. AMA Policy D-20.992. Routine HIV Screening. Available at: searchpf.ama-assn.org/SearchML/searchDetails.action?uri=%2FAMADoc%2Fdirectives.xml-0-488.xml. Retrieved January 28, 2017.

d. American College of Obstetricians and Gynecologists. Routine Human Immunodeficiency Virus Screening.

Committee Opinion No. 596.*Obstet Gynecol.* 2014, **123**: 1137–9. Available at: www.acog.org/Resources-And-Publications/Committee-Opinions/Committee-on-Gynecologic-Practice/Routine-Human-Immunodeficiency-Virus-Screening. Retrieved January 28, 2017.

References

1. Palella, F.J. Jr, Deloria-Knoll, M., Chmiel, J.S. et al. Survival benefit of initiating antiretroviral therapy in HIV-infected persons in different CD4+ cell strata. *HIV Outpatient Study Investigators.* Ann Intern Med. 2003, **138**:620–6.

2. Centers for Disease Control and Prevention, Association of Public Health Laboratories. *Laboratory Testing for the Diagnosis of HIV Infection Updated Recommendations.* Atlanta, GA: CDC; Silver Spring, MD: APHL, 2014. Available at: http://stacks.cdc.gov/view/cdc/23447. Retrieved June 27, 2014.

3. Bentsen, C., McLaughlin, L., Mitchell, E. et al. Performance evaluation of the bio-rad laboratories GS HIV combo Ag/Ab EIA, a 4th generation HIV assay for the simultaneous detection of HIV p24 antigen and antibodies to HIV-1 (groups M and O) and HIV-2 in human serum or plasma. *J Clin Virol.* 2011, **52**(Suppl 1): S57–61.

4. Guttmacher Institute. *An Overview of Minors' Consent Law. State Policies in Brief.* New York, NY: Guttmacher Institute, 2013. Available at: www.guttmacher.org/state center/spibs/spib_OMCL.pdf. Retrieved January 28, 2017.

5. American College of Obstetricians and Gynecologists. Prenatal and perinatal human immunodeficiency virus testing: Expanded recommendations. *Committee Opinion No. 635*Obstet Gynecol. 2015, **125**:1544–7.

6. American College of Obstetricians and Gynecologists. Human immunodeficiency virus. *ACOG Committee Opinion No. 389.* Obstet Gynecol. 2007, **110**:1473–8.

Chapter 33

Sexually Transmitted Infections

Kevin A. Ault

Why Screen?

Sexually active women may be exposed to a variety of common sexually transmitted infections (STIs). *Chlamydia trachomatis* is an obligate intracellular bacterium. It can infect the columnar epithelium of the urethra, cervix, endometrium, and fallopian tubes. It is a common STI, especially among young adults and adolescents. There are approximately 1 million cases of *Chlamydia* annually in the United States, making *Chlamydia* the most common bacterial infection reported to the Centers for Disease Control and Prevention (CDC). Over the past two decades, rates of *Chlamydia* have gradually increased (Figure 33.1). This is likely due to increased screening and reporting. Rates of 3–19 percent in young women aged 15–24 have been reported [1]. Clinical diseases such as cervicitis and pelvic inflammatory disease (PID) are associated with chlamydial infections. Long-term gynecological sequelae such as ectopic pregnancy and tubal factor infertility are associated with prior infection with *Chlamydia trachomatis*. *Neisseria gonorrhoeae* is a gram-positive bacterium, and it also will infect the epithelial surfaces of the lower genital tract. Clinically, gonorrhea causes similar diseases to *Chlamydia*, such as cervicitis, PID, and tubal factor infertility. Gonorrhea is less prevalent than *Chlamydia*. Data from the CDC indicate a prevalence of 0–5 percent in young adult women [1]. Historically, *N. gonorrhoeae* has quickly developed antibiotic resistance to commonly used antibiotics. Herpes simplex virus (HSV) is a common viral STI. Up to 50 million Americans are infected by HSV-2 [2]. However, because HSV infections are symptomatic, routine screening is not recommended. *Trichomonas vaginalis* is another common STI that can cause symptomatic vaginal discharge but little other morbidity. Other chapters cover human immunodeficiency virus (HIV), Hepatitis B, and Hepatitis C screening and prevention.

Rationale for Screening

Screening for *Chlamydia* and gonorrhea is a potential strategy for improving women's health for multiple reasons: (1) *Chlamydia* and gonorrhea are common asymptomatic infections; (2) these infections are associated with adverse outcomes; (3) sensitive and specific screening tests are available; and (4) effective and inexpensive antibiotic regimens are available. In contradistinction to bacterial STIs such as *Chlamydia*, there is no curative treatment for HSV. Screening programs for *Chlamydia* have been well studied. A randomized trial of screening for *Chlamydia* in young women in Seattle, Washington, showed a 56 percent reduction in PID rates [3]. A retrospective analysis of *Chlamydia* screening in British Columbia, Canada, found PID hospitalization rates decreased by 80 percent and ectopic pregnancy by 50 percent during the 17-year period after the screening program was implemented [4]. There are no studies that show screening helps decrease transmission to uninfected partners.

Factors That Affect Screening

The CDC has identified several special populations for STI screening based upon epidemiologic risk factors.

Age: Consistent epidemiological evidence shows the highest rates of infection in adolescent and young adults and supports routine screening for *Chlamydia* and gonorrhea.

Persons in correctional facilities: The higher prevalence of STIs among incarcerated women supports raising the age for *Chlamydia* and gonorrhea screening to 35 or younger. Screening for syphilis is indicated on the basis of disease prevalence in the facility and local community.

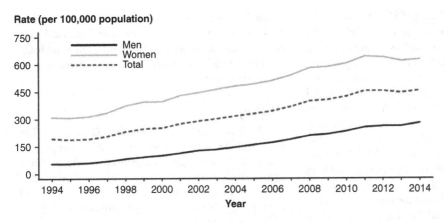

Figure 33.1 Rates of *Chlamydia trachomatis* Infection in the United States, 1994–2014. Data from the Centers for Disease Control and Prevention

Source: Centers for Disease Control and Prevention. Sexually Transmitted Disease Surveillance 2014. *Atlanta, GA: US Department of Health and Human Services, 2015. Available at: www.cdc.gov.*

BOX 33.1 Additional Factors That Indicate Increased Risk for Chlamydia and Gonorrhea Infections [1,2]

New sex partner, more than one sex partner, a sex partner with concurrent partners, or a sex partner who has a sexually transmitted infection (STI)
Inconsistent condom use
Previous or coexisting STI
Exchanging sex for money or drugs
Known high-prevalence population such as incarcerated women, military recruits, and women receiving care at public STI clinics

---

Women who have sex with women (WSW): While STI transmission may follow different patterns in WSW, clinicians should offer screening according to current guidelines.

Transgender individuals: Risk assessment should focus on current anatomy and sexual behaviors.

Recommend Guidelines and Where to Find Them

A sexual history and assessment for STI exposure should be a part of each well-woman visit. Age-based screening for *Chlamydia* and gonorrhea in adolescent and young adult women is consistent with CDC guidelines and the recommendations of the Well-Woman Task Force (WWTF) [a-b]. The current recommendation for *Chlamydia* screening is to test sexually active women aged 24 and younger on an annual basis. Screening recommendations for gonorrhea parallel the recommendations for *Chlamydia* [b, c]. Asymptomatic women over the age of 24 should be screened for both of these bacterial infections if they have one or more of the risk

factors summarized in Box 33.1. *Chlamydia* and gonorrhea screening are also endorsed by the US Preventive Services Task Force (USPSTF) [c]. Currently, there are no organizations that endorse routine screening for asymptomatic genital HSV infection [d]. According to CDC guidelines, screening asymptomatic women for syphilis is not recommended unless a sexual partner is known to be infected. Additionally, CDC does not endorse routine screening of nonpregnant adolescents or women who are asymptomatic for trichomonas, bacterial vaginosis, human papillomavirus, Hepatitis A virus, and Hepatitis B virus [a]. Guidelines for HIV and Hepatitis infection are discussed further in the preceding chapters. The CDC provides a useful table summarizing sexually transmitted disease (STD) screening recommendations at www.cdc.gov/std/tg 2015/screening-recommendations.htm. The WWTF adopted the CDC and USPSTF guidelines.

How to Screen

Three mobile applications for smart phones are available to support STI screening. The American College of Obstetrics and Gynecology (ACOG) has an application that allows users to search for specific topics such as "*Chlamydia*." Search results will show relevant ACOG documents. The USPSTF has an application named "ePSS." Screening recommendations are based on the clinical information entered at the initial screen, and this information includes gender, age, pregnancy status, and a few other variables. Clinicians may find the USPSTF application useful; there is considerable overlap with the WWTF recommendations. The CDC has an application based on the 2015 CDC STD Guidelines. This application is best for searching for antibiotic treatments for STIs.

There are multiple available tests for detecting *Chlamydia* and gonorrhea. "Nucleic acid amplification tests" (NAATs) target and amplify key bacterial nucleic acid sequences unique to the specific microorganism [5]. NAATs are a vast improvement over prior methods of culture or antigen detection. This improved sensitivity makes NAATs the best test for screening for *Chlamydia* and gonorrhea. These tests can be performed on urine or endocervical samples.

Additional screening is warranted in women seeking evaluation and treatment for STIs. According to the CDC, all such persons should be offered screening for HIV infection, irrespective of their risk status. Hepatitis B vaccine should be routinely offered to all unvaccinated women who seek evaluation or treatment for STIs, along with immediate prevaccination serologic testing to determine susceptibility and the need to complete the vaccination series. The preceding chapters provide additional information on screening methods for HIV and Hepatitis B.

Testing for *T. vaginalis* may be offered to women with vaginal discharge and asymptomatic women with risk factors (multiple-sex partners, exchanging sex for payment, illicit drug use, or a history of STI). The CDC recommends using highly sensitive and specific tests for detecting trichomonas. NAATs are favored due to their sensitivity being three to five times higher than wet-mount microscopy. Screening for bacterial vaginosis and HSV infection is not recommended in asymptomatic patients [a].

New Developments Likely to Affect Future Guidelines

A 2014 review article concluded that vaginal specimens were the "preferred specimen type" for *Chlamydia* and gonorrhea screening [5]. Patient-collected vaginal swabs have the same sensitivity as endocervical samples and may be more sensitive than urine samples.

The USPSTF guidelines for herpes screening are currently under review.

Billing

The ICD-10 code for screening for STIs is Z11.3. This code excludes screening for HIV and human papillomavirus. Another potentially useful code is Z20.2, exposure to infections with a predominantly sexual mode of transmission. The CPT codes for NAAT testing for *Chlamydia* and gonorrhea is 87491 and 87591, respectively.

Illustrative Cases

A healthy 20-year-old female comes in for her first well-woman visit. She is sexually active using condoms. She has one lifetime male partner.

A sexual history and assessment for STI exposure should be a part of each well-woman visit. In addition, this patient would fall into the guidelines for age-based screening. There are also several important STI-related counseling messages that should be discussed, including that condoms reduce the risk of STI.

Screen now? Yes for *Chlamydia* and gonorrhea, as well as HIV

Next screening: Annually until age 24

A healthy 28-year-old female was last seen 6 months ago for a well-woman exam. Since that time, she has three male partners, and she does not use condoms consistently. She wants to be "tested for everything" because one of her partners was recently seen at a local health department for an unknown STI. On examination, there is no vaginal discharge or cervicitis.

This patient has a number of risk factors for STI including multiple recent partners, inconsistent condom use, and possible contact with an infected partner.

Screen now? Yes for *Chlamydia* and gonorrhea, as well as HIV and trichomonas. She should also be offered Hepatitis B vaccination if unvaccinated. The CDC does not recommend screening for syphilis unless the sexual partner is known to be infected and does not recommend screening for HSV or bacterial vaginosis in asymptomatic women.

Next screening: Depending on risk factors

A 55-year-old parous woman is seen for a well-woman visit. Her last menstrual period was 6 years ago. She has well-controlled hypertension. She has not been sexually active for 4 years. Previously, she had vaginal dryness and painful intercourse when sexually active. The patient would like to be sexually active with a new male partner, but is concerned about pain. On examination, there are atrophic changes and yellow discharge.

Patient does not have risk factors for STI.
Screen now? No
Next screening: Depending on risk factors

Guidelines

a. Workowski, K.A. and Bolan, G.A. Sexually transmitted diseases treatment guidelines, 2015. *MMWR Recomm Rep.* 2015, **64**(No. RR-3):1–138.

b. Conry, J.A. and Brown, H. Well-Woman Task Force: Components of the Well-Woman Visit. *Obstet Gynecol.* 2015, **126**(4):697–701.

c. LeFevre, M.L. on behalf of US Preventive Services Task Force. Screening for chlamydia and gonorrhea: US preventive services task force recommendation statement. *Ann Intern Med.* 2014, **161**(12):902–10.

d. US Preventive Services Task Force. Screening for genital herpes recommendation statement. Available at: www .uspreventiveservicestaskforce.org/Page/Document/Re commendationStatementFinal/genital-herpes-screening. Retrieved April 25, 2016.

References

1. Centers for Disease Control and Prevention. *Sexually Transmitted Disease Surveillance 2014.* Atlanta, GA: US Department of Health and Human Services, 2015. Available at: www.cdc.gov. Retrieved January 28, 2017.

2. Satterwhite, C.L., Torrone, E., Meites, E. et al. Sexually transmitted infections among US women and men: Prevalence and incidence estimates, 2008. *Sex Transm Dis.* 2013, **40**(3):187–93.

3. Scholes, D., Stergachis, A., Heidrich, F.E. et al. Prevention of pelvic inflammatory disease by screening for cervical chlamydial infection. *N Engl J Med.* 1996, **334**(21):1362–6.

4. Rekart, M.L., Gilbert, M., Meza, R. et al. Chlamydia public health programs and the epidemiology of pelvic inflammatory disease and ectopic pregnancy. *J Infect Dis.* 2013, **207**(1):30–8.

5. Papp, J.R., Schachter, J., Gaydos, C.A., and Van Der Pol, B. Recommendations for the laboratory-based detection of *Chlamydia trachomatis* and *Neisseria gonorrhoeae* – 2014. *MMWR.* 2014, **63**(RR02):1–19.

Skin Cancer

34

Meghan L. Valentine

Why Is Screening and Prevention Important?

Skin cancer is the most common type of cancer in the United States [1], with current estimates that one in five Americans will develop skin cancer in their lifetime [2]. An estimated 5.4 million cases of nonmelanoma skin cancer (NMSC) are diagnosed in 3.3 million people annually [3]. Of these cases, approximately two-thirds are basal cell carcinoma (BCC) and one-quarter are squamous cell carcinoma (SCC) [4]. Both SCC and BCC are highly curable if detected early. In contrast, melanoma, which accounts for less than 2 percent of skin cancer cases, is responsible for the majority of skin cancer deaths [5]. The incidence of melanoma among white Americans has been increasing for the past 30 years, from 8.7 per 100,000 persons in 1975 to 28.1 per 100,000 persons in 2012. It is estimated that in 2015, melanoma will account for 74,000 cases of newly diagnosed skin cancer, with 9,940 associated deaths [6].

Rationale for Screening and Prevention

Exposure to ultraviolet radiation (UVR) is a major risk factor for skin cancer, and exposure reduction is an important strategy for skin cancer risk reduction. Behavioral counseling on sun-protective behaviors appears most effective in adolescents and young adults. Both traditional cancer prevention and appearance-focused messages, which stress the effect of UVR on skin, have been shown to be effective in this population [7].

Early detection is another appealing strategy. Screening entails either a whole or partial body examination, focused on detection of melanoma and NMSC. The main purpose of screening is to detect cancers earlier, allowing earlier treatment and

reduction in skin cancer morbidity and mortality. While skin cancer diagnosed at an earlier stage, especially in the case of melanoma, is associated with improved survival, research has not shown a correlation between early detection and all-cause skin cancer morbidity and mortality [a]. Additionally, prior research has shown that most primary care physicians report insufficient training to feel confident in their skills to perform whole-body skin examinations [8]. Therefore, whole-body skin examination at the time of well-woman exam is not recommended.

Factors That Affect Screening

Exposure to UVR: Increasing intermittent (or recreational) sun exposure, as opposed to total or chronic exposure, appears to be associated with increased risk of all types of skin cancer [4]. Timing of exposure to UVR is significant, with increased exposure during childhood and youth contributing more to one's lifetime risk of skin cancer than after age 35 [7]. Excessive UVR through sun exposure or tanning bed use also raises risk.

Phenotypic characteristics: Fair skin, light eye and hair color, freckles, and tendency to sunburn easily elevate risk [4].

Diseases or treatments that suppress the immune system [4]

Family history of melanoma [9]

Nevi: Increased number of dysplastic nevi or total number of nevi >50 increase risk [9].

Previous history of NMSC [9]

Recommended Guidelines and How to Find Them

Multiple US professional organizations have published guidelines on skin cancer prevention and screening. The majority of the guidelines reiterate those of the US Preventive Services Task Force (USPSTF) [a], with a few exceptions.

The USPSTF recommends counseling children and adolescents aged 10–24 who have fair skin about minimizing their exposure to UVR. For adults older than 24 years, they cite insufficient evidence to assess the balance of benefits and harms of behavioral counseling. They recommend against both clinician-performed skin cancer screening and patient skin self-examination. These guidelines are publicly available on the USPSTF website.

The Well-Woman Task Force (WWTF) similarly recommends counseling adolescents and young adults, aged 13–24, about minimizing their exposure to UVR and recommends against whole-body examination [b]. However, in contrast to the USPSTF, the WWTF recommends that women of all ages be encouraged to use sunscreen regularly and avoid artificial tanning. The American College of Obstetricians and Gynecologists (ACOG) parallels these recommendations with the exception of not making a statement on whole-body examination [c].

The American Academy of Family Physicians (AAFP) has adopted the USPSTF guidelines [d] and endorses these recommendations on their website. The American Academy of Pediatrics (AAP) published a policy statement in 2011 [e], recommending clinicians incorporate advice about UVR exposure into counseling for all children, especially children at high risk of developing skin cancer. The AAP, in contrast to the AAFP or USPSTF, recommends skin examination as part of a complete physical examination in teenagers, citing high rates of melanoma in this age group. The American Academy of Dermatology (AAD) [f] notably does not provide guidance on clinician-performed skin cancer screening and, however, has offered free skin cancer screening clinics since 1985 [9]. The American Cancer Society (ACS) has no specific recommendation for skin cancer screening, other than a cancer-related check-up by a physician, which may include a skin examination, during a periodic health examination for people aged 21 and older [g].

How to Screen

While all patients should receive similar counseling regardless of risk status, risk factors can guide clinicians on which patients may require a stronger emphasis on sun-protective behaviors. Counseling should be performed on adolescent girls and women of all ages. Since UVR exposure during childhood and youth has shown to have the highest impact on lifetime risk of skin cancer, behavioral interventions may be particularly important in this age group.

Primary prevention of skin cancer focuses on behavioral counseling on sun-protective behaviors. These behavioral interventions include avoidance of mid-day sun (10 a.m. to 3 p.m.), wearing protective clothing and broad-rimmed hats, applying sunscreen with a sun-protection factor (SPF) of 15 or greater, and avoiding indoor tanning [4]. Sunglasses should be worn to protect the skin around the eyes [5]. Patients should be counseled on avoidance of indoor tanning and sun lamps. Based on an extensive review of scientific evidence, the International Agency for Research on Cancer classified ultraviolet-emitting tanning devices as "carcinogenic to humans," showing a higher risk of melanoma in those who regularly use sunbeds [10].

Effective counseling interventions are generally of low intensity and performed during the well-woman visit. Interventions may use cancer prevention or appearance-focused messages as a motivational tool. Appearance-focused messages include self-guided booklets, videos on photoaging, UV facial photography, or 30-minute peer counseling sessions [7]. For adolescent women, appearance-focused methods have shown to be most effective in reducing artificial UVR exposure via indoor tanning [4].

Several organizations that focus on sun safety or skin cancer prevention have created age-appropriate educational materials, many of which include appearance-based messages. (Examples from the National Cancer Institute can be found at http://rtips.cancer .gov/rtips.) The Community Preventive Services Task Force also has a number of resources related to skin cancer prevention through advocacy and interventions that target child care centers; outdoor occupational, recreational, and tourism settings; primary and middle schools; and communities. These resources can be found at www.thecommunityguide.org/can cer/index.html.

Routine whole-body skin examination or patient skin self-examination is not recommended by the WWTF. Lesions brought to the provider's attention by the patient or incidentally noted can be described with either the ABCDE mnemonic or the ugly duckling approach. The ABCDE mnemonic is an acronym used to detect characteristics of melanoma. ABCDE stands for: (A) asymmetry (one half of nevus does not match the other half of the nevus); (B) border irregularity (edges of nevus are ragged, notched, or blurred); (C) color (pigmentation of the nevus is not uniform, with variable degrees of tan, brown, or black); (D) diameter >6 mm; and (E) evolving (nevus is changing over time). The ugly duckling approach assesses which nevi do not look like the others within a cluster of nevi [9]. Any suspicious lesion should be referred to a dermatologist.

New Developments Likely to Affect Future Recommendations

The USPSTF published a draft of their updated recommendations on skin cancer screening in December 2015 [9]. The draft recommendation is unchanged from their previous 2009 recommendation, citing insufficient evidence to assess the balance of benefits and harms of visual skin cancer screening in adults. The draft is currently closed for comment and under review for final publication.

The World Health Organization, American Medical Association, and AAD all support legislation to ban the use of artificial tanning devices by people younger than 18 years [e]. In an effort to reduce additional UVR exposure in adolescents, several US states have initiated legislation to ban the use of tanning beds for persons less than 18 years of age [9]. Legislative efforts focus both on age limitations and written-consent processes. Currently, more than 60 percent of US states regulate tanning facilities for minors, and regulatory efforts are increasing [e].

Further primary care–oriented counseling trials, which promote sun-protective behaviors, are needed to assess success of interventions, especially in young women. Additionally, further research is needed on the benefits and harms of whole-body screening and its effect on reducing adverse health outcomes.

Billing

The appropriate CPT evaluation and management code should be used for billing established (99394–99397) and new (99384–99387) patient well visits. Behavioral counseling regarding sun-protective interventions is covered under the ICD-10 code Z71.89, counseling on health and promotion of disease prevention. The skin cancer screening examination is covered under the ICD-10 code Z12.83, encounter for screening for malignant neoplasm of the skin or screening examination for skin cancer. Alternatively, the wellness diagnosis Z01.419 may be used.

Illustrative Cases

A healthy 17-year-old presents for her annual well-adolescent exam in January. On examination, you note that her skin is unusually tan for this time of year. On questioning, she admits to using an indoor tanning bed on a weekly basis.

The recommendation from all major guidelines is to provide counseling on sun-protective behaviors. The patient should be informed on the harms of excessive UVR exposure during adolescence and increased risk of skin cancer. Counseling should include discussion of risk-reducing behaviors including avoiding indoor tanning, avoiding mid-day sun (10 a.m. to 3 p.m.), wearing protective clothing and broad-rimmed hats, applying sunscreen with an SPF of 15 or greater, and wearing sunglasses when outdoors.

Behavioral counseling: Yes

Skin cancer whole-body examination: No

A healthy 55-year-old woman presents for an annual well-woman exam. Her coworker was recently diagnosed with melanoma and she is concerned regarding her risk of skin cancer. She is wondering if there is a screening exam for melanoma that can be performed.

It is important to inform the patient that melanoma rates increase with age [9]. She should be counseled to avoid artificial tanning and to use sunscreen with an SPF of 15 or greater on a regular basis. At this time, multiple professional organizations including the USPSTF, ACOG, WWTF, and AAFP recommend against routine whole-body screening examinations. If she notes a suspicious lesion, she should schedule an appointment with a dermatologist.

Behavioral counseling: Yes

Skin cancer whole-body examination: No

Next counseling: Next well-woman visit

A 45-year-old healthy woman presents for a well-woman exam.

While counseling the patient on preventive health measures, discussion of sun-protective behaviors should be addressed. She should be encouraged to regularly use sunscreen when outdoors and to avoid artificial tanning.

Behavioral counseling: Yes

Skin cancer whole-body examination: No

Next counseling: Next well-woman visit

Guidelines

a. US Preventive Services Task Force. Screening for skin cancer: US Preventive Services Task Force recommendation statement. *Ann Intern Med.* 2009, **150** (3):188–93.

b. Conry, J.A. and Brown, H. Well-Woman Task Force: Components of the Well-Woman Visit. *Obstet Gynecol.* 2015, **126**(4):697–701.

c. American College of Obstetricians and Gynecologists. *Guidelines for Adolescent Health Care [CD-ROM]*, 2nd edition. Washington, DC: American College of Obstetricians and Gynecologists, 2011.

d. AAFP Clinical Preventive Service Recommendation: Skin Cancer. Available at: www.aafp.org/patient-care/ clinical-recommendations/all/skin-cancer.html. Retrieved January 4, 2016.

e. Council on Environmental H, Section on D, Balk SJ. Ultraviolet radiation: A hazard to children and adolescents. *Pediatrics.* 2011, **127**(3):588–97.

f. American Academy of Dermatology. *Clinical Guidelines.* Schaumburg, IL: American Academy of Dermatology. Available at: www.aad.org/education/clinical-guide lines. Retrieved January 4, 2016.

g. American Cancer Society. *American Cancer Society Guidelines for the Early Detection of Cancer Atlanta.* Atlanta, GA: American Cancer Society. Available at: www.cancer.org/healthy/findcancerearly/cancerscree ningguidelines/american-cancer-society-guidelines- for-the-early-detection-of-cancer. Retrieved January 4, 2016.

References

1. Guy, G.P., Jr., Thomas, C.C., Thompson, T. et al. Vital signs: Melanoma incidence and mortality trends and projections – United States, 1982–2030. *MMWR Morb Mortal Wkly Rep.* 2015, **64**(21):591–6.

2. Stern, R.S. Prevalence of a history of skin cancer in 2007: Results of an incidence-based model. *Arch Dermatol.* 2010, **146**(3):279–82.

3. Rogers, H.W., Weinstock, M.A., Feldman, S.R., and Coldiron, B.M. Incidence estimate of nonmelanoma skin cancer (keratinocyte carcinomas) in the US population, 2012. *JAMA Dermatol.* 2015, **151**(10):1081–6.

4. Lin, J.S., Eder, M., and Weinmann, S. Behavioral counseling to prevent skin cancer: A systematic review for the US Preventive Services Task Force. *Ann Intern Med.* 2011, **154**(3):190–201.

5. American Cancer Society. *Cancer Facts & Figures.* Atlanta, GA: American Cancer Society, 2015.

6. Howlader, N.N.A., Krapcho, M., Garshell, J. et al. *SEER Cancer Statistics Review* 1975–2012. Bethesda, MD: National Cancer Institute.. Available at: http://seer .cancer.gov/csr/1975_2012. Retrieved January 4, 2016.

7. Moyer, V.A.; Force USPST. Behavioral counseling to prevent skin cancer: US Preventive Services Task Force recommendation statement. *Ann Intern Med.* 2012, **157**(1):59–65.

8. Wise, E., Singh, D., Moore, M. et al. Rates of skin cancer screening and prevention counseling by US medical residents. *Arch Dermatol.* 2009, **145**(10):1131–6.

9. US Preventive Services Task Force. Draft Recommendation Statement: Skin Cancer: Screening. November 2015. Available at: www .uspreventiveservicestaskforce.org/Page/Document/dr aft-recommendation-statement168/skin-cancer- screening2. Retrieved on January 4, 2016.

10. Beauty and the beast. *Lancet Oncol.* 2009, **10**(9):835.

Chapter 35

Cervical Cancer

David Chelmow

Why Screen?

In 2014, there were an estimated 12,360 new cases of cervical cancer, and 4,020 women died of the disease in the United States [1]. These figures are truly tragic, as cervical cancer is particularly amenable to primary prevention through vaccination, and secondary prevention through screening with Pap and human papillomavirus (HPV) testing. Cervical cancer screening remains the model for successful cancer prevention. Whenever cervical screening is introduced into a population, cervical cancer incidence falls [2]. Advances in understanding of cervical cancer pathogenesis combined with results of new studies have led to further improvements in cervical screening and iterative revisions to major society guidelines. The move away from annual Pap testing has been a prime motivator for the reexamination of the well-woman visit and inspiration for the Well-Woman Task Force (WWTF). While no longer required annually, cervical screening remains a key component of well-woman care.

Rationale for Screening

The success of cervical cancer screening relies on several important characteristics of cervical cancer pathogenesis. Cervical cancer is caused by high-risk types of HPV. There is a long lag time between infection and development of cancer, and there are readily detectable premalignant states usually present for years prior to the development of malignancy. Cervical cytology (Pap testing) detects squamous intraepithelial lesions, and HPV testing detects HPV infection, two important strategies for detecting cervical cancer precursors and allowing intervention to prevent cancer. These interventions generally excise or ablate the cervical transformation zone, where these premalignant lesions occur. Loop electrical excision procedure (LEEP) in the office setting is most frequently performed, although cryotherapy and cold knife and laser conization can also be used.

Unfortunately, there are some important factors that complicate screening. Infection with high-risk HPV types is extremely common, and most infected women will never develop cancer. The bulk of women infected with HPV get transient infection manifested by either no cytologic abnormality or low-grade lesions. These infections have extremely small cancer risk, and treatment of this very large group of women would have little benefit. In a much smaller group of women, viral DNA incorporates into the cellular host genome leading to true malignant potential manifested by high-grade cellular changes detectable by cytology and biopsy [3]. Even in this group with high-grade lesions, some will regress and progression to cancer is slow. Data on risk come from a widely condemned unethical, unapproved experiment, where women with carcinoma in situ were followed without intervention. Approximately one-third developed cervical cancer over 30 years of follow-up [4]. Diagnostic procedures, particularly colposcopy, are uncomfortable and generate significant cost, and therapeutic procedures, particularly LEEP, may increase the risk of preterm delivery [5].

The challenge of cervical screening is to detect the lesions that are truly cancer precursors allowing treatment to prevent cancer, while minimizing the number of women with transient infection who need evaluation and treatment. In particular, it is critical to avoid unnecessary treatment of lesions without significant malignant potential. New observational and randomized trial data have allowed iterative refinement of cervical screening in the form of a series of revisions to major society guidelines incorporating HPV testing and extending screening intervals. The resulting guidelines balance the tension between maximizing detection and minimizing unnecessary intervention.

Factors That Affect Screening

Immune status: Cervical cancer is caused by HPV. As a viral infection, host immune factors are important determinants of risk. Women with compromised immune systems are at higher risk for premalignant lesions and more rapid progression from infection to cancer and are specifically excluded from current major society guidelines. Women with HIV have different screening guidelines. Other forms of immunocompromise are also excluded, although criteria for immunocompromise are not specifically outlined. In general, it is meant to include women with significant immunocompromise, such as organ transplant or high-dose chronic steroids. Women with common problems such as diabetes, which have a minimal impact on immunity, should follow the regular screening guidelines.

DES exposure: Women with prenatal diethylstilbestrol (DES) exposure are at risk for rare clear cell cancers of the vagina. They are specifically excluded from standard screening guidelines and are best managed by providers with expertise in this area.

Age: Cervical cancer risk varies significantly with age. Risk is so low that screening women under age 21 is not effective in preventing cervical cancer and can lead to many unnecessary interventions. All major guidelines except those for HIV-infected women specifically recommend against screening women under age 21. HPV infection rates also vary by age. Infection is common at all ages but is particularly common under age 30. The high rate of HPV infection in younger women limits the use of HPV testing for screening, so screening with co-testing is not currently recommended in women under age 30. Age also plays into cessation of screening. The long lag time between new infection and development of cancer prevents screening older women with adequate prior negative screening from making appreciable impact on cancer prevention. A woman newly infected with HPV after age 65 is unlikely to develop cervical cancer in her lifetime. Limitations in interpreting cytology in the context of atrophic changes limit effectiveness of screening in older women, making screening more likely to be harmful than beneficial and leading to recommendations to cease screening in women over age 65 with adequate prior normal screening.

Hysterectomy: Cervical cancer arises from the cervix. Surgical removal of the cervix prevents cervical cancer. Vaginal cancer can occur, but is tremendously rare and not prevented by screening. All current guidelines recommend cessation of screening in patients who have had hysterectomy with cervical removal, provided they have not had recent high-grade lesions. Supracervical hysterectomy with retention of the cervix requires continued screening.

Symptoms: Cervical cancer screening is intended for women without symptoms. Women with symptoms such as bleeding need to be evaluated with appropriate diagnostic testing, not screening methods.

Visible lesions: Some patients with cervical cancer will have normal screening tests. Visible cervical abnormalities require diagnostic testing, typically cervical biopsy. Evaluation of visible lesions with screening tests is not appropriate.

Prior abnormalities: Prior cervical abnormalities raise the risk of cervical cancer precursors and cancer. Patients with abnormalities need evaluation and either treatment or close follow-up until documented resolution. Management depends on the specific lesion and is outlined in guidelines by the American Society for Colposcopy and Cervical Pathology (ASCCP) [e]. Patients should not return to routine screening until follow-up has been completed as outlined in the ASCCP guidelines. Patients who have been treated for CIN-2 or -3 require screening for 20 years after treatment of the lesion, even if it extends screening past age 65.

Things that don't affect screening: The American Cancer Society (ACS) guidelines are meant to be implemented as written to the women to which they apply, which are essentially all women with a cervix who are not HIV infected, prenatally DES exposed, or significantly immunocompromised. The guidelines should not be altered for age at first intercourse, smoking, vaccination, or other common potential risk factors.

Recommended Guidelines and How to Find Them

In the United States, the leading cervical screening guidelines [a] have been maintained and iteratively revised by ACS in conjunction with ASCCP and the American Society for Clinical Pathology (ASCP). The consensus conference included representatives from 25 major organizations. Most major organizations, including the American College of Obstetricians and Gynecologists (ACOG), [b] have adopted these guidelines, as did the WWTF. The ASCCP has developed an excellent app that covers both screening and management of abnormal tests, and is available from their website (www.asccp.org). The US Preventive Services Task Force (USPSTF), which uses a different development process, made recommendations that are identical to the ACS guidelines except that they do not express a preference between co-testing and cytology alone for women aged 30–65 [c]. Both source documents are publicly available on the ASCCP and USPSTF websites. Guidelines for the management of HIV-infected women are covered in the guidelines from the Department of Health and Human Services AIDSinfo website [d].

How to Screen

Screening requires direct visualization of the cervix through a speculum. Blindly collected specimens are not acceptable. Lubrication of the speculum increases patient comfort, but some lubricants include inhibiting substances that may interfere. While both conventional Pap tests and liquid-based media are acceptable, liquid-based media is much more frequently used in the United States as it allows use of HPV for co-testing and triage of abnormal cytology [b].

Screening of usual women (women without prenatal DES exposure, HIV infection, or immunocompromise) should be performed per the ACS/ASCCP/ASCP guidelines (Table 35.1), which vary with age and presence of a cervix. Women under age 21 should not be screened. Women aged 21–29 should be screened with cervical cytology alone every 3 years. Women aged 30–65 should be screened with co-testing every 5 years (preferred). Women in this age group can also be screened with cytology alone every 3 years (acceptable). Women over age 65 should stop screening provided they have had adequate prior screening and no history of CIN-2 or higher in the past 20 years.

Women with HIV, immunocompromise, or DES exposure fall outside these guidelines. In general, screening with annual cytology alone starting at age 21 is appropriate for women who were exposed to DES in utero [b]. Guidelines for HIV-infected women [d] were revised after the conclusion of the Task Force Report. The revised guidelines specify beginning screening within 1 year of the onset of sexual activity but no later than age 21. Women under age 30 should be screened with cytology alone. After three consecutive annual normal tests, cytology can be performed every 3 years. Women aged 30 and older can be screened with either every 3-year cytology (once they have had three consecutive annual normal tests) or co-testing. While management of women with other forms of immunocompromise is not specified, it is reasonable to extrapolate these guidelines. Abnormal screening tests should be managed per the ASCCP consensus guidelines [e].

New Developments Likely to Affect Future Guidelines

In April 2014, the Food and Drug Administration (FDA) approved an additional indication for a previously approved HPV test to allow its use for primary screening in women aged 25 and older. This approval was based largely on data from a large US-based study of HPV primary screening [6] which validated a triage algorithm for positive tests. Interim guidance was developed by a panel convened by ASCCP and the Society of Gynecologic Oncology (SGO) [f]. The interim guidance panel noted "because of equivalent or superior effectiveness, primary HPV screening can be considered as an alternative to current cytology-based cervical cancer screening methods." Primary HPV screening is not currently recommended by ACS and USPSTF but will be considered in future revisions. Because of reasonable test characteristics, particularly in comparison to cytology alone, it is likely that primary HPV testing will be incorporated into future guidelines.

Longer term, greater use of HPV vaccination will hopefully lead to decreased incidence of cervical cancer precursors, which would adversely affect the specificity of cervical cytology, and could lead to recommendations with increased preference for HPV-based testing. Given the poor uptake of HPV vaccination in the

Table 35.1 Screening Methods for Cervical Cancer: Joint Recommendations of the American Cancer Society, the American Society for Colposcopy and Cervical Pathology, and the American Society for Clinical Pathology

Population	Recommended Screening Method	Comments
Women younger than 21 years	No screening	
Women aged 21–29 years	Cytology alone every 3 years	
Women aged 30–65 years	Human papillomavirus and cytology co-testing (preferred) every 5 years Cytology alone (acceptable) every 3 years	Screening by HPV testing alone is not recommended*
Women older than 65 years	No screening is necessary after adequate negative prior screening results**	Women with a history of CIN 2, CIN 3, or adenocarcinoma in situ should continue routine age-based screening for at least 20 years
Women who underwent total hysterectomy	No screening is necessary	Applies to women without a cervix and without a history of CIN 2, CIN 3, adenocarcinoma in situ, or cancer in the past 20 years
Women vaccinated against HPV	Follow age-specific recommendations (same as unvaccinated women)	

CIN: cervical intraepithelial neoplasia; HPV: human papillomavirus.
Modified from Saslow, D., Solomon, D., Lawson, H.W., Killackey, M. et al. American Cancer Society, American Society for Colposcopy and Cervical Pathology, and American Society for Clinical Pathology screening guidelines for the prevention and early detection of cervical cancer. *J Low Genit Tract Dis.* 2012, 16:175-204. Modified with the permission of ASCCP © American Society for Colposcopy and Cervical Pathology.
* After the Joint Recommendations were published, a test for screening with HPV testing alone was approved by the US Food and Drug Administration. Providers using this test should follow the interim guidance developed by the American Society for Colposcopy and Cervical Pathology and the Society for Gynecologic Oncology. (Huh, W.K., Ault, K.A., Chelmow, D., Davey, D.D. et al. Use of primary high-risk human papillomavirus testing for cervical cancer screening: Interim clinical guidance. *Obstet Gynecol.* 2015, 125:330–7.)
** Adequate negative prior screening results are defined as three consecutive negative cytology results or two consecutive negative co-test results within the previous 10 years, with the most recent test performed within the past 5 years. Women with a history of CIN 2 or higher should continue screening for a total of 20 years after spontaneous regression or appropriate management of CIN 2, CIN 3, or adenocarcinoma in situ, even if it extends the screening past age 65 years.

United States, it will unfortunately be some time in the future before this problem needs addressing.

Billing

Cervical screening is typically covered under the ICD-10 code Z01.419, encounter for gynecological examination (general) (routine) without abnormal findings. Other possible codes include Z12.4, encounter for screening for malignant neoplasm of cervix, and Z77.9 other contact with and (suspected) exposures hazardous to health. While HPV testing as part of co-testing is not specified in the descriptive language, it is typically covered under the same codes. Medicare requires special Healthcare Common Procedure Coding System (HCPCS) codes: G0101 for the screening pelvic and clinical breast examination and Q0091

for obtaining the Pap specimen. While in the past cervical screening was covered annually, Medicare specifies coverage no more frequently than every 2 years, and some private payers now have similar requirements. As screening within the guidelines is no more frequent than every 3 years, this should not cause problems. Patients where more frequent screening is appropriate (most frequently HIV-infected patients) are typically billed with the Z77.9 code.

Illustrative Cases

A healthy 17-year-old presents for a well-adolescent visit. She has been sexually active since age 15. Her mother told her to "ask for a Pap smear."

Recommendations from all major guidelines are to not initiate cervical screening until age 21 except in women with HIV infection. HPV infection is common in this age group and cervical cancer vanishingly rare. Screening adolescents is not effective. It is an opportune time to address HPV vaccination for primary prevention. The vaccine is recommended through age 26. While its effect may have been diminished by exposure to HPV through her prior sexual activity, it will likely still decrease her risk.

Screen now? No

Next screening: Age 21

A healthy 25-year-old G0 presents for a well-woman visit. Her last screen was at age 21, and was normal. She is without symptoms.

She is overdue for screening and should have cervical cytology. Both the USPSTF and ACS agree on recommendations for 21- to 29-year-olds and recommend screening every 3 years with cervical cytology. This patient's last screen was 4 years ago, so she requires screening. As she is younger than age 26, HPV vaccination for primary prevention is recommended if not already administered. Because of the high prevalence of HPV and the low risk of cancer, incorporation of HPV testing into screening is not currently recommended because of concerns that its use will lead to large increases in colposcopy and cervical treatment with little impact on cancer prevention.

Screen now? Yes

Next screen if normal: Age 28

A 45-year-old woman with hypertension presents for a well-woman visit. She smokes 1 pack per day. She was last screened with cervical cytology alone 3 years ago. She denies history of abnormal cervical screening. She has had five lifetime sexual partners.

Both the ACS and USPSTF allow screening with cytology every 3 years in women aged 30–65. As this woman was screened 3 years ago with cytology, she is due for her next screen. According to the USPSTF, both screening with cytology every 3 years and co-testing every 5 years are acceptable. ACS notes that both are acceptable but that co-testing is preferred. In several studies cited in the ACS guideline document [a], 5-year co-testing achieved lower cancer rates than 3-year cytology after two rounds of testing without significantly increasing need for additional testing.

Her smoking does not affect screening recommendations, although she should be counseled about smoking cessation.

Screen now? Yes (co-test preferred, can screen with cytology alone if co-test not available)

Next screen if normal: Age 50 (or 48 with cytology alone)

A 32-year-old HIV-positive woman presents for a well-woman visit. She was recently diagnosed with HIV. Prior screening was sporadic, but she reports no history of abnormal tests.

Women with immunocompromise from HIV or other causes fall outside the ACS and USPSTF screening guidelines. Guidelines for HIV-infected women [d] have recently been revised and are now age based. Women aged 30 or older can be followed with every 3-year cytology once they have had three consecutive normal annual tests or with every 3-year co-testing.

Screen now? Yes – screen with co-test

Next screen if normal: 3 years if co-test normal

A 60-year-old woman presents for an annual well-woman visit. She is new to your practice. She had a hysterectomy at age 47 for bleeding from fibroids. She never had any abnormal screening tests, and recalls being told that "everything was OK" with the specimen at her postop visit. Her prior provider was performing annual vaginal pap tests, all of which had been normal. On inspection of the vagina, the cervix is surgically absent.

Both the ACS and USPSTF recommend discontinuing screening after surgical removal of the cervix. Vaginal cancer occurs, but is exceedingly rare, and there is no reason to think screening for it is effective. Conversely, cytology obtained from atrophic vagina can be difficult to interpret and lead to unnecessary further testing. Both guidelines make exceptions for women with prior cervical cancer or CIN-2 or worse diagnosis in the preceding 20 years. Neither set of guidelines makes specific recommendations for what to do for these women. ACOG [b] suggests continued screening with cytology alone every 3 years in women with cervical cancer ever or CIN-2+ in the last 20 years. While this patient was able to describe her screening history, difficulty obtaining prior records or inability to document prior negative screening is not a reason for continuing screening after surgical removal of the cervix.

Screen now? No

Next screen: N/A

A 67-year-old woman presents for a well-woman visit. She reports having a LEEP for CIN-3 at age 55. She was followed closely afterwards, and has had two normal co-tests in the 10 years prior to age 65, with the most recent at age 62.

This woman is at higher risk because of her CIN-2+. Risk of recurrence does not fully decline for 20 years after treatment of a high-grade lesion. ACS guidelines [a] recommend continuing screening for 20 years after spontaneous regression or appropriate management of the lesion. As this patient is 5 years after her last co-test, she should be screened, preferably with co-testing. She requires continued screening until age 75.

In a woman without prior history of a high-grade abnormality, two normal co-tests after age 55 with the most recent within 5 years of age 65 would have met criteria for discontinuing screening. For women with adequate prior normal screening, risk of developing cervical cancer after age 65 is low enough that both USPSTF and ACS recommend discontinuing screening. Once screening is discontinued, it should not be restarted.

Guidelines

Usual Risk Women

a. Saslow, D., Solomon, D., Lawson, H.W. et al. American Cancer Society, American Society for Colposcopy and Cervical Pathology, and American Society for Clinical Pathology screening guidelines for the prevention and early detection of cervical cancer. *CA Cancer J Clin.* 2012, **62**:147–72. Available at: www.asccp.org/Guidelines/Screening-Guidelines. Retrieved December 30, 2016.

b. American College of Obstetricians and Gynecologists. Cervical cancer screening and prevention. Practice Bulletin No. 168. *Obstet Gynecol.* 2016, **128**:e111–30. Available at: www.acog.org/Resources-And-Publications/Practice-Bulletins-List. Retrieved December 30, 2016.

c. Moyer, V.A. Screening for cervical cancer: US Preventive Services Task Force recommendation statement. U.S. Preventive Services Task Force. *Ann Intern Med.* 2012, **156**:880–91. Available at: www.uspreventiveservicestaskforce.org/uspstf/uspscerv.htm. Retrieved December 30, 2016.

Women with HIV Infection

d. Panel on Opportunistic Infections in HIV-Infected Adults and Adolescents. Human Papillomavirus Disease in: Guidelines for the prevention and treatment of opportunistic infections in HIV-infected adults and adolescents: Recommendations from the Centers for Disease Control and Prevention, the National Institutes of Health, and the HIV Medicine Association of the Infectious Diseases Society of America. Available at: https://aidsinfo.nih.gov/guidelines/html/4/adult-and-adolescent-oi-prevention-and-treatment-guidelines/343/hpv Retrieved December 30, 2016.

Management of Abnormal Screening Tests

e. Massad, L.S., Einstein, M.H., Huh, W.K. et al. 2012 Updated consensus guidelines for the management of abnormal cervical cancer screening tests and cancer precursors. *Obstet Gynecol.* 2013, **121**:829–46 and *J Lower Gen Tract Dis.* 2013, **17**:S1–27.

Interim Guidance for Primary HPV Screening

f. Huh, W.K., Ault, K., Chelmow, D. et al. Use of primary high risk human papillomavirus testing for cervical cancer screening: Interim clinical guidance. *J Lower Genital Tract Dis Obstet Gynecol.* 2015, **125**:330–7, and *Gynecol Oncol.* 2015, **136**:178–82. Available at: www.sgo.org/wp-content/uploads/2012/09/HPV-Guidance-Doc-Article_main.pdf. Retrieved December 30, 2016.

References

1. Howlader, N., Noone, A.M., Krapcho, M. et al. editor. *SEER Cancer Statistics Review, 1975–2011.* Bethesda, MD: National Cancer Institute, April 2014. Available at: http://seer.cancer.gov/csr/1975_2011/, based on November 2013 SEER data submission, posted to the SEER website.

2. Gustafsson, L., Pontén, J., Zack, M., and Adami, H.O. International incidence rates of invasive cervical cancer after introduction of cytological screening. *Cancer Causes Control.* 1997, **8**(5):755–63.

3. Wright, T.C. Jr and Schiffman, M. Adding a test for human papillomavirus DNA to cervical-cancer screening. *N Engl J Med.* 2003, **348**:489–90.

4. McCredie, M.R., Sharples, K.J., Paul, C. et al. Natural history of cervical neoplasia and risk of invasive cancer in women with cervical intraepithelial neoplasia 3: A retrospective cohort study. *Lancet Oncol.* 2008, **9**: 425–34.

5. Kyrgiou, M., Koliopoulos, G., Martin-Hirsch, P. et al. Obstetric outcomes after conservative treatment for intraepithelial or early invasive cervical lesions: systematic review and meta-analysis. *Lancet.* 2006, **367**: 489–98.

6. Wright, T.C., Stoler, M.H., Behrens, C.M. et al. Primary cervical cancer screening with human papillomavirus: End of study results from the ATHENA study using HPV as the first-line test. *Gynecol Oncol.* 2015, **136**(2): 189–97.

Chapter 36

Colorectal Cancer

Marygrace Elson

Why Screen?

Colorectal cancer (CRC) is the third leading cause of cancer death in women in the United States after lung and breast cancer. It accounts for 10 percent of new cancer cases and 9 percent of cancer deaths in US women [1]. CRC screening reduces mortality from advanced disease by early detection as well as detection and removal of adenomatous polyps at risk of progressing from adenoma to carcinoma. It is estimated that as many as 60 percent of CRC deaths could be prevented if all men and women aged 50 and older were routinely screened [2]. Despite evidence that screening is effective, only about half of US women are up to date with screening for CRC. The screening rate is even less in individuals who are uninsured.

Rationale for Screening

CRC screening aims to detect and allow removal of premalignant polyps before they become cancer and to detect existing cancers at an earlier stage, facilitating earlier initiation of treatment and higher cure rates.

Available screening tests can be divided into two groups (Table 36.1): tests that focus on prevention by detecting both premalignant adenomatous polyps and cancer, allowing prevention and early detection, and tests that focus on early cancer detection alone. The first group includes colonoscopy and sigmoidoscopy. Tests in the second group detect cancer by identifying blood in the stool. These tests include high-sensitivity fecal occult blood testing (FO BT) and fecal immunochemical testing (FIT) for globin. Given the potential advantages of prevention over early detection, the American Cancer Society (ACS) joint guidelines clearly express a preference for these tests if resources are available and the patient is willing to undergo an invasive test.

Table 36.1 Tests for Colorectal Cancer Screening and Prevention
Screening Tests That Detect Both Adenomatous Polyps and Cancer

Test	Interval (Years)	Reduction in CRC Mortality	Comparison to Colonoscopy for Cancer Detection	Discussion Points
Colonoscopy	10	83%		Requires complete bowel preparation Examines entire colon Adenoma removal can possibly prevent CRC Requires conscious sedation (will need a driver and will miss a day of work) Risks: perforation, bleeding, cardiovascular complications (2.8/1,000 procedures) Dependent on endoscopist skill
Flexible sigmoidoscopy	5	60%–70% for left-sided lesions	Detects approximately 45% of cancers compared to colonoscopy	Requires complete or partial bowel preparation Left colon only Colonoscopy recommended for follow up of positive findings

Table 36.1 (cont.)

Test	Interval (Years)	Reduction in CRC Mortality	Comparison to Colonoscopy for Cancer Detection	Discussion Points
				No or minimal sedation required Risks: perforation
Computed tomography colonography	5	Undetermined	Similar sensitivity to colonoscopy for cancers	Requires complete bowel preparation Polyps <6 mm may not be visualized Colonoscopy recommended for follow up of positive findings Dependent on radiologist skill Possible small radiation-related risk
Double-contrast barium enema	5	Undetermined	Detects 30%–50% of cancers found at colonoscopy	Requires bowel preparation Colonoscopy recommended follow-up of positive findings In most locations has been replaced by CTC

Screening Tests That Detect Cancer Alone

Test	Interval (Years)	Reduction in CRC Mortality	Comparison to Colonoscopy for Cancer Detection	Discussion Points
Fecal occult blood testing	1	15%–33%		Peroxidase reaction to heme UGI bleeding can cause false positives Dietary exclusions Multiple stool specimens obtained at home Colonoscopy usual follow-up test
Fecal immunochemical test	1	74%	Detects 60%–90% of cancers found at colonoscopy	Detects globin Colonoscopy if test is positive
Stool high-sensitivity DNA testing (sDNA)	Every 1 or 3 years	Undetermined	Undetermined	Multitargeted testing for associated mutations Colonoscopy if test is positive

Source: Data from Levin, B., Lieberman, D.A., McFarland, B. et al., Screening and surveillance for the early detection of colorectal cancer and adenomatous polyps, 2008: A joint guideline from the American Cancer Society, the US Multi-Society Task Force on Colorectal Cancer, and the American College of Radiology. *Gastroenterology.* 2008, 134:1570–95; National Cancer Institute. Colorectal cancer screening (PDQ®). Available at: www.cancer.gov/cancertopics/pdq/screening/colorectal/HealthProfessional. Retrieved April 9, 2014; Telford, J.J., Levy, A.R., Sambrook, J.C., Zou, D., and Enns, R.A. The cost-effectiveness of screening for colorectal cancer. *CMAJ.* 2010, 182: 1307–13; and National Cancer Institute. Colorectal Screening for Health Professionals: Summary of Evidence. Available at: www.cancer.gov/types/colorectal/hp/colorectal-screening-pdq

CTC: computerized tomography colonography; CRC: colorectal cancer

Women have a higher risk of developing right-sided (proximal) colon cancer than men. Proximal colon cancers are more aggressive than left-sided (distal) colon cancers. Proximal colonic tumors are more often flat, while distal colonic tumors are commonly polypoid and more easily detected [3]. Proximal tumors are more common in African Americans than in whites [4]. Tests that screen the proximal colon may be particularly important in women, especially African American women.

Factors That Affect Screening

Personal preferences: Sociocultural barriers, fears, and personal preferences may significantly affect which of the many very different options are acceptable to an individual patient. Avoiding inconvenience or loss of work, fear of pain, concern about cost, or modesty are common impediments to undergoing colonoscopy. A history of abuse can be a significant barrier [1].

Availability of options: Not all recommended screening options may be available in a specific region or within a particular patient's means or insurance coverage.

Age: Colon cancer risk increases with age.

Race: African Americans have a higher colon cancer risk, leading to recommendations to begin screening at age 45 instead of age 50 [4].

Family history: Women with a single first-degree relative with CRC or advanced adenoma at age younger than 60 or two first-degree relatives with CRC or advanced adenomas (>1 cm in size, high-grade dysplasia, or villous component) are at increased risk. These women should begin screening at age 40 or 10 years younger than age at diagnosis of the youngest affected relative [5].

Hereditary nonpolyposis colorectal cancer (HNPCC): Women with HNPCC have significantly increased lifetime risks of CRC.

Familial adenomatous polyposis (FAP): Women with FAP or at risk of FAP based on family history have significant increased lifetime risk of CRC and typically undergo prophylactic colectomy.

Inflammatory bowel diseases: Individuals with inflammatory bowel disease, Crohn's disease, or ulcerative colitis are at increased risk for CRC.

Recommended Guidelines and How to Find Them

The Well-Woman Task Force recommendations for CRC screening [a] represent an evidence-based consensus between multiple major guidelines. The ACS, the US Multi-Society Task Force on Colorectal Cancer, and the American College of Radiology developed joint guidelines published in 2008 [b].

The American College of Obstetricians and Gynecologists published a Committee Opinion consistent with the joint work group recommendations [3] ['(c)']. The US Preventive Services Task Force (USPSTF) revised their guidelines after publication of the WWTF recommendations. The 2016 guidelines have minor differences from the joint guidelines, and allow any of the validated screening methods. [d]

How to Screen

An individualized risk assessment for CRC should be performed in adults, including family history [a].

CRC screening should begin at age 50 in average-risk women and age 45 in average-risk African American women. Routine screening is not recommended for women aged 76–85, but individual considerations may support screening in some patients following shared, informed decision-making. Screening is not recommended after age 85 [1] ['(a)']. The USPSTF recommends that the decision to screen in women ages 76 to 85 "should be an individual one, taking into account the patient's overall health and prior screening history." [c].

USPSTF recommended screening methods are:

- Colonoscopy every 10 years
- FOBT or FIT annually
- Flexible sigmoidoscopy every 5 years
- Computer tomography colonography (CTC) every 5 years
- FIT DNA, every 1 or 3 years
- Flexible sigmoidoscopy every 10 years, plus FIT every year

FOBT from a single digital office examination should not be performed due to an unacceptable sensitivity of only 4.9 percent [b].

Providers should discuss recommended CRC screening options with the patient to identify the method she is most likely to accept and complete. There are numerous differences (Table 36.1) that may be important to the individual patient's decision. She should be counseled regarding locally available options as well as options available with travel or referral. As pragmatically stated in the USPSTF report "the best screening test is the one that gets done" [4].

Patients with HNPCC should begin screening at age 20–25 with colonoscopy every 2 years until age 40 and annually thereafter. Patients with FAP should undergo annual screening with colonoscopy or flexible sigmoidoscopy until colectomy is appropriate. Women with strong family history as evidenced by a single first-degree relative with CRC or advanced adenoma at age younger than 60 or two first-degree relatives with CRC or advanced adenomas (>1 cm in size, high-grade dysplasia, or villous component) should begin screening at age 40 or 10 years younger than age at diagnosis of the youngest affected relative [5].

New Developments Likely to Affect Future Recommendations

Many options currently exist for colorectal screening. The single most pressing needs are adequate studies to better understand the differences in benefits and harms between the methods, and optimizing less invasive methods to make screening more acceptable to patients.

Video capsule endoscopy ("pillcam") uses a noninvasive capsule after colon preparation. Colonoscopy is required for findings. It is presently not cost-effective, but cost may decrease in the future [3]. Peripheral blood testing for circulating tumor cells or messenger RNA (mRNA) is another emerging technology with potential for the future.

Epidemiologic and genetic studies focusing on gender and ethnic differences may lead to more specific CRC screening guidelines for different population groups as well as for individuals with other associated risks such as inflammatory bowel disease, heavy smoking, or obesity.

Billing

Z12.11 is the ICD-10 code for "encounter for screening for malignant neoplasm of colon" and can be used to code for home FOBT and FIT tests returned to the laboratory.

Illustrative Cases

A 40-year-old woman comes to the office for well-woman exam. She is healthy, with body mass index (BMI) 24 kg/m², exercises regularly, and takes a diet that is high in fiber and low in fat. Her father had a small adenoma removed from his descending colon at age 65.

She is at average risk and should begin screening at age 50. Her father was >60 at his diagnosis, so she does not meet criteria for a strong family history. She should be encouraged to continue her healthy habits and report any change in family history.

Screen now? No

Next screening: Age 50

A 54-year-old woman comes to the office for her well-woman visit. She has well-controlled hypertension, BMI 26 kg/m², is somewhat sedentary, and underwent menopause at age 51. She has no known family history of CRC. Her internist has recommended screening colonoscopy. Over the last 3 years, she has twice scheduled the procedure and then canceled it. On further questioning, she states that she is very fearful about the procedure as her best friend had rectal bleeding after her colonoscopy requiring hospitalization.

She is overdue to initiate screening for CRC. She should be counseled regarding her multiple screening options, and partner in the decision regarding the most appropriate screening method for her. In particular, she should be counseled about noninvasive alternatives such as annual FIT or FOBT. She should be counseled that if she has a positive result, colonoscopy would be recommended for evaluation.

Screen now? Yes

Next screen if FOBT/FIT normal: 1 year

A 52-year-old woman presents for a well-woman visit. She is transferring to your care. She is healthy, underwent menopause at age 49, and is up to date with mammography and cervical screening. When asked about colorectal screening, she says that her prior gynecologist always does a digital rectal exam checking for occult blood at the time of her pelvic examination and she has had negative hemoccult tests every time. She asks if you will perform this screen during her examination.

In-office single FOBT is ineffective for CRC screening. She should be counseled regarding effective CRC screening options.

Screen now? Yes

Next screen if normal: 10 years if colonoscopy. Appropriate interval if other CRC screening is performed.

A 22-year-old woman comes to the office for her first pelvic examination. She is a healthy college student with regular withdrawal menses on oral contraceptives. Family history reveals that her mother was very recently diagnosed with colon cancer at age 45. Your patient doesn't know any more details. Her physical examination is within normal limits.

Her mother has a very early diagnosis of colon cancer. If possible, she should find out more about her mother's diagnosis and whether any special testing was done of her mother's tumor. If her mother has a genetically linked type of cancer (such as HNPCC) she may be a candidate to begin screening for CRC now [a].

Screen now? Yes, if HNPCC diagnosed, otherwise no.

Next screen: If does not have HNPCC, initiate screening at age 35, 10 years before age at diagnosis of her mother. If other family members are diagnosed with colon cancer in the interim, screening should begin 10 years earlier than the age of the youngest family member's diagnosis.

Guidelines

Usual Risk Women and Women at Increased Risk

a. Conry, J.A. and Brown, H. Well-Woman Task Force: Components of the Well-Woman Visit. *Obstet Gynecol.* 2015, **126**(4):697–701.

b. Levin, B., Lieberman, D., McFarland, B. et al. Screening and surveillance for the early detection of colorectal cancer and adenomatous polyps, 2008: A Joint Guideline from the American Cancer Society, the US Multi-Society Task Force on Colorectal Cancer, and the American College of Radiology. *Gastroenterology.* 2008, **134**:1570–95 and *CA Cancer J Clin.* 2008, 58:130–60.

c. American College of Obstetricians and Gynecologists. Colorectal cancer screening strategies. Committee Opinion #609. *Obstet Gynecol.* 2014, **124**(4):849–55.

d. Screening for colorectal cancer: US Preventive Services Task Force recommendation statement. US Preventive Services Task Force. JAMA2016;315-2564-2575. Available at: http://www.uspreventiveservicestaskforce.org/Page/Document/UPdateSummaryFinal/colorectal-cancer-screening2?ds=1&s=colorectal cancer screening referenced 6/25/16.

References

1. Krishnan, S. and Wolf, J. Colorectal cancer screening and prevention in women. *Women's Health.* 2011, 7: 213–26.

2. He, J. and Efron, J. Screening for colorectal cancer. *Adv Surg.* 2011, **45**:31–44.

3. Kim, S., Paik, H., Yoon, H. et al. Sex- and gender-specific disparities in colorectal cancer risk. *World J Gastroenterol.* 2015, **21**:5167–75.

4. Dimou, A., Syrigos, K., and Saif, M. Disparities in colorectal cancer in African-Americans vs whites: Before and after diagnosis. *World J Gastroenterol.* 2009, 15(30):3734–43.

5. Rex, D., Johnson, D., Anderson, J. et al. American College of Gastroenterology guidelines for colorectal cancer screening 2008. *Am J Gastroenterol.* 2009, **104**:739–50.

Chapter 37

Ovarian Cancer

Beth Cronin

Why Screen?

In the United States in 2010, an estimated 21,880 women were diagnosed with epithelial ovarian cancer (EOC), and 13,850 died of the disease. For women diagnosed with early-stage disease, 5-year survival rates are as high as 95 percent. Advanced-stage disease is associated with a very poor prognosis, with 5-year survival rates as low as 30 percent. EOC is diagnosed in advanced stages approximately 70–80 percent of the time. Given this large discordance in survival rates, a screening test to identify women in early stages could clearly be beneficial. The lifetime risk of developing ovarian cancer is 1.2–1.4 percent for a woman of general population risk and 12–46 percent for women with a known genetic or strong family history. Given these large differences, it may be appropriate to approach screening differently based on risk.

Rationale for Screening and Prevention

Despite significant effort, no screening methods studied to date appear effective for average-risk women. Part of the problem is that ovarian cancer is likely not a single disease, and cancers that present at an advanced stage may be biologically different than those diagnosed early. Until recently, it was thought that ovarian cancer had its sole origin in the ovaries. However, recent studies support two different types of EOC:

- Type 1: a low-grade, slow-growing type originating in the ovaries
- Type 2: a high-grade, rapidly growing cancer likely originating from intraepithelial lesions outside the ovary, generally the fallopian tube

In general, particularly effective screening tests identify a precursor lesion that can be treated before invasive disease develops, like identification of cervical intraepithelial neoplasia in screening and prevention of cervical cancer. Unfortunately, there are no known precursor lesions for ovarian cancer, so research has focused on early detection of invasive disease. The transition time between early- and late-stage disease is unclear, which creates uncertainty as to whether earlier detection will even improve mortality outcomes [1]. Given the low prevalence of ovarian cancer of 1 case per 2,500 women, there are definite risks of causing unnecessary harm when screening general-population-risk women.

Serum marker screening, particularly CA-125, has been extensively studied. While early studies demonstrated that levels were increased in approximately 80 percent of women with EOC, follow-up studies showed poor rates of sensitivity and specificity in women with early-stage disease. CA-125 is not useful as a screening test in women at general population risk because it is affected by many other benign conditions, including endometriosis, pregnancy, pelvic inflammatory disease, leiomyomas, menstruation, and adenomyosis. The high frequency of these conditions, particularly in premenopausal women, leads to many false positives.

Transvaginal ultrasound (TVUS) can be used to identify changes in ovarian size and morphology before ovarian malignancy is symptomatic and could theoretically be used as a screening tool. TVUS can be impacted by sonographer abilities, and it has been difficult to identify which specific markers accurately predict early-stage EOC. Screening trials with TVUS have demonstrated positive predictive value (PPV) ranging from 1 to 27 percent, so it is not recommended for routine screening in low-risk women [a].

Two recent large trials involving almost 300,000 women attempted to validate screening methods but were unable to demonstrate improvements in mortality. They examined use of TVUS combined with CA-125 with different cutoffs and follow-up algorithms, but neither demonstrated a survival benefit [2, 3].

The Gynecologic Oncologic Group study, GOG-0199, demonstrated a 2.6 percent rate of invasive or intraepithelial ovarian, tubal, or peritoneal neoplasm at the time of risk-reducing surgery in high-risk women [4]. They analyzed 966 asymptomatic women over age 30 years who were undergoing risk-reducing bilateral salpingo-oophorectomy (BSO). Overall, they identified 25 cases of invasive or intraepithelial ovarian/tubal/peritoneal neoplasms, but none were found in the 387 women with negative BRCA mutation testing and normal CA-125 levels. Fifty-six percent of the women diagnosed with a neoplasm had either intraepithelial lesions or stage I or II malignancy, all diagnoses with significantly better prognoses than typically diagnosed stage III or IV disease. These studies demonstrate that occult cancers are found in high-risk women and support the idea that risk-reducing surgery should be offered and recommended to those women with genetic mutations. Future work is ongoing to determine the optimal age to recommend this surgery to best balance risk reduction and minimization of morbidity associated with surgical menopause as well as whether a staged procedure with initial bilateral salpingectomy followed by oophorectomy at later age would be equally protective.

Factors That Affect Screening and Prevention

Symptoms: Ovarian cancer has been billed as a "silent disease," but women diagnosed with EOC often report a history of nonspecific symptoms, including abdominal or pelvic pain as well as bloating, urinary symptoms, and early satiety. These symptoms are often persistent but difficult for many women to pinpoint. An ovarian cancer symptom index was developed in an attempt to guide screening for early-stage disease. Early studies demonstrated a sensitivity of 56.7 percent for early-stage disease and 79.5 percent for late-stage disease, with specificity of 86.7 percent for women under age 50 and 90 percent for those older than 50 years [5]. Unfortunately, further studies did not confirm these findings. Although this symptom index did not demonstrate clear use for universal screening, women presenting with these symptoms should be further evaluated.

BRCA mutations: Women with BRCA1 or BRCA2 germ line mutations in cancer susceptibility genes have a 46 percent lifetime risk of developing EOC, tubal, or peritoneal carcinoma. BRCA1 and BRCA2 mutations account for approximately 15 percent of ovarian carcinomas and a high proportion of fallopian and peritoneal carcinomas.

Hereditary nonpolyposis colorectal cancer (HNPCC): Women with DNA mismatch repair gene mutations, associated with HNPCC, have a 9–12 percent lifetime risk of developing ovarian cancer.

Recommended Guidelines and How to Find Them

The US Preventive Services Task Force (USPSTF) clearly states that screening for ovarian cancer is not recommended for women who do not have a known genetic mutation that increases their risk of ovarian cancer [b]. This recommendation has been adopted by the Well-Woman Task Force (WWTF) as well. For women at general population risk, the American College of Obstetricians and Gynecologists (ACOG) has written committee opinions on the early detection of EOC [a] and salpingectomy for prevention of ovarian cancer [c], which can be accessed through the ACOG website. Both the Society of Gynecologic Oncology (SGO) [d] and ACOG [e] have released guidelines to help practitioners best determine which patients warrant referral for genetic counseling and testing. Guidelines for management of patients at high risk for Hereditary Breast/Ovarian Cancer (HBOC) syndromes can be found at National Comprehensive Cancer Network (www.nccn.org) [f].

How to Screen

Women of general population risk, without family history prompting referral for genetic counseling and consideration of HBOC mutation testing, should not undergo routine screening for ovarian cancer.

At the well-woman visit, the review of systems should include questions that may detect symptomatic low-risk women. These symptoms include pelvic or abdominal pain, bloating, urinary urgency or frequency, and early satiety. If these symptoms are new or lasting more than 12 days a month, appropriate evaluation based on symptom descriptions and physical examination findings should be performed.

Family history should be obtained at the well-woman visit to identify women who would benefit from genetic counseling and possible HBOC mutation testing. Routine testing for BRCA mutation is not recommended for women without personal or family history consistent with increased risk of mutation. A thorough family history is an important first step in screening for familial cancer syndromes, and the SGO guidelines can be used to identify who should be offered referral to genetic counseling [d]. Recommendations for testing for HBOC are made based on further family history. Testing should be deferred in adolescents, as the medical or psychosocial benefits of the test will not be present until adulthood as ovarian cancer is so rare in adolescents.

Women with BRCA1, BRCA2, or HNPCC mutations should be offered risk-reducing surgery. A BSO is currently recommended by age 40 or after childbearing is completed for BRCA1 or BRCA2 carriers. Those women with HNPCC mutation should be offered risk-reducing hysterectomy and BSO between 35 and 40 years if childbearing is completed.

If high-risk women choose to defer risk-reducing surgery, they should be offered surveillance for ovarian cancer with serial CA-125 and TVUSs. There is limited data on whether to recommend annual or every 6-month screening intervals. Prospective validation of the screening methodology and interval is yet to be completed [f]. Consideration can be given for applying these guidelines for high-risk women to those with family histories of EOC, but not documented genetic mutations, as it is possible that there are yet unidentified genetic links that increase risk for EOC.

New Developments Likely to Affect Future Recommendations

Tubal ligation appears to have a protective effect against the development of ovarian cancer. ACOG has recently published a committee opinion supporting bilateral salpingectomy at the time of hysterectomy or as an alternative sterilization method to reduce future risk of malignancy [c]. While further confirmatory studies are needed, bilateral salpingectomy at time of hysterectomy or sterilization appears to be safe and not lead to increased complications.

Small studies have not shown diminished ovarian function after salpingectomy. Stronger confirmatory data may change future guidance from offering salpingectomy to specifically recommending it.

The UK Collaborative Trial of Ovarian Cancer Screening (UKCTOCS) recently published its results evaluating a comparison between a multimodal screening arm with pattern of CA-125 over time interpreted using risk of ovarian cancer calculation (ROCA) which triaged to repeat CA-125 versus repeat plus TVUS, and annual TVUS screenings with triage based on findings. These two arms were compared to a no screening arm. They demonstrated relative reductions in mortality in the two screening arms (15 percent in the multimodal group and 11 percent in the TVUS group), but they were not statistically significant. They plan to continue the study with further follow-up to assess if the mortality reduction identified is valid [3].

Recent studies have also identified additional genes that may be associated with increased ovarian cancer risk. The number of associated genes will likely continue to rise as technology improves and more research is performed, which will hopefully in turn lead to better screening options for patients [6].

Billing

Given that ovarian cancer screening is not recommended in the general-population-risk patient, it will typically not be covered by an average-risk patient's insurance. The ICD-10 code for ovarian cancer screening is Z12.73: encounter for screening for malignant neoplasm of ovary. Most insurance companies will cover a TVUS and CA-125 in high-risk women. It is important to verify coverage, as some insurers will not cover all tests, for example, Doppler examination for screening. The applicable billing code for patients being referred for genetic counseling and screening based on family history is Z84.81.

Illustrative Cases

A 15-year-old G0 presents for her well-adolescent visit. She is sexually active and would like contraception. She states that her mother, aged 39, was diagnosed with EOC 3 months ago and is doing well on chemotherapy. She thinks her maternal grandmother also died of breast cancer, but she is not sure as this was before she was born.

Given her mother's diagnosis of EOC, and likely premenopausal breast cancer in her maternal grandmother, her mother should undergo genetic counseling and likely testing for *BRCA* mutations. If these were negative, further consideration for HNPCC or Peutz-Jeghers syndromes may be considered. The results of her mother's testing would further dictate future screening and testing recommendations [e]. The WWTF recommends that consideration for genetic screening should be deferred in adolescents as the benefits of the test information are not seen until adulthood, given the rarity with which ovarian cancer is seen in adolescents. The weight of this knowledge in an adolescent is often too great.

Genetic screening now? No

When should screening begin? First test mother to determine her risk

A 35-year-old G3P3 presents for a well-woman visit. Her good friend was recently diagnosed with EOC and has been telling her that everyone should be screened to prevent this cancer.

An in-depth family history should be obtained. In the absence of familial risk factors for ovarian cancer, screening is not indicated. No studies have shown that screening average-risk women with either laboratory markers or ultrasound has reduced mortality from ovarian cancer.

Screen now? No

Screen ever? Not unless significant family history

A 36-year-old G2P2 presents for a well-woman visit. She had two uncomplicated vaginal deliveries followed by a tubal ligation. She has had no other surgeries nor does she have any medical problems. She states that her mother was diagnosed with ovarian cancer 6 months ago. Based on her family history of an immediate family member having the diagnosis of ovarian cancer, she and her mother were referred for genetic counseling. A BRCA1 mutation was found.

BRCA1 carriers have a 46 percent lifetime risk for the development of ovarian cancer [d]. Based on this increased risk, a BSO is recommended by age 40 or after childbearing. Although she has had a tubal ligation, prophylactic BSO is still recommended. If she chooses not to have a BSO, she should undergo serial testing with CA-125 and TVUS at least yearly, if not every 6 months [f].

Screen now: Patient should be offered prophylactic BSO. If she declines, CA-125 and TVUS is indicated.

Next screen: Patient should continue CA-125 and TVUS every 6–12 months until she undergoes prophylactic BSO

A 56-year-old G3P3 presents for a well-woman visit. She is up to date on cervical cancer screening and colonoscopies. She denies family history of breast, ovarian, or colorectal malignancies.

In a woman with a negative family history, no screening for ovarian cancer is indicated. Discussion of warning symptoms and signs for which she should contact the office is warranted.

Screen now: No

Next screen: She should have her family history and review of symptoms updated at each well-woman visit. In the absence of high-risk factors developing, no future screening is indicated.

Guidelines

Screening Recommendations for General Population

a. Moyer, V.A. Screening for ovarian cancer. US Preventive Services Task Force Reaffirmation recommendation statement. US Preventive Services Task Force. *Ann Intern Med.* 2012, **157**:900–4. Available at: www.uspreventiveservicestaskforce.org/Page/Document/RecommendationStatementFinal/ovarian-cancer-screening. Retrieved February 11, 2016.

b. American College of Obstetricians and Gynecologists. The role of the obstetrician-gynecologist in the early detection of epithelial ovarian cancer. Committee Opinion No. 477. *Obstet Gynecol.* 2011, **117**:742–6.

Recommendations for Prophylactic Surgery

c. American College of Obstetrics and Gynecology. Salpingectomy for ovarian cancer prevention. Committee Opinion No. 620. *Obstet Gynecol.* 2015, **125**: 279–81.

Guidelines for Familial Cancer Risk Assessment

d. Lancaster, J.M., Powell, C.B., Chen, L.M., and Richardson, D.L. Society of Gynecologic Oncology statement on risk assessment for inherited gynecologic cancer predispositions. *Gynecol Oncol.* 2015, **136** (1):3–7.

e. American College of Obstetricians and Gynecologists. Hereditary cancer syndromes and risk assessment.

Committee Opinion No. 634. *Obstet Gynecol.* 2015, **125**: 1538–43.

Screening Recommendations for High-Risk Women

f. National Comprehensive Cancer Network. Genetic/familial high-risk assessment: breast and ovarian. Available at: www.nccn.org/professionals/physician_gls/pdf/genetics_screening.pdf. Retrieved January 25, 2016.

References

1. Clarke-Pearson, D.L. Clinical practice. Screening for ovarian cancer. *N Engl J Med.* 2009, **361**(2):170–7.

2. Buys, S.S., Partridge, E., Black, A. et al. Effect of screening on ovarian cancer mortality: The prostate, lung, colorectal and ovarian (PLCO) cancer screening randomized controlled trial. *JAMA.* 2011, **305**(22): 2295–303.

3   Jacobs, I.J., Menon, U., Ryan, A. et al. Ovarian cancer screening and mortality in the UK Collaborative Trial of Ovarian Cancer Screening (UKCTOCS): A randomised controlled trial. *Lancet.* Published online December 17, 2015.

4. Sherman, M.E., Piedmonte, M., Mai, P.L. et al. Pathologic findings at risk-reducing salpingo-oophorectomy: Primary results from Gynecologic Oncology Group Trial GOG-0199. *J Clin Oncol.* 2014, **32**(29):3275–83.

5. Goff, B.A., Mandel, L.S., Drescher, C.W. et al. Development of an ovarian cancer symptom index: Possibilities for earlier detection. *Cancer.* 2007, **109**(2): 221–7.

6. Norquist, B.M., Harrell, M.I, Brady, M.F. et al. Inherited mutations in women with ovarian carcinoma. *JAMA Oncol.* 2016, **2**(4):482–90.

Breast Cancer

Eduardo Lara-Torre

Why Screen and Prevent?

Breast cancer is the most common non-cutaneous cancer in women, accounting for 27 percent of all cancers [1]. It is the second leading cause of death from cancer, exceeded only by lung cancer. The overall lifetime risk of developing breast cancer is one in eight, and risk steadily increases with age. Breast screening allows diagnosis of cancer at an early stage (less than 2 cm), which is associated with improved survival at 5 (89–98 percent) and 10 years (90 percent) [2]. Early diagnosis also minimizes the need for radical surgery and extensive radiation and chemotherapy needed for the treatment of advanced disease. Although uncomfortable, mammography is widely accepted among women across all socioeconomic levels. For populations at significant increased risk, interventions are available to prevent or delay the occurrence of cancer. Targeted prevention using medications (chemoprevention) is clearly beneficial for some women, and information on the optimal agents and populations who will benefit most is evolving rapidly.

Rationale for Screening and Prevention

Breast self-awareness is generally defined as women's awareness of the normal appearance and feel of their breasts. It is different from breast self-examination. With breast self-awareness, the patient should be encouraged to be alert for changes in their breast, and if they note changes, they should contact their health care provider for further evaluation. Recommendations for breast self-awareness stem from the desire to optimize the diagnosis of cancers not detected by mammography. Up to 50 percent of breast cancers diagnosed in women younger than 50 years of age and up to 70 percent of those older than 50 are detected by women themselves [1,3].

Both breast self-examination and clinical breast examination rely on the ability to palpate an abnormal growth in the breast. Unfortunately, lesions typically need to be 2 cm in size or larger to be palpable and are unlikely to be detected when smaller. Most palpable masses are not cancer, but rather benign pathology such as fibroadenomas or fibrocystic changes. Although the concept of examining the breast to detect small masses had good intentions, most studies show no benefit in cancer diagnosis or survival [3]. A decade of research summarized in Cochrane reviews on both self-examination and clinical examination did not find any benefit [4–6]. To the contrary, these examinations lead to an increase in unnecessary interventions, including biopsies, without impacting on cancer diagnosis or survival rates. For this reason, most guidelines discourage performing these techniques for breast cancer screening.

Mammography has the potential to diagnose breast cancer prior to it being palpable or otherwise clinically apparent, which is extremely important as early diagnosis increases the success of treatment. Screening mammography is unequivocally effective for reducing death from breast cancer. Estimates of relative mortality reduction with screening varied by study type, from median 15 percent with modeling studies, 19 percent from randomized controlled trials, and larger estimates from observational studies (25–54 percent) [7]. The older the woman, the fewer patients need to be screened to prevent one cancer death. At ages 40–49, it takes 735 patients to reduce the mortality by 40 percent, while for those aged 60–69 it takes only 355. Over a 10-year period, screening 10,000 women aged 60–69 will result in 21 fewer breast cancer deaths, screening women aged 50–59 will result in eight fewer breast cancer deaths, and screening women aged 40–49 will result in three fewer deaths [5]. While the number needed to screen is higher in younger women so are the years of life saved by screening [8].

As with other screening tests, interpretation of mammography needs to balance achieving the highest rate of detection with an acceptable rate of false positives. In the United States across all ages, screening digital mammography has a sensitivity of 77–95 percent and a specificity of 94–97 percent. Some negative screens will be false negatives, with the potential for causing false reassurance and individuals delaying rescreening. Many abnormal mammograms will lead to additional testing including further imaging and biopsies which will not contribute to early cancer detection. The probability of a call back over a 10-year period is 40 percent with biennial and 60 percent with annual screening. The probability of biopsy is 4 percent with biennial and 7 percent with annual screening. This additional testing can cause stress and anxiety for patients [9].

Other potential harms of screening include overdiagnosis and radiation exposure. Overdiagnosis refers to cancers detected by screening that would not have led to clinically relevant disease and would not have ever been detected if the screening had not been performed. Estimates of overdiagnosis vary. The Cancer Intervention and Surveillance Modeling Network (CISNET) estimates as high as one in eight women diagnosed with biennial screening will be overdiagnosed, while other estimates are lower. Overdiagnosis increases with frequency of screening and earlier initiation of screening. Cumulative mammography-related radiation exposure can lead to new malignancies of the breast and non-breast cancer. With lifetime biennial screening starting at 50, there may be three breast cancers associated with radiation exposure for every 10,000 screenings, resulting in 0.5 deaths. If screening starts at 40, this number increases to 4 cancers per 10,000 screenings, resulting in one death [5].

Organizations making guideline recommendations for mammography generally used the same evidence and agree on the benefits and harms. Nonetheless, they came to a variety of recommendations about age of initiation, interval to repeat studies, and age to stop screening. These differences stem from their applying different weights to the potential harms, particularly the need for additional testing. To a large degree, balancing benefits and harms is an individual decision, which requires shared decision-making to determine appropriate recommendations for individual patients.

In the United States, Selective Estrogen Receptor Modulators (SERMs) are approved for the prevention of breast cancer. Tamoxifen was proven effective as adjuvant therapy in the treatment of breast cancer. The effective prevention of recurrence led to research on primary prevention. The initial data showed a 38 percent overall reduction in invasive breast cancer and a 48 percent reduction in estrogen receptor (ER)-positive cancers in women at high risk of breast cancer, which persisted over 10 years. Raloxifene is also effective for the prevention of invasive breast cancer in high-risk women. In the largest comparative study, raloxifene showed a 50 percent reduction in invasive breast cancer. The main difference between the two includes reduced incidence of noninvasive cancer with tamoxifen balanced against less risk of uterine cancer and thromboembolic disease with raloxifene [g].

Factors That Affect Screening and Prevention

Personal preferences: Much of the difference between recommendations for mammography relates to balance between benefits and harms, particularly the need for additional testing. Patient anxiety, aversion to additional testing, and desire to achieve additional breast cancer protection are important factors for guiding shared decision-making for choosing between different screening guidelines.

Personal history of breast biopsies: Having a negative biopsy is associated with increased risk in the future, likely because of risks related to the findings that prompted the biopsies.

Genetic predisposition (BRCA mutations): The estimated lifetime risk for patients with a BRCA1 mutation is 65 percent and with BRCA2 mutation is 45 percent [10]. These mutations account for 3 percent–5 percent of all breast cancers.

Age: Breast cancer risk increases with age, from 1 in 1,760 at age 20 to 1 in 27 at age 70.

Age of first menses and first birth: Menarche before the age of 12 increases the risk of breast cancer slightly, likely because of the longer lifetime estrogen exposure. Risk also increases depending on the age at first birth in those with none or one relative with breast cancer. If they have two or more relatives with cancer, their risk decreases with age of first birth.

Family history: There is an increase in risk in women with one or more first-degree relatives with breast cancer.

Ethnicity: Non-Hispanic white and non-Hispanic blacks have the highest risk of breast cancer. Those of Asian Pacific descent have lower risk [2].

Breast density: High breast density is associated with increased risk of breast cancer. Increased density makes reading screening images more difficult and can lead to false negative and false positive studies.

Personal history of cancer: Patients with a history of ductal carcinoma in situ (DCIS) or lobular carcinoma in situ (LCIS), as well as those who received chest radiation, are at increased risk of developing invasive breast cancer.

Other factors: Not breast-feeding, alcohol consumption, increased height, history of ovarian or endometrial cancer, and obesity all increase risk.

Recommended Guidelines and How to Find Them

The American College of Obstetricians and Gynecologists (ACOG), American Cancer Society (ACS), US Preventive Services Task Force (USPSTF), National Comprehensive Cancer Network (NCCN), American College of Radiology (ACR), and numerous other organizations all make recommendations for breast cancer screening in average-risk patients and chemoprevention for high-risk patients. The scope of each guideline varies as do specific recommendations. The Well-Woman Task Force (WWTF) recommendations were based on the guidelines that were in place at the time of the meeting [a]. Since that time, there have been significant updates to the USPSTF [b] and ACS [c] guidelines, with important implications for the original WWTF recommendations.

Encouragement of breast self-awareness has been removed from several of the guidelines that were reviewed by the WWTF. At present, only NCCN specifically recommends breast self-awareness [d]. It is reasonable to encourage patients to report new symptoms or changes in their breasts to their providers. Both the ACS and the USPSTF explicitly no longer recommend breast self-examination. While

the WWTF stated that it could be offered as part of breast self-awareness, it seems unlikely that they would have made this recommendation in light of the revised recommendations from ACS and USPSTF. Similarly, both ACS and USPSTF explicitly recommend against clinical breast examination. Given these recommendations and the supportive data for minimal improvement in breast cancer detection and large increase in additional testing, the original WWTF recommendation regarding clinical breast examination is no longer applicable, and clinical breast examination is not necessary in asymptomatic average-risk women.

Table 38.1 summarizes the most widely accepted mammography guidelines. Many other organizations adopt one of these society's recommendations. For instance, the American Academy of Family Practice [e] adopted the USPSTF guidelines. All guidelines clearly recognize the effectiveness of mammography but differ in recommendations for age to start, whether to perform every 1 or 2 years, and age to stop screening. At one extreme, ACR [f] and NCCN recommend annual screening starting at age 40. At the other extreme, USPSTF recommends every 2-year screening between ages 50 and 75, although it allows initiating screening as early as age 40 with shared decision-making. ACS guidelines are intermediate. The differences between guidelines have generated much controversy. In January 2016, ACOG convened a conference of the major guideline-issuing organizations to attempt to reach consensus recommendations; the final report from the conference is not yet available.

The WWTF reviewed older guidelines and concluded:

- For women aged 40 and older, the decision to start or terminate regular screening mammography should be individualized and should take into account patient context, including an assessment of breast cancer risk, comorbidities, and the patient's values regarding specific benefits and harms of screening. (Strong)
- Routine screening mammography should occur by age 50 years. (Strong)
- The frequency of routine screening should take into account patient context and should be either annual or biennial. (Qualified)

While derived from older guidelines, the Task Force recommendations encompass the range of current guidelines and provide a useful framework for

Table 38.1 Mammography Screening Guidelines for Average-Risk Women

Organization	Age to Initiate Screening	Interval	Age to Stop Screening
American Cancer Society	Start at age 45. Should have opportunity to start at age 40	Ages 45–54: annually. Ages 54 and older: transition to biennial screening or have opportunity to continue screening annually	Continue as long as overall health good and life expectancy is 10-years or longer
American College of Radiology	Start at age 40	Annual	Continue as long as a woman has a life expectancy of more than 5–7 years on the basis of age and health status, is willing to undergo additional testing, and would be treated for breast cancer if diagnosed
National Comprehensive Cancer Network	Start at age 40	Annual	Consider severe comorbid conditions limiting life expectancy and whether therapeutic interventions are planned. Upper age limit for screening is not yet established
US Preventive Services Task Force	Start at age 50. Women may consider beginning screening in their forties	Biennial	Evidence is insufficient to assess the additional benefits and harms of screening mammography in women aged 75 or older, so no recommendation for or against screening

using shared decision-making and incorporating patient values to make individual screening recommendations within the scope of any of the major current guidelines. Within this framework, screening average-risk women should start no earlier than age 40 and no later than age 50 and should occur every 1 or 2 years. Providers should guide patients in their decisions about when to initiate mammography and annual or biennial screening by helping patients assess their priorities in avoiding additional testing and other potential adverse consequence of screening and their desire to maximize reduction in breast cancer risk. Patients desiring maximal protection against breast cancer and tolerant of call backs and biopsies should opt for beginning screening in their early 40s and annual testing. Women who want reasonable protection while minimizing additional testing should start later and consider biennial testing.

USPST, ACS, NCCN, and the Task Force all recommend chemoprevention for women at high risk for breast cancer. The NCCN guidelines provide the most specific recommendations for chemoprevention, including recommendations for eligibility and administration.

How to Screen and Prevent

At the well-woman visit, the review of systems should include questions about breast symptoms including pain, discharge, and masses. Women with symptoms need appropriate diagnostic evaluation. Family history should be reviewed, and the patient referred for genetic counseling and testing if a genetic predisposition is suspected (see the chapter on Genetic Testing).

Recommendations for screening are intended for average-risk women, and chemoprevention is reserved for high-risk women, so breast cancer risk should be assessed. A number of validated tools are available for risk assessment including the Gail model and the National Cancer Institute's Breast Cancer Assessment Tool [11]. These tools stratify risk and provide a percentage risk estimate. Separate screening

Table 38.2 Tools for Breast Cancer Risk Assessment

Tool	Available at	Indication	Main Difference
National Cancer Institute (Gail model)	www.cancer.gov/bcrisktool	Regular-risk women	Is not appropriate for patients with significant genetic risk or other high-risk factors such as precancer or radiation
IBIS Breast Cancer Risk Evaluation Tool	www.ems-trials.org/riskevaluator/	Women with a history of LCIS	Increases accuracy for invasive breast cancer risk assessment
Chest Radiation Effects in Breast Cancer	http://jnci.oxfordjournals.org/content/97/19/1428.full.pdf	Women with history of chest radiation for Hodgkin's lymphoma	Better assesses the risk associated with radiation
BOADICEA Model	http://ccge.medschl.cam.ac.uk/boadicea/	Women with BRCA1 or BRCA2 mutations	Better estimates increased risk from genetic carrier states

IBIS: International Breast Cancer Prevention Studies; LCIS: Lobular Carcinoma in situ; BOADICEA: Breast and Ovarian Analysis of Disease Incidence and Carrier Estimation Algorithm

guidelines for high-risk women are available from NCCN. More advanced tools are available (Table 38.2) and may be useful for special circumstances [12–14].

Average-risk women should not undergo routine clinical breast examination nor do they require education in breast self-examination. Breast self-awareness counseling is reasonable. Physicians should encourage women of all ages to understand the normal appearance and "feel" of their breasts and to report any changes to their health care providers.

Starting at age 40, average-risk women should be counseled regarding mammograms. All the screening recommendations in Table 38.1 are effective at reducing risk of mortality from breast cancer. Providers should engage in shared decision-making with patients to determine individual screening most appropriate for their values and concerns. In conducting this discussion, providers should assess patient risk, comorbidities, anxiety over breast cancer and additional testing, and individual goals. Patients who want to minimize their breast cancer mortality risk and will tolerate the potential for call backs and additional testing are more appropriate for guidelines with earlier initiation and more frequent screening. Women who are willing to accept a slight increase in breast cancer risk to decrease risk of call backs or additional testing will do better with guidelines that test less frequently and start later. Decisions to end

screening should be based on the patient's quality of life, life expectancy, and willingness to initiate treatment if cancer is diagnosed. Screening average-risk women should start no earlier than age 40 and no later than age 50. It should occur every 1 or 2 years. It should cease at age 75, when a patient would no longer act on the screening results, or when life expectancy is unlikely to exceed 7–10 years.

Chemoprevention of breast cancer is indicated when the 5-year actuarial breast cancer risk as estimated by the modified Gail model (available at: www.cancer.gov/bcrisktool/Default.aspx) is 1.7 percent or greater or lifetime risk is 20 percent or greater. Additional indications include a known genetic predisposition or a pedigree suggestive of predisposition. The patient's menopause status determines which prophylaxis is recommended. For premenopausal patients over age 35, tamoxifen 20 mg daily for 5 years is recommended and provides protection that extends up to 10 years. The use of other agents is currently under investigation in clinical trials, and their use is not recommended. For postmenopausal women, tamoxifen 20 mg daily for 5 years and raloxifene 60 mg daily for 5 years are both effective. Although tamoxifen seems to have better long-term prevention past the initial 5 years, the risks associated with its use (including endometrial stimulation and hyperplasia) may make raloxifene a better alternative for some patients. Exemestane 25 mg daily and anastrozole 1 mg daily for 5 years have both shown significant risk reductions in invasive breast cancer and are alternatives for chemoprevention [g].

New Developments Likely to Affect Future Guidelines

There are currently significant controversies in mammography recommendations. New data may help inform the recommendations and promote a consensus among the multiple stakeholder organizations. In the interim, current recommendations require shared decision-making for individual patients. Shared decision-making is complicated by absence of effective tools to help patients understand the benefits, harms, and balance between benefits and harms of screening. Effective counseling tools will likely become available.

Further refinement of risk assessment is likely through personalized medicine, which will allow individualization of screening and prevention. Further refinement of screening technology may decrease falsely abnormal screens, as well as improve testing in women where current technologies have limitations, for instance women with dense breasts.

Another main area of research is the development of new agents to prevent cancer. Many drugs including fenasteride, exemestane, Non Steroidal Anti-inflammatory drugs (NSAIDs), statins, metformin, tibolone, and other SERMs are currently under investigation.

Billing

Breast cancer screening is typically covered under the ICD-10 code Z01.419, encounter for gynecological examination (general) (routine) without abnormal findings. Other possible codes include Z12.39, encounter for screening for malignant neoplasm of breast, and Z12.31, encounter for screening mammogram for breast cancer. Code Z53.20 may be used when a patient declines screening during a visit. Medicare has a special HCPCS code, G0101, for a clinical breast examination. Medicare specifies coverage no more frequently than every 2 years. In patients with significant risk factors (Z91.89) such as family history (Z80.3), genetic predisposition (Z15.01), or personal history of cancer (Z85.3), screening may be covered more often and allows for annual visits and multiple imaging modalities including magnetic resonance imaging (MRI).

ICD-10 does not have a specific code for chemoprevention of breast cancer. Codes may be used for patients with significant risk factors (Z91.89) such as family history (Z80.3), genetic predisposition (Z15.01), and general chemoprevention (Z41.8).

Illustrative Cases

A healthy 35-year-old Caucasian woman presents for a well-woman visit. She requests education regarding her risk for breast cancer and her options for screening. She has no family or personal history of breast cancer. Her menses started at age 13 and she had one child at age 25. She has never had a breast biopsy.

Online risk assessment tools can be used to better understand risk. Once risk is determined, counseling is individualized. In this case, the patient has the same risk as the general population. This patient can be counseled about breast awareness. Initiation of mammograms can be offered starting at age 40 depending on the patient's concerns and preferences but should be started no later than age 50. Screening intervals of every 1 or 2 years should also be determined with shared decision-making.

Screen now? No

Next screen: Initiate screening between ages 40 and 50

A healthy premenopausal 45-year-old Caucasian woman presents for a well-women visit. She reports having two first-degree relatives with breast cancer before the age of 50. She had a biopsy of her breast in her 30s for a benign condition. Her menarche was at age 11 and she has no children. She is concerned about cancer and requests education on screening and prevention of cancer. She has never had a mammogram.

This patient is at high risk. Using the National Cancer Institute online risk calculator, her lifetime risk is 32 percent. Patients with a risk higher than 20 percent may benefit from alternative screening modalities, genetic testing and counseling, and chemoprevention. The NCCN guidelines for high-risk women recommend a yearly mammogram, clinical breast examination, and encouragement of breast awareness. Referral for genetic counseling is indicated. Testing of available family members for predisposing genetic mutations like BRCA may be helpful. She can be offered testing if her relatives are not available. She meets eligibility requirements for chemoprevention and should be offered tamoxifen chemoprophylaxis. More frequent screening, including clinical breast examinations every 6 months and annual MRI 6 months after mammography, may also be beneficial.

Screen now? Yes
Next screen: 6 months

A healthy 75-year-old African American patient presents for a well-woman visit. She has no chronic medical conditions. She is active with yoga and swimming. She takes no medications. She has had mammograms every other year since age 50 and all have been normal. She had menarche at age 15, three children in her twenties, and has never had a breast biopsy. She has no personal or family history of breast cancer. She wonders if she should stop her mammograms now that she has reached the age of 75.

The decision to discontinue breast cancer screening, as with other screening decisions, should be individualized. Patients should make decisions about continuing screening based on overall health status, risk, and intent to undertake interventions to treat any conditions that are diagnosed. Life expectancy and quality of life should also inform this decision. At some point, patients may decide that the diagnosis of cancer at advanced age, combined with limitations in overall health, may lead to decisions to not pursue treatment. At present, few studies include older women. The decision should be reviewed at each visit; screening should be readdressed as the patient ages and their overall health deteriorates.

Screen now? Per patient preference
Next screen: Review decision annually

Guidelines

a. American College of Obstetricians and Gynecologists. Well-Woman-Task Force recommendations for screening. Available at: www.acog.org/About-ACOG/ACOG-Departments/Annual-Womens-Health-Care/Well-Woman-Recommendations. Retrieved March 12, 2016.

b. Breast Cancer Screening. US Preventive Services Task Force. Available at: www.uspreventiveservicestaskforce.org/Page/Document/UpdateSummaryFinal/breast-cancer-screening1?ds=1&s=. Retrieved March 21, 2016.

c. Breast Cancer Screening Guidelines. American Cancer Society. Available at: www.cancer.org/cancer/breastcancer/moreinformation/breastcancerearlydetection/breast-cancer-early-detection-acs-recs. Retrieved March 21, 2016.

d. Breast Cancer Screening Guidelines. National Comprehensive Cancer Network. Available at: www.nccn.org/professionals/physician_gls/pdf/breast-screening.pdf. Retrieved March 21, 2016.

e. Breast Cancer Screening. American Academy of Family Physicians. Available at: www.aafp.org/patient-care/clinical-recommendations/all/breast-cancer.html. Retrieved March 21, 2016.

f. Lee, C.H., Dershaw, D.D., Kopans, D. et al. Breast cancer screening with imaging: Recommendations from the society of breast imaging and the ACR on the use of mammography, breast MRI, breast ultrasound, and other technologies for the detection of clinically occult breast cancer. *J Am Coll Radiol.* 2010, 7:18–27.

g. Breast Cancer Risk Reduction Guidelines. National Comprehensive Cancer Network. Available at: www.nccn.org/professionals/physician_gls/pdf/breast_risk.pdf. Retrieved March 20, 2016.

References

1. American College of Obstetricians and Gynecologists. Breast cancer screening. Practice Bulletin No. 122. *Obstet Gynecol.* 2011, **118**:372–82.

2. American Cancer Society. *Breast Cancer Facts and Figures: 2015–2016.* Atlanta, GA: American Cancer Society, 2015. Available at: www.cancer.org/research/cancerfactsstatistics/cancerfactsfigures2016/index. Retrieved February 12, 2016.

3. Weiss, N.S. Breast cancer mortality in relation to clinical breast examination and breast self-examination. *Breast J.* 2003, **9**(Suppl 2):S86–9.

4. Kösters, J.P. and Gøtzsche, P.C. Regular self-examination or clinical examination for early detection of breast cancer. *Cochrane Database Syst Rev.* 2003, (**2**):CD003373.

5. Siu, A.L.; US Preventive Services Task Force. Screening for breast cancer: US Preventive Services Task Force recommendation statement. *Ann Intern Med.* 2016. doi:10.7326/M15–2886. [Epub ahead of print]

6. Thomas, D.B., Gao, D.L., Ray, R.M. et al. Randomized trial of breast self-examination in Shanghai: Final results. *J Natl Cancer Inst.* 2002, **94**:1445–57.

7. Oeffinger, K.C., Fontham, E.T., Etzioni, R. et al.; American Cancer Society. Breast cancer screening for women at average risk: 2015 guideline update from the American Cancer Society. *JAMA.* 2015, **314**:1599–614.

8. Mandelblatt, J.S., Stout, N.K., Schechter, C.B. et al. Collaborative modeling of the benefits and harms associated with different US breast cancer screening strategies. Benefits and harms of US breast cancer screening strategies. *Ann Intern Med.* 2016, **164**: 215–25.

9. US Preventive Services Task Force. Screening for breast cancer: US Preventive Services Task Force final recommendations. Available at: www.uspreventiveservicestaskforce.org/Page/Document/

RecommendationStatementFinal/breast-cancer-screening1. Retrieved April 7, 2016.

10. Antoniou, A., Pharoah, P.D., Narod, S. et al. Average risks of breast and ovarian cancer associated with BRCA1 or BRCA2 mutations detected in case series unselected for family history: A combined analysis of 22 studies. *Am J Hum Genet.* 2003, **72**:1117–30.

11. National Cancer Institute's Breast Cancer Assessment Tool. Available at: www.cancer.gov/bcrisktool. Retrieved February 12, 2016.

12. IBIS Breast Cancer Risk Evaluation Tool. Available at: www.ems-trials.org/riskevaluator/. Retrieved February 12, 2016.

13. Travis, L.B., Hill, D., Dores, G.M. et al. Cumulative absolute breast cancer risk for young women treated for Hodgkin lymphoma. *J Natl Cancer Inst.* 2005, **97**: 1428–37.

14. BOADICEA Model for Breast Cancer Risk Assessment. University of Cambridge. Available at: http://ccge.medschl.cam.ac.uk/boadicea/. Retrieved February 12, 2016.

Chapter 39

Genetic Screening for Cancer

Vanessa H. Gregg

Why Screen?

Breast cancer is common, with a lifetime risk of about 12 percent in the general population. According to Surveillance, Epidemiology and End Results (SEER) data through 2012, breast cancer is the most common type of cancer, with an estimated 231,840 new cases of female breast cancer and 40,290 women dying of the disease in 2015 [1].

Several factors increase the risk for breast cancer, including breast density as assessed by mammography, hormonal variables, and family history. Women with family history of breast cancer can be at dramatically increased risk for breast and other types of cancers. In addition to breast cancer, the risk of ovarian, endometrial, colon, and other malignancies can be elevated based on family history of these types of cancer.

There are a number of genetic mutations that have been associated with breast, ovarian, uterine, and colon cancers (Table 39.1). Mutations in the BRCA1 and 2 cancer susceptibility genes are the most well known. Women with certain BRCA1 and 2 mutations are at significantly increased risk for breast and ovarian cancers. In addition, mutations in DNA repair genes responsible for Lynch syndrome, Cowden syndrome, Li-Fraumeni syndrome, and others can cause a significantly increased risk of a variety of cancers. Mutations in these genes are inherited in an autosomal dominant fashion, meaning that women are at increased risk of developing an associated cancer if they inherit only one mutated gene. Identifying high-risk family pedigrees can lead to life-changing genetic diagnostics and treatments.

Rationale for Screening

There have been major advances in DNA sequencing technologies since 2005. As a result, genetic testing is readily available for germ line mutations that increase the risk for a variety of cancers, including breast, ovarian, uterine, and colon cancers [2].

In appropriately identified women, genetic screening for hereditary predisposition to malignancy can be a life-saving diagnostic tool. Specific guidelines exist for a variety of genetic cancer syndromes. Genetic counseling and testing can identify specific genetic mutations that are associated with some types of cancer. Women who are identified to be at increased risk can receive targeted screening, medical therapies, and surgical interventions to reduce or eliminate cancer risk.

Hereditary Breast and Ovarian Cancer (HBOC)

Five to ten percent of all breast cancers are hereditary. Of all hereditary breast cancers, 30–50 percent are attributable to mutations in BRCA1 and BRCA2. It is estimated that about 10 percent of ovarian cancers are also due to mutations in BRCA1 and 2. The diagnosis of a mutation in BRCA1 or 2 encompasses a large number of different mutations in these tumor suppressor genes. Mutations in the BRCA1 and 2 genes are inherited in an autosomal dominant fashion [a].

In addition to the 10 percent of ovarian cancers due to BRCA1 and 2 mutations, an additional 10 percent of ovarian cancers are likely attributable to other genetic cancer susceptibility genes, including Lynch syndrome mutations and other mutations.

Lynch Syndrome

Lynch syndrome, also known as hereditary nonpolyposis colorectal cancer syndrome, is the most common hereditary type of colorectal cancer, with a population prevalence estimated to be as high as 1 in 440. Lynch syndrome is associated with a group of genetic mutations in genes that are responsible for DNA mismatch repair. Approximately 2–3 percent

Table 39.1 Hereditary Cancer Syndromes

Hereditary Cancer Syndrome	Genetic Mutation	Prevalence	Most Commonly Associated Cancers	Comments
BRCA1 and BRCA2	Mutation in tumor suppressor genes	1 in 500 (higher in certain ethnic groups)	Breast, ovarian, prostate, male breast, pancreatic, melanoma	
Lynch	DNA mismatch repair. MLH1, MSH2, MSH6, PMS2 and EPCAM	1 in 440 to 1 in 3,000 prevalence	Endometrial, colon, ovarian	Other cancer types include brain, urinary tract, pancreas, biliary tract, and other intestinal cancers
Li-Fraumeni	p53 gene mutation	Rare	Breast, sarcoma, brain, adrenocortical, bone	68%–93% lifetime risk of developing cancer
Cowden	PTEN mutation	1 in 200,000	Breast, thyroid, uterine, renal, colon	Other clinical features include hamartomas and classic mucocutaneous findings. 20%–50% lifetime risk of breast cancer

Source: Data from Guidelines [f, a, & b] and References [3, 4]

of colorectal cancers occur in individuals with this syndrome [b]. The inheritance pattern for Lynch syndrome is autosomal dominant. There are several different genes associated with this syndrome, and the most prevalent are MLH1, MSH2, MSH6, PMS2, and EPCAM. Testing for Lynch syndrome can be performed either by doing a blood test to look for these genetic mutations or by testing for altered function in tumor tissues. Tumor testing is often the first step and can be performed through several different testing approaches [c].

Women with Lynch syndrome are at significantly increased risk for colon, uterine, and ovarian cancers. Women with Lynch syndrome have a lifetime incidence of endometrial cancer that has been estimated to be as high as 60 percent. Lynch syndrome carriers have a lifetime incidence of colorectal cancer as high as 80 percent. Other associated malignancies include ovary, brain, urinary tract, pancreas, biliary tract, and other intestinal cancers [b].

Factors that Affect Screening

Adolescents and young adults: The cancers that are caused by these genetic mutations typically occur in adulthood, so no harm would be expected by delaying testing until full adulthood and mature decision-making capacity. There are some important exceptions to this recommendation, such as a family history of extremely early-onset malignancy, potential emotional stress of waiting for testing, or rare cases in which an adolescent girl may be at risk of inheriting two copies of the same genetic mutation with more significant health consequences. Such cases should be handled through specialists with expertise in this area [d, e, c].

Ethnic background: Certain ethnic groups may be at increased risk for genetic cancer susceptibility. There are founder populations with a high concentration of certain genetic mutations. For example, women of Ashkenazi Jewish ancestry have a much higher prevalence of BRCA1 and 2 mutations, with a population prevalence of about 1 in 40 individuals [f, a].

Prior genetic testing in the family: A woman may present for care with documentation of a cancer genetic mutation having already been identified in her family. The woman's statistical probability of having a mutation will be significantly altered by the presence of a mutation in the family, and the approach to genetic testing will be different [f, a].

Women with no family history of cancer: Absence of family history of cancer, particularly in women outside at-risk ethnicities, places them at average risk for a genetic cancer susceptibility [d].

Recommended Guidelines and How to Find Them

A number of organizations provide guidelines for genetic screening for cancers. The Well-Woman Task Force (WWTF) derived their recommendations from a consensus of these recommendations. They made a strong recommendation that:

> All women should receive a family history evaluation as a screening tool for inherited risk of cancer. If their personal or family history is associated with an increased risk of potentially harmful mutations, they should be referred for genetic counseling, if genetic counseling services are available; and be offered genetic testing.
>
> Routine genetic counseling or BRCA testing is not recommended for women who do not have a personal or family history associated with an increased risk of potentially harmful mutations in BRCA1 or BRCA2.

These recommendations stem largely from the US Preventive Services Task Force (USPSTF) recommendations [d], which were also endorsed by the American Academy of Family Physicians (AAFP) [g]. They provide a grade B recommendation that is more specific as to which cancers warrant referral and specify that validated screening tools be used:

> The USPSTF recommends that primary care providers screen women who have family members with breast, ovarian, tubal, or peritoneal cancer with 1 of several screening tools designed to identify a family history that may be associated with an increased risk for potentially harmful mutations in breast cancer susceptibility genes (*BRCA1* or *BRCA2*). Women with positive screening results should receive genetic counseling and, if indicated after counseling, BRCA testing.

The American College of Obstetricians and Gynecologists (ACOG) [f] recommends routine hereditary cancer risk assessment by obtaining a family cancer history with referral as necessary.

More specific guidance is available from several specialty organizations. ACOG provides additional recommendations for HBOC [a] which recommend genetic risk assessment for women with greater than an approximately 20–25 percent chance of having an inherited predisposition to breast and ovarian cancers and that it may be helpful for women with greater than an approximately 5–10 percent chance of developing these malignancies. In addition, ACOG has published separate recommendations for Lynch syndrome [h]. The National Comprehensive Cancer Network (NCCN) provides guidelines for determinations of appropriateness for genetic testing and clinical management based on personal and family histories that are widely accepted and are followed by clinicians and genetic counselors. These guidelines are updated annually. They provide separate guidelines for HBOC and for colon cancer [e, c]. The American Gastroenterological Association Institute has a guideline on the diagnosis and management of Lynch syndrome, which includes guidance regarding the groups who need to be referred for further evaluation and management strategies for confirmed Lynch syndrome patients [b].

The Task Force recommendations are consistent with other guidelines including the NCCN and the USPSTF in recommending that testing for cancer genetic syndromes should be delayed until the age of adulthood or until an adolescent has mature decision-making capabilities.

How to Screen

All women of reproductive age and beyond should have family history obtained and regularly updated as a screening tool for inherited risk for cancer. This should be performed at all well-woman visits. Family history should include information about both maternal and paternal ancestry and should include at least first- and second-degree relatives. Cancer history should include types of cancers and ages at diagnosis. Ethnicity of the lineage is also important [d, f].

There are multiple tools available to assist in the obtaining and maintaining of family history information in the medical record. Many electronic medical

BOX 39.1 Family History Suspicious for Hereditary Breast and Ovarian Cancer

- Breast cancer diagnosed prior to age 50
- Bilateral breast cancer
- Family history of both breast and ovarian cancers
- Breast cancer in one or more male relatives
- Family member or members with two primary types of cancer known to be associated with BRCA1 and 2
- Triple negative breast cancer
- Ashkenazi Jewish ancestry

Source: [d, f, a, e]

BOX 39.2 Family History Suspicious for Lynch Syndrome

- Endometrial cancer prior to age 50
- Suspicious cases of colorectal cancer by Amsterdam or revised Bethesda guidelines, including early-onset colorectal cancer or families with multiple affected family members*

* See criteria from NCCN [c] for details

Source: [f, h, c]

records (EMRs) include a Family History section, including the ability to enter specific cancer types, age of onset, and family lineage information. There are additional resources available online through the National Human Genome Research Institute at www .genome.gov/11510372. There are several risk assessment models available to calculate a woman's risk of breast cancer. The Gail model, the Tyrer-Cuzick model, and the Claus model, as well as the probability model BRCAPRO, are tools that can be used to assess risk [3].

If personal or family history is suggestive of a hereditary predisposition to cancer, a woman should be referred to a genetic counselor or a clinician with expertise in hereditary cancer syndromes. Such providers can offer both further risk assessment and testing for cancer-causing gene mutations.

There are several family history pedigree features suspicious for HBOC. When family history suggests any of these patterns, the patient should be referred for genetic counseling and possible testing [d, a–c] (Boxes 39.1 and 39.2).

Genetic testing for mutations in BRCA1 and BRCA2 should not be undertaken unless there is a significant personal or family history to support that testing. A woman at average risk for breast cancer, without personal or family history of breast, ovarian or other malignancies, should not undergo testing for these or other cancer genetic mutations [d].

If a woman presents with documentation of a cancer genetic mutation having already been identified in her family, she should be referred for genetic counseling. Site-specific testing can be performed to identify whether she is a carrier for that specific genetic mutation. Such testing is much less expensive than a comprehensive search for all of the potential genetic mutations [f, e] [3].

Genetic counselors are an excellent resource for counseling and testing for women who may have an inherited genetic cancer susceptibility. Both the American College of Medical Genetics and Genomics (www.acmg.net) and the National Society of Genetic Counselors (www.nsgc.org) have websites with information regarding recommendations for genetics referral as well as searchable lists of genetic counselors by geographic area.

New Developments Likely to Affect Future Recommendations

Cancer genetics is an evolving field. As DNA testing technologies continue to improve, more genetic tests have become available and are much less expensive.

BOX 39.3 Useful Billing Codes for Hereditary Cancer Syndromes

Family history of cancer:

Breast: Z80.3

Ovary: Z80.41

Uterus: Z80.49

Cervix: Z80.49

Personal history of cancer:

Breast: Z85.3

Ovary: Z85.43

Cervix: Z85.41

Uterus: Z85.42

Endometrial: Z85.42

Genetic susceptibility to cancer:

Breast: Z15.01

Ovary: Z15.02

Endometrium: Z15.04

Other/Lynch: Z15.09

Cancer screenings:

Breast (mammogram): Z13.31

Breast (other): Z12.39

Cervix: Z12.4

Vagina: Z12.72

Ovary: Z12.73

Other genitourinary organs: Z12.79

At one time, it was necessary to choose a single genetic mutation for which to test, as it was cost prohibitive to test for multiple mutations at the same time. Now, it is possible to order cancer genetic panels, including testing for multiple genetic mutations, at a similar cost to what was once the cost for a single genetic mutation test. As a result, more women will opt for a panel test and more information will be obtained more quickly. One of the issues that arise from panel testing is that mutations may be identified about which little clinical information is known. Women will have to work closely with genetic counselors and care providers to understand how to interpret test results. Mutations that were once thought to be very rare may be identified with more frequency.

Billing

Major insurance carriers have criteria for coverage of genetic counseling and testing based on the patient's

personal and family histories. The criteria can vary and be challenging to navigate. In some areas, insurers may require that testing be ordered through a genetic counselor for the testing to be covered by insurance. BRCA1 and 2 testing may be grouped under preventive medicine and therefore covered at a better rate than other types of medical testing. The Federal Genetic Information Nondiscrimination Act was passed in 2008. This act prohibits health insurers from discrimination based on genetic predisposition. It also prohibits employers from using genetic information as a factor in making decisions regarding hiring, firing, or promotion. A number of ICD-10 codes are useful for billing (Box 39.3).

Illustrative Cases

A 30-year-old healthy woman presents for a well-woman visit. In obtaining her family history, you learn that her paternal aunt had breast cancer at age 30. In addition, her paternal grandmother died of ovarian cancer at age 50. She reports that no genetic testing has been done in the family.

This patient should be referred for genetic counseling and possible genetic testing for HBOCs. Her family history is suspicious for HBOC syndrome due to a combination of both breast and ovarian cancers occurring in the same genetic lineage as well as early-onset breast cancer in her paternal aunt. BRCA mutations can be inherited from both maternal and paternal lineages.

The patient should check the family history details with her family prior to meeting with the genetic counselor. Details about types of cancer, ages of onset, as well as information about cancer-unaffected relatives, can help to refine the risk assessment. Many genetic counselors will follow NCCN guidelines as well as insurance authorization criteria to determine whether a patient is an appropriate candidate for genetic testing.

Ideally, the genetic testing would be performed on a cancer-affected family member. If her paternal aunt is alive, that aunt would be the best candidate for genetic testing. If the aunt is deceased, another option would be to test the patient's father, as he is genetically more similar to the cancer-affected aunt than is your patient.

The interpretation of genetic test results can be confusing, so the testing must be handled by a genetic counselor or a provider who is well versed in the interpretation of the test results. Genetic testing results must be interpreted in the context of what is already known about the family. If this patient has genetic testing herself, in the absence of definitive genetic information about her cancer-affected family members, the patient's results would be termed "uninformative negative." An uninformative negative is reassuring as no mutation has been identified, but the patient is still considered to be at increased risk for developing breast and ovarian cancer due to the unexplained cancers in her family. The NCCN website provides definitions for commonly used genetic terms, including uninformative negative, inconclusive, true-negative, and true-positive genetic test results [d, f, a, e].

Counsel and screen now? Yes

Next screen? Depends on results of genetic counseling and testing

A healthy 30-year-old woman presents for a well-woman visit. She reports no personal or family histories of cancer. She expresses concern about developing breast cancer, as she has a neighbor who was just diagnosed with early-onset breast cancer. She has read about BRCA1 and 2 mutations and wonders if she should be tested to see if she is a carrier.

The patient should be advised that breast cancer is common, and all women have some risk of developing breast cancer. The prevalence for a BRCA1 or 2 mutation in the general population is about 1 in 500 or less. In the absence of any family history, cancer genetic testing is not recommended [d], [3].

Screen now? No

Next screen? Reassess patient risk at each well-woman visit

A healthy 25-year-old woman presents for a well-woman visit. She reports that her mother's sister was recently diagnosed with ovarian cancer. As part of her treatment planning, the maternal aunt had genetic testing and was found to carry a BRCA2 mutation. There is no other family history of cancer. Your patient wants to know what she should do with this new family history information.

This asymptomatic 25-year-old woman should be offered referral for genetic counseling and possible testing. She should take a copy of her maternal aunt's BRCA2 mutation test results with her to her appointment. The patient can opt for site-specific testing for the known genetic mutation identified in her family. Another option would be for her mother to first pursue the testing, and then the patient would be tested only if her mother is positive for the identified mutation.

Further recommendations would then be made based on test results. If the patient tests positive, she would be advised to follow guidelines from NCCN and ACOG regarding surveillance and risk management, including options for chemoprevention and prophylactic surgery. If the patient does not carry the BRCA2 mutation, then she is considered to be at normal population-level risk for breast and ovarian cancers [f, a, e].

Counsel and screen now? Yes

Next screen? Depends on results of genetic counseling and testing

A healthy 30-year-old woman presents for a well-woman visit. She reports that her mother was recently diagnosed with colon cancer at the age of 60. She reports that some kind of testing was done on her mother's tumor and her mother says she may need to be screened early for colon cancer.

The next step for management is referral to a genetic counselor. The patient should get additional information from her mother to confirm whether Lynch syndrome has been diagnosed. If so, the patient can pursue testing to determine whether she also has Lynch syndrome. If she tests positive, she is at significantly increased risk for uterine and colon cancers as well as other malignancies. She would then require high-risk surveillance and would be a candidate for chemoprevention and possible prophylactic surgery, under the care of a provider or team of providers with expertise with this syndrome [a, b].

Counsel and screen now? Yes

Next screen? Depends on results of genetic counseling and testing

Guidelines

a. American College of Obstetricians and Gynecologists. Hereditary breast and ovarian cancer syndrome. ACOG Practice Bulletin No. 103. *Obstet Gynecol.* 2009, 113:957–66.

b. Rubenstein, J.H., Enns, R., Heidelbaugh, J., and Barkun, A. American Gastroenterological Association Institute guideline on the diagnosis and management of Lynch syndrome. *Gastroenterology.* 2015, **149**:777–82.

c. NCCN Clinical Practice Guidelines in Oncology. NCCN Guidelines: Genetic/Familial High-Risk Assessment: Colorectal. Available at: www.nccn.org/professionals/physician_gls/pdf/genetics_colon.pdf. Retrieved May 20, 2016.

d. Moyer, V.A. Risk assessment, genetic counseling, and genetic testing for BRCA-related cancer in women: US Preventive Services Task Force recommendation statement. US Preventive Services Task Force. *Ann Intern Med.* 2014, **160**:271–81. Available at: www.uspreventiveservicestaskforce.org/Page/Document/UpdateSummaryFinal/brca-related-cancer-risk-

assessment-genetic-counseling-and-genetic-testing. Retrieved May 19, 2016.

e. NCCN Clinical Practice Guidelines in Oncology. NCCN Guidelines: Genetic/Familial High-Risk Assessment: Breast and Ovarian. Available at: www.nccn.org/professionals/physician_gls/pdf/genetics_screening.pdf. Retrieved May 20, 2016.

f. American College of Obstetricians and Gynecologists. Hereditary cancer syndromes and risk assessment. Committee Opinion No. 634. *Obstet Gynecol.* 2015, **125**: 1538–43.

g. American Academy of Family Physicians. *Breast Cancer: Clinical Preventive Service Recommendation.* Leawood, KS: AAFP, 2015. Available at: www.aafp.org/patient-care/clinical-recommendations/all/breast-cancer.html. Retrieved May 19, 2016.

h. American College of Obstetricians and Gynecologists. Lynch syndrome. Practice Bulletin No. 147. *Obstet Gynecol.* 2014, **124**:1042–54.

References

1. Howlader, N., Noone, A.M., Krapcho, M. et al., editors. *SEER Cancer Statistics Review, 1975–2012.* Bethesda, MD: National Cancer Institute. Available at: http://seer.cancer.gov/csr/1975_2012/ (http://seer.cancer.gove/csr/), based on November 2014 SEER data submission, posted to the SEER web site, April 2015. Retrieved May 21, 2016.

2. Caskey, C., Gonzalez-Garay, M., Pereira, S., and McGuire, A. Adult genetic risk screening. *Annu Rev Med.* 2014, **65**:1–17.

3. Stuckey, A.R. and Onstad, M.A. Hereditary breast cancer: An update on risk assessment and genetic testing in 2015. *Am J Obstet Gynecol.* 2015, **213**(2):161–5.

4. Rich, T.A., Woodson, A.H., Litton, J., and Arun, B. Hereditary breast cancer syndromes and genetic testing. *J Surg Oncol.* 2015, **111**:66–80.

Depression

Tiffany A. Moore Simas

40

Why Screen?

Depression is the most common psychiatric disorder in the United States. In 2014, almost 16 million adults ≥18 years (6.7 percent) and an additional almost 3 million adolescents aged 12–17 (11.4 percent) had at least one major depressive episode in the prior year. Beginning with menarche and carrying through menopause, the rates of depression in women are at least double those of men. Adolescent girls (16.2 percent) have greater than three times the rate (5.3 percent) of their male counterparts; adult women (8.2 percent) have almost double the rate as men (4.8 percent) [1]. The highest-risk time for most women revolves around childbearing; 15 percent of pregnant and postpartum women experience perinatal depression [2] with rates being as high as 40 percent in socioeconomically disadvantaged and adolescent populations. Depression is associated with decreased quality of life, increased disability and impairment, adverse pregnancy outcomes, and increased mortality including suicide. The effects of depression extend beyond individual women to their children, families, and employers. The economic consequences to individuals and society are substantial.

Rationale for Screening

Unless directly asked, few patients in primary care settings discuss symptoms of depression. Rather than describing mood symptoms, women more often report nonspecific symptoms such as headache or pain. Without screening, only about 50 percent of patients with major depression are identified [3].

Risk factors for depression include genetic (e.g., family history, female gender), neuroendocrine (e.g., menstrual, perinatal, and menopausal hormonal alterations), environmental, social (e.g., poor social support, childhood traumas), and medical history including prior psychiatric history. Knowledge of these numerous risk factors is helpful but does replace the need for screening.

Validated depression screening instruments are available, relatively easy to administer, inexpensive, and are acceptable to patients. The performance of available tools when used as screening instruments (i.e., as part of systematic screening during routine health evaluations, not prompted by risk factors, signs, or symptoms) would significantly increase detection rates from 50 [3] to 90 percent [4].

There are effective treatments for depression, including psychotherapy, pharmacotherapy, and combinations of both. Early treatment initiation is associated with better response rates, making early recognition through screening desirable. Even the most severe forms of depression can be treated.

Factors That Affect Screening

Perinatal period (pregnancy and postpartum):
Many of the signs and symptoms associated with a depression diagnosis are also common physiological or emotional responses to the unique neuroendocrine, physical, and psychosocial adjustments of pregnancy and caring for an infant. One in seven women experience depression in the perinatal period [2]. Approximately, one-third of women enter pregnancy with a depressive disorder, another one-third have onset in pregnancy, and the last one-third have postpartum onset.
The *Diagnostic and Statistical Manual of Mental Disorders*, fifth edition (DSM-5) considers postpartum onset to occur within the 4 weeks following delivery [5]; however, many extend this period to include the first postpartum year [2]. Baby blues, a temporary condition characterized by a mother having sudden onset of significant mood swings, is common and

occurs in up to 85 percent of women. Women experiencing baby blues may screen positive for perinatal depression. Distinction between the two conditions may only be possible in retrospect; baby blues typically occurs right after childbirth, usually in the first week and is mostly self-limited (peak at 3–5 days, resolution often 10–12 days postpartum). Postpartum depression is independent of baby blues, but baby blues should be recognized as a risk factor for depression with postpartum onset.

Age: The extremes of reproductive age can affect screening for depression. Once reaching puberty, adolescent girls have twice the risk of depression as compared to boys. Hormonal factors and mood changes related to menstruation play a role; additionally, sociocultural factors likely also affect depression development in girls of this age group. Similarly, hormonal fluctuations and sleep disturbances in the transition to menopause can trigger depression, with symptoms generally improving with menopause. Depression in elderly women can often go unrecognized and thus untreated. Some view depression as a natural part of aging especially in the context of other chronic medical illnesses, the natural loss of family and friends, and social transitions. Depression in older persons can more prominently include memory problems (pseudodementia) and somatic complaints. It may additionally be a side effect of medications used to treat hypertension, heart attacks, stroke, hip fractures, or macular degeneration, for example.

Recommended Guidelines and How to Find Them

The Well-Woman Task Force (WWTF) depression screening recommendations [6] were predominantly based on the evidence-based recommendations of the US Preventive Services Task Force (USPSTF) [a, b]. Evidence-informed guidelines from numerous other stakeholder medical societies also informed the WWTF consensus recommendations; these included the American Medical Association (AMA) [c], American Academy of Pediatrics (AAP) [d], American Academic of Family Physicians (AAFP) [e], Association of Women's

Health Obstetric and Neonatal Nurses (AWHONN) [f], American Congress of Obstetricians and Gynecologists (ACOG) [g, h], American College of Nurse Midwives (ACNM) [i], and the Preconception Health and Health Care Committee (PCHHC) [j]. These various guideline recommendations ranged from universal [d, f, i, j] to risk-based screening [c], and to screening only when staff-assisted supports are in place to ensure accurate diagnosis, treatment, and follow-up [a, b, e, g, h]. Variability in recommendations is consistent with concerns that screening enhances detection, but in isolation does not improve treatment initiation, engagement, or clinical outcomes. In accordance, the WWTF had uniform expert agreement that

> Patients should not be denied recommended screening because of any limitation of local resources. Rather, providers should have plans for referral, even if it means the patient will have to travel outside her community. Providers are encouraged to develop initial management skills that are within the scope of their specialty and practice to meet local patient needs. Patients should be counseled about limitations in local resources at the time of testing. [6]

The final WWTF recommendations are consistent across all age categories: women should be screened for depressive disorders using a validated instrument at annual visits and in the postpartum period. Since the publication of the WWTF guidelines, the USPSTF updated their depression screening guidelines for adults aged 18 and older; screening for depression is recommended in the general adult population, including pregnant and postpartum women [k].

Depression screening should also be performed when clinically indicated such as in the presence of risk factors or other signs and symptoms.

How to Screen

Diagnoses and criteria: Depressive disorders share common features of sad, empty, or irritable mood, accompanied by somatic and cognitive changes that are associated with distress and/or impairment in social, occupational, educational, or other important functional areas. Specific depressive disorders differ in duration, timing, and presumed etiology. Depressive disorders, to be considered for persons aged 12 and older, are defined in DSM-5 [5] and include:

- major depressive disorder (MDD)
- persistent depressive disorder (dysthymia)
- premenstrual dysphoric disorder
- substance/medication-induced depressive disorder
- depressive disorder due to another medical condition
- other specified depressive disorder
- unspecified depressive disorder

MDD is the most common of the depressive disorders. MDD is characterized by having five (or more) of the following symptoms for most of the day nearly every day for a minimum of two consecutive weeks, and as a baseline change. At least one of the symptoms must be:

- Depressed mood (in adolescents, this can be irritable mood)

  or

- Loss of interest or pleasure in most or all activities

  Other additional symptoms include the following:

- Change in weight or appetite
- Insomnia or hypersomnia
- Psychomotor agitation or retardation
- Fatigue or loss of energy
- Feelings of worthlessness or guilt
- Poor concentration or indecisiveness
- Recurrent thoughts of death or suicide

Screening tools: Numerous screening instruments exist to query individual patients about depression-associated somatic and cognitive changes that increase risk of a depression diagnosis. Most instruments can be self-administered, in relatively short time, and are then scored by the clinical care team and considered with regards to established cut-points. Utilization and accuracy of screening instruments have been studied in primary care settings as the venues in which most depression care is delivered, and thus the appropriate context for screening.

A literature synthesis of validated case-finding instruments utilized to identify depression in primary care settings noted a median sensitivity of 85 percent (range 50–97 percent) and a median specificity of 74 percent (range 51–98 percent) [4]. With consideration of these performance characteristics, the authors went on to describe that in a setting with a major depression prevalence rate of 10 percent and in which a clinician sees 100 patients, 32 patients with a positive screening score would be encountered.

Of the original 100, 10 would have major depression in which 9 would have been correctly identified by screening (true positives) and 1 would have been missed (false negative) thus resulting in a 90 percent detection rate. Of the 32 screen positive patients, 23 (72 percent) would not meet criteria for major depression (false positives) [4].

Given the significant risk of misclassification related to the low positive predictive value of a positive screen in primary care settings [4], follow-up with a diagnostic interview is necessary [3,4]. It is worthwhile noting that many patients with false positive screening results for major depression would meet criteria for other psychiatric diagnoses such as dysthymia, premenstrual dysphoric disorder, and others [4].

First-line depression treatment is relatively low risk and thus the potential for harm with false positives is relatively minimal and is decreased further with subsequent diagnostic evaluations. Screening is generally supported and well tolerated; however, screening does not necessarily translate into treatment engagement due to multilevel barriers.

Screening in the general population: Table 40.1 lists information on six instruments of easy to average literacy levels, not requiring scoring calculators, and evaluated in at least one study including a minimum of 100 subjects [4,7]. Although there are numerous others, the Beck Depression Inventory (BDI), Center for Epidemiologic Studies Depression Scale (CES-D), and Zhung Self-Rating Depression Scale (SDS) are among the most thoroughly evaluated instruments in primary care settings and can be used to rate depression severity in addition to monitoring therapy response [7]. The Geriatric Depression Scale (GDS) has been evaluated in populations aged 60 and older and thus may be preferred by clinicians caring for older women; however, its performance lacks evidence of superiority over instruments developed for general primary care populations. On the opposite end of the age spectrum, the most common screening instruments utilized in adolescents are the Patient Health Questionnaire for Adolescents (PHQ-A) and the Beck Depression Inventory-Primary Care Version [8].

Screening in pregnancy and postpartum: Table 40.2 lists information on seven instruments used to screen pregnant and postpartum women [2]. The Edinburgh Postnatal Depression Scale (EPDS)

Table 40.1 Depression Screening Instruments and Performance for Major Depressive Disorder

Instrument	Items (N)*	Score Range	Usual Cut-Point†	Literacy Level‡	Administration Time (minutes)	Monitor Severity or Response	Link to Instrument PDF
BDI	21, 13; 7	0–63	10–19 Mild 20–29 Moderate ≥30 Severe	Easy	2–5	Yes	http://mhinnovation.net/sites/default/files/downloads/innovation/research/BDI%20with%20interpretation.pdf
CES-D	20, 10	0–60	≥16	Easy	2–5	Yes	www.actonmedical.com/documents/cesd_long.pdf
GDS¶	30, 15	0–30	≥11	Easy	2–5	Yes	http://neurosciencecme.com/library/rating_scales/depression_geriatric_long.pdf
PHQ-2	2	0–2	≥1	Average	<1	No	www.cqaimh.org/pdf/tool_phq2.pdf
PHQ-9	9	0–27	(See details in link for scoring) 0–4 None 5–9 Mild 10–14 Moderate 15–19 Major 20–27 Severe	Average	<2	Yes	www.cqaimh.org/pdf/tool_phq9.pdf
SDS	20	25–110 (sum / 80 × 100)	50–59 Mild 60–69 Moderate ≥70 Severe	Easy	2–5	Yes	http://healthnet.umassmed.edu/mhealth/ZungSelfRatedDepressionScale.pdf

BDI: Beck Depression Inventory; CES-D: Center for Epidemiologic Studies Depression Scale; CI: Confidence Interval; Dx: Diagnosis; GDS: Geriatric Depression Scale; PHQ: Patient Health Questionnaire; SDS: Zhung Self-Rating Depression Scale

* These numbers refer to different versions of the same instrument and are listed from most to least number of items

† Cut-point is given for the instrument with the greatest number of items

‡ Easy (third- to fifth-grade reading level), average (sixth- to ninth-grade reading level)

¶ Evaluated only in populations aged 60 and older

Source: Modified from Williams, J.W. Jr, Pignone, M, Ramirez, G, and Perez Stellato, C. Identifying depression in primary care: a literature synthesis of case-finding instruments. *Gen Hosp Psychiatry.* 2002, 24(4):225–37, with permission from Elsevier to utilize content in the table (www.journals.elsevier.com/general-hospital-psychiatry/).

Table 40.2 Depression Screening Tools in Pregnant and Postpartum Populations

Screening Tool	Number of Items	Time to Complete (minutes)	Sensitivity and Specificity	Spanish Available
Edinburgh Postnatal Depression Scale	10	<5	Sensitivity 59%–100%, Specificity 49%–100%	Yes
Postpartum Depression Screening Scale	35	5–10	Sensitivity 91%–94%, Specificity 72%–98%	Yes
Patient Health Questionnaire 9	9	<5	Sensitivity 75%, Specificity 90%	Yes
Beck Depression Inventory	21	5–10	Sensitivity 47.6%–82%, Specificity 85.9%–89%	Yes
Beck Depression Inventory II	21	5–10	Sensitivity 56%–57%, Specificity 97%–100%	Yes
Center for Epidemiologic Studies Depression Scale	20	5–10	Sensitivity 60%, Specificity 92%	Yes
Zung Self-Rating Depression Scale	20	5–10	Sensitivity 45%–89%, Specificity 77%–88%	No

Source: With permission from American College of Obstetricians and Gynecologists. Screening for perinatal depression. ACOG Committee Opinion No. 630. *Obstet Gynecol.* 2015, 125:1268–71.

and the Postpartum Depression Screening Scale (PDSS) were developed specifically for and validated in perinatal populations [9]. Other instruments were developed for the general population and have been validated in perinatal populations (e.g., BDI, PHQ-2, and PHQ-9) [9].

Screening non-English-speaking women: Numerous validated depression screening instruments are available in non-English languages, thus consideration should be given to using instruments translated into the patient's preferred language. It should be noted that no translated instruments are tested or studied as well as their English-language counterparts.

Clinical interview for screen positive patients: Patients scoring above a specific threshold on a screening instrument require more thorough evaluation with a clinical interview for definitive diagnosis. The diagnostic interview is standardly done in the primary care setting without routine referrals. Symptoms are evaluated with regards to their intensity, duration, influence on daily functioning, and the context in which they occur (e.g., perinatal onset, cyclic occurrence following ovulation and remitting within few days of menses), in addition to the role of other medical conditions, substance use, and recent

significant losses (e.g., bereavement, financial ruin) [5]. Additionally, suicide risk and previous episodes of mania are critical to assess prior to establishing a treatment plan, especially if it involves medication. A thorough review of systems to evaluate other medical conditions that may present as depression (e.g., hypothyroidism, diabetes mellitus) or may increase risk of depression (e.g., autoimmune disorders, malignancy) may warrant additional testing. Depression often co-occurs with other conditions like substance use disorder and thus additional screening for other conditions may be merited. There are no laboratory tests, imaging studies, or pathologic tissue examinations that can aide in the diagnosis.

New Developments Likely to Affect Future Recommendations

Since the publication of the WWTF guidelines, the USPSTF put forth updated recommendations in January 2016 with regards to screening for depression in adults aged 18 and older. The updated guidelines were notable for recommending screening in the general adult population, including both pregnant and postpartum women [k]. Identified gaps in existing evidence and thus areas of needed future research were numerous and included but were not limited to (1) accuracy of screening instruments in non-English and non-Spanish languages, (2) timing and optimal screening intervals in all populations, (3) accuracy of screening in pregnancy and associated treatment harms and benefits, (4) postpartum antidepressant treatment harms and benefits, and importantly, (5) identification of and ways to address barriers to adequate depression care systems [k].

The USPSTF is anticipated to issue updated recommendations regarding screening for depression in children and adolescents. It is likely that screening will be recommended for adolescents aged 12–18 when adequate diagnosis, treatment, and monitoring systems exist [8].

Although there are no current biological screening tests, it is conceivable with advances in personalized and genomic medicine that neuroendocrine and genetic testing will be available in the future.

Billing

Depression screening in a primary care population is covered under ICD-10 code Z13.89, encounter for screening for other disorder. This code covers a wide array of screening activities including but not limited to alcoholism, behavioral disorder, genitourinary condition, congenital anomaly, and many others.

Medicare requires special HCPCS codes: G0444 (annual depression screening, 15 minutes).

Depression screening in a postpartum population is covered under ICD-10 code Z39.2 (Routine Postpartum follow up – Screening for Postpartum Depression). Given global payment of pregnancy and postpartum care, utilization of this code may facilitate tracking but is unlikely to represent additional reimbursement.

When a depressive disorder is diagnosed, there are numerous additional codes for specific diagnoses and with qualifiers related to primary or recurrent episodes, presence of associated symptoms including psychoses, severity, and evidence of partial or full remission.

Illustrative Cases

A healthy 31-year-old woman presents for a well-woman visit with no complaint.

The WWTF recommends annual screening for depressive disorders, using a validated instrument.

Table 40.3 Links to Depression Screening Tools for Pregnant and Postpartum Populations

Instrument	Link to Instrument PDF
Edinburgh Postnatal Depression Scale (EPDS)	www.fresno.ucsf.edu/pediatrics/downloads/edinburghscale.pdf
Postpartum Depression Screening Scale (PDSS)	(requires purchase)
Patient Health Questionnaire 9 (PHQ-9)	www.cqaimh.org/pdf/tool_phq9.pdf
Beck Depression Inventory (BDI)	http://mhinnovation.net/sites/default/files/downloads/innovation/research/BDI%20with%20interpretation.pdf
Beck Depression Inventory II (BDI-II)	(requires purchase)
Center for Epidemiologic Studies Depression Scale (CES-D)	www.actonmedical.com/documents/cesd_long.pdf
Zung Self-Rating Depression Scale (SDS)	http://healthnet.umassmed.edu/mhealth/ZungSelfRatedDepressionScale.pdf

Screen now? Yes

Next screening: At next annual examination (and when clinically indicated)

A healthy 25-year-old woman presents for her routine postpartum visit with questions about contraception, and returning to full physical activity following her cesarean delivery.

The WWTF recommends screening postpartum for depression using a validated instrument. Consideration should be given to use of a screening instrument that has been validated in postpartum populations (Tables 40.2 and 40.3).

Screen now? Yes

Next screening: At next annual examination (and when clinically indicated)

A 22-year-old primigravida at 9 weeks gestational age is attending her first prenatal care visit. She has a medical history significant for depression with a suicide attempt when she was an adolescent. Other than experiencing fatigue and some weight gain, she reports feeling well and is not currently being managed for depression with either pharmacologic or nonphar-macologic treatments.

Women with a depression history are at increased risk for perinatal depression and thus screening at this time is clinically indicated in order to establish a baseline or identify an unrecognized recurrence. Additionally, since the WWTF consensus, the USPSTF has published updated guidelines that recommend screening in pregnancy. One in seven women experience depression in the perinatal period; approximately, one-third of these women enter pregnancy with a depressive disorder, another one-third have onset in pregnancy, and the last one-third have postpartum onset. As this patient is pregnant, consideration should be given to use of a screening instrument that has specifically been validated in pregnancy (Tables 40.2 and 40.3), as many normal changes and experiences of pregnancy resemble depression symptoms.

Screen now? Yes

Next screening: If screen positive, a diagnostic evaluation is merited and additional screening could be performed in pregnancy and postpartum to monitor severity, response, or progression. If this patient has a negative screen, additional screening could be performed later in pregnancy based on history and clinical indication. Minimally, a postpartum screen should be performed.

A 27-year-old woman presents for her fourth visit in 2 years with a complaint of pelvic pain unrelated to menstruation.

Depression is a common comorbidity in chronic pain syndromes, and depression can present with somatic complaints. In addition to an appropriate history, physical examination, and evaluation for physical etiologies of pelvic pain, she should be screened for depression with a validated instrument. The majority of primary care patients with depression present with somatic symptoms including headache, fatigue, chronic pain, and others. The WWTF recommendations focus on screening during routine visits (e.g., annual and postpartum examinations), regardless of age; however, screening should be considered when risk factors such as chronic pelvic pain are identified.

Screen now? Yes.

Next screening: At annual examination and other encounters based on clinical situation

A 60-year-old woman with known medical comorbidities of chronic hypertension and coronary artery disease presents to a well-woman visit with complaints

of fatigue, weight gain, loss of concentration, and sadness.

The WWTF recommends screening yearly for depression with a validated tool at the well-woman visit. This woman is also demonstrating symptoms of depression and thus would merit screening based on symptoms. As her symptoms also overlap with those of hypothyroidism, a thyrotropin measurement would be indicated. Some experts recommend a thyrotropin measurement in all women over the age of 50 due to the increased prevalence of hypothyroidism [7]. If laboratory evaluation of thyroid function is consistent with hypothyroidism, treatment of this underlying condition with thyroid hormone supplementation may be sufficient to treat the depression. If she does not have evidence of thyroid disease, her depression screen is positive, and her subsequent diagnostic evaluation for depression is positive, then primary treatment of depression is merited.

There are numerous medical conditions including malignancies, diabetes mellitus, autoimmune disorders, coronary heart disease, and disorders of the central nervous system (e.g., stroke) that are associated with an increased prevalence of depression. Diagnostic testing for these conditions should be dictated by the presence of clinical symptoms, and treatment should be directed at both the medical condition and depression when co-occurring. Of note, some medications including steroids and those used to treat hypertension, heart attacks, stroke, hip fractures, or macular degeneration, for example, are associated with depression.

Screen now? Yes

Next screening: At follow-up evaluation

Guidelines

a. Screening for depression in adults: US Preventive Services Task Force recommendation statement. US Preventive Services Task Force. *Ann Intern Med.* 2009, **151**:784–92.

b. Screening and treatment for major depressive disorder in children and adolescents: US Preventive Services Task Force recommendation statement US Preventive Services Task Force [published erratum appears in Pediatrics 2009;123:1611]. *Pediatrics.* 2009, **123**:1223–8.

c. American Medical Association. *Guidelines for Adolescent Preventive Services (GAPS): Recommendations Monograph.* Chicago, IL: American Medical Association, 1997.

d. American Academy of Pediatrics. *Recommendations for Preventive Pediatric Health Care.* Elk Grove Village, IL: American Academy of Pediatrics, 2014. Available at: www.aap.org/en-us/professionalresources/practice-support/Periodicity/Periodicity%20Schedule_FINAL.pdf. Retrieved January 22, 2016.

e. American Academy of Family Physicians. *Depression: Clinical Preventive Service Recommendation.* Leawood, KS: American Academy of Family Physicians, 2015. Available at: www.aafp.org/patient-care/clinical-recommendations/all/depression.html. Retrieved January 22, 2016.

f. Association of Women's Health, Obstetric and Neonatal Nurses. *The Role of the Nurse in Postpartum Mood and Anxiety Disorders.* Washington, DC: Association of Women's Health, Obstetric and Neonatal Nurses, 2008. Available at: www.awhonn.org/awhonn/binary.content.do?name=Resources/Documents/pdf/5_PMAD.pdf. Retrieved January 22, 2016.

g. American College of Obstetricians and Gynecologists. *Guidelines for Adolescent Health Care [CD-ROM],* 2nd edition. Washington, DC: American College of Obstetricians and Gynecologists, 2011.

h. American College of Obstetricians and Gynecologists. *Guidelines for Women's Health Care,* 4th edition. Washington, DC: American College of Obstetricians and Gynecologists, 2014.

i. American College of Nurse Midwives. *Depression in Women. Position Statement.* Silver Spring, MD: American College of Nurse Midwives, 2013. Available at: www.midwife.org/ACNM/files/ACNMLibraryData/UPLOADFILENAME/000000000061/Depression%20in%20Women%20May%202013.pdf. Retrieved January 22, 2016.

j. Jack, B.W., Atrash, H., Coonrod, D.V., et al. The clinical content of preconception care: An overview and preparation of this supplement. *Am J Obstet Gynecol.* 2008, **199**:S266–79.

k. Siu A.L. et al. Screening for depression in adults: US Preventive Services Task Force recommendation statement. *JAMA.* 2016, **315**(4)380–7.

References

1. Center for Behavioral Health Statistics and Quality, *Behavioral Health Trends in the United States: Results from the 2014 National Survey on Drug Use and Health (HHS Publication No. SMA 15–4927, NSDUH Series H-50).* Health and Human Services, Editor, 2015. Available at: www.samhsa.gov/data/. Retrieved January 7, 2016.

2. American College of Obstetricians and Gynecologists. Screening for perinatal depression. Committee Opinion #630. *Obstet Gynecol.* 2015, **125**(5): 1268–71.

3. Mitchell, A.J., Vaze, A., and Rao, S. Clinical diagnosis of depression in primary care: A meta-analysis. *Lancet.* 2009, **374**(9690):609–19.

4. Williams, J.W., Jr., Pignone, M., Ramirez, G., and Perez Stellato, C. Identifying depression in primary care: A literature synthesis of case-finding instruments. *Gen Hosp Psychiatry.* 2002, **24**(4):225–37.

5. American Psychiatric Association. *Diagnostic and Statistical Manual of Mental Disorders,* 5th edition. Arlington, VA: American Psychiatric Publishing, 2013.

6. Conry, J.A. and Brown, H. Well-Woman Task Force: Components of the well-woman visit. *Obstet Gynecol.* 2015, **126**(4):697–701.

7. Williams, J.W., Noel, P.H., Cordes, J.A., Ramirez, G., and Pignone, M. Chapter 19: Is this Patient Clinically Depressed? In: *The Rational Clinical Examination – Evidence-Based Clinical Diagnosis.* New York, NY: McGraw-Hill, 2009.

8. US Preventive Service Task Force (USPSTF). *Draft Recommendation Statement: Depression in Children and Adolescents: Screening.* 2015 [cited 2016 February 24, 2016]. Available at: www.uspreventiveservicestaskforce.org/Page/Document/draft-recommendation-statement116/depression-in-children-and-adolescents-screening1.

9. Myers, E.R., Aubuchon-Endsley, N., Bastian, L.A. et al. AHRQ Comparative Effectiveness Review 106. Efficacy and Safety of Screening for Postpartum Depression. Rockville, MD: Agency for Healthcare Research and Quality (US), 2013.

Chapter 41

Domestic and Intimate Partner Violence

Kavita Shah Arora

Why Screen?

More than one in three women in the United States have experienced intimate partner violence (IPV) at some point in their lifetime, accounting for almost 5 million incidents of physical or sexual assault annually [1]. The true prevalence is likely higher given the barriers to disclosure. While specific risk factors exist, it is important to note that IPV occurs in every race, religion, ethnicity, sexual orientation, socioeconomic status, and gender. IPV is associated with short-term emotional and physical consequences including reproductive coercion (partner behavior intended to maintain power and control related to reproductive health) and longer-term sequelae including depression, rape, transmission of sexually transmitted infections (STIs), lasting emotional and physical impairment, and death. The high prevalence and serious public health consequences of IPV justify screening as a core part of women's health care.

Rationale for Screening

Women facing IPV seldom disclose this to their physicians without being asked. Patients may report nonspecific symptoms or no symptoms at all during health care visits. Obstetrician-gynecologists are uniquely situated to screen for IPV in light of the trust developed during long-term relationships where many sensitive reproductive health issues are discussed. Key messages, resources, and referrals made after positive screening facilitate patient access to social and legal services and improve patient safety. Screening is crucial given that 76% of interventions result in at least one statistically significant benefit to the patient, whether reduction in violence, improvement in physical and emotional health, among others [2].

Factors That Affect Screening

Age: IPV during adolescence leads to a high rate of unintended pregnancy, STIs, tobacco use,

mental health problems including suicide attempts, and may produce lifelong physical and psychological ramifications. IPV and elder abuse exist along a continuum given the likelihood that the victim knows the perpetrator (often a partner or an adult child). While abuse can be physical, sexual, or emotional, it can also encompass financial exploitation, abandonment, and neglect.

Disability: Women with physical and developmental disabilities are at increased risk for IPV given the reliance on their caretakers. Financial control, medication sabotage, and withholding of support devices and services are distinct methods of abuse toward those with disabilities.

Pregnancy: Reproductive coercion can lead to unintended pregnancy through rape, sabotage of birth control methods, and other physical or emotional pressure tactics. IPV is associated with poor reproductive outcomes, including poor maternal weight gain, infection, stillbirth, preterm delivery, and low birth weight. Pregnancy and the postpartum period are often also associated with escalation of physical violence including homicide. Therefore, the American College of Obstetrics and Gynecology (ACOG) recommends IPV screening in each trimester of pregnancy and postpartum, before resuming annual screening.

Recommended Guidelines and How to Find Them

The Well-Woman Task Force (WWTF) encountered some inconsistency regarding the interpretation of the strength and quality of data available to generate evidence-based guidelines for IPV screening. For example, the Institute of Medicine recommends screening and counseling adolescents and women regarding past and current abuse but does not recommend a specific screening interval [a]. The US Preventive Services Task Force makes a Grade B recommendation to screen women of childbearing age and to refer screen-positive women to intervention services [b]. The American Academy of Pediatrics recommends at least annual screening but cautions that more frequent screening may be required if clinical circumstances suggest additional risk factors such as pregnancy and multiple visits for STI testing [c]. The American Academy of Family Physicians recommends screening women of childbearing age without a specified screening interval and also notes that there is insufficient evidence to assess screening of adults who are no longer of childbearing age [d]. ACOG recommends periodic screening in all women with increased frequency during obstetric care [e]. The final WWTF focused on the care of nonpregnant women and made a recommendation for annual screening as well as provision of or referral for intervention services [f].

How to Screen

Screening should always be done privately. Self-administered, computerized, and physician-led screening methods are equally effective. In order to properly frame the screening interview, it is recommended to state that screening is universally practiced by the clinician and review the confidential nature of the screening. IPV screening can be easily universalized, normalized, and destigmatized by making it part of a patient's standard medical history. The use of culturally sensitive, nonjudgmental, and nonstigmatizing terms is important. For women who do not communicate in English as their primary language, it is important to use a translator who is not a family member and to be sensitive to language barriers and cultural norms. Sample screening questions are available through ACOG [3], the Agency for Healthcare Research and Quality (AHRQ) [2], and the Family Violence Prevention Fund [1]. There are various validated screening tools available, many of which are well studied in asymptomatic women such as the four-question HITS (hurt, insult, threaten, scream) with a sensitivity >86 percent and specificity >91 percent [2]. Finally, access to information and support services can be improved if all staff receives IPV

training and hotline numbers are displayed privately in examination rooms and restrooms. Positive screening should be immediately followed by assessing safety, formulating a safety contract, and offering information and resources such as local domestic violence agencies, shelters, crisis hotlines, law enforcement, and legal aid, which are available through the National Domestic Violence hotline. It is also important that physicians are aware of the relevant state and federal laws and regulations surrounding IPV in order to remain in compliance [4].

New Developments Likely to Affect Future Guidelines

While the prevalence of IPV in the lesbian, gay, bisexual, and transgender (LGBT) population is estimated to be similar to that of the general population, the manifestations, ramifications, and screening strategy may differ [5]. New information to help optimize screening of LGBT patients could potentially lead to specific recommendations which are different from the current recommendations.

Billing

IPV screening is typically covered under the ICD-10 code Z01.419, encounter for gynecological examination (general) (routine) without abnormal findings. If a patient screens positive, counseling regarding abuse can be covered under Z65.8, other problems related to psychosocial circumstances. An examination following abuse is covered by T74.11XA, adult physical abuse, confirmed, initial encounter or T74.21XA, adult sexual abuse, confirmed, initial encounter. An examination following alleged rape should be coded Z04.41.

Illustrative Cases

A healthy 16-year-old woman presents for a well-adolescent visit. She has been sexually active since age 14. She is accompanied by her mother.

After initial discussion with the patient's mother present, it is important to ask the patient to discuss her medical history with her privately. Once the mother has left the room, the recommended annual IPV screening should be completed. IPV is common in this age group and it is also an excellent time to discuss safe sex practices.

Screen now? Yes

Next screening: Age 17 unless other clinical risk factors

A 35-year-old woman in a same-sex relationship presents to your office to establish care. She screens positive for IPV.

The WWTF recommends annual screening for this patient, although research is developing regarding the optimal screening strategy, manifestations, and consequences of IPV in the LGBT population. As this patient has screened positive, further discussion should identify the nature of the abuse, a safety contract should be made, and resources given for support. Close follow-up care is prudent.

Screen now? Yes

Next screening: N/A. Now that the patient has screened positive, follow-up visits will focus on her safety and access to resources.

A 65-year-old woman who is wheelchair bound due to a recent cerebrovascular event presents to your office for a routine annual examination. She is accompanied by her adult son.

This patient should be screened for IPV as well as elder abuse. It is important to include screening questions that address the patient's ability to access and control her finances, support services such as wheelchair or cane, and whether she is receiving adequate care and attention from her caregivers.

Screen now? Yes

Next screening: Age 66 unless other clinical risk factors

A healthy 28-year-old woman presents for a new obstetric patient visit at 28 weeks of pregnancy. She is accompanied by her partner who is translating for her.

This patient is at higher risk for IPV given both her pregnancy and the late presentation to care. It is important that the partner be asked to leave the room and a medical translator be used to screen for IPV in a culturally competent and sensitive manner. She should also receive standard pregnancy care, including STI screening and assessment of fetal gestation/growth. ACOG recommends heightened screening in pregnancy including at the new obstetric visit, once every trimester, and at the postpartum visit.

Screen now? Yes

Next screening: Late third-trimester as well as postpartum visits

Guidelines

a. Committee on Preventive Services for Women. *Clinical Preventive Services for Women: Closing the Gaps.* Washington, DC: Institute of Medicine, 2011. Available at: www.nap.edu/download.php?record_id=13181. Retrieved January 21, 2016.

b. Moyer, V.A. Screening for intimate partner violence and abuse of elderly and vulnerable adults: US Preventive Services Task Force recommendation statement. US Preventive Services Task Force. *Ann Intern Med.* 2013, **158**:478–86.

c. Tanski, S., Garfunkel, L.C., Duncan, P.M., Weitzman, M., editors. *Performing Preventive Services: A Bright Futures Handbook.* Elk Grove Village, IL: American Academy of Pediatrics, 2010. Available at: http://brightfutures.aap.org/continuing_education.html. Retrieved January 21, 2016.

d. American Academy of Family Physicians. *Intimate Partner Violence and Abuse of Elderly and Vulnerable Adults. Clinical Preventive Service Recommendation.* Leawood, KS: American Academy of Family Physicians, 2013. Available at: www.aafp.org/patient-care/clinical-recommendations/all/domestic-violence.html. Retrieved January 21, 2016.

e. American College of Obstetricians and Gynecologists. Intimate partner violence. Committee Opinion No. 518. *Obstet Gynecol.* 2012, **119**:412–7.

f. Conry, J.A. and Brown, H. Well-Woman Task Force: Components of the Well-Woman Visit. *Obstet Gynecol.* 2015, **125**(4):697–701.

References

1. Black, M.C., Basile, K.C., Breiding, M.J. et al. *The National Intimate Partner and Sexual Violence Survey (NISVS): 2010 Summary Report.* Atlanta, GA: National Center for Injury Prevention and Control, Centers for Disease Control and Prevention, 2011. Available at: www.cdc.gov/ViolencePrevention/pdf/NISVS_Report2010-a.pdf. Retrieved January 21, 2016.

2. Intimate Partner Violence Screening. Agency for Healthcare Research and Quality. 2015 Available at: www.ahrq.gov/professionals/prevention-chronic-care/healthier-pregnancy/preventive/partnerviolence.html#practices. Retrieved January 21, 2016.

3. American College of Obstetricians and Gynecologists. Intimate partner violence. Committee Opinion No. 518. *Obstet Gynecol.* 2012, **119**:412–7.

4. Chamberlain, L. and Levenson, R. *Family Violence Prevention Fund. Reproductive Health and Partner Violence Guidelines: An Integrated Response to Intimate Partner Violence and Reproductive Coercion.* San Francisco, CA: Family Violence Prevention Fund, 2010. Available at: www.futureswithoutviolence.org/userfiles/ file/HealthCare/Repro_Guide.pdf. Retrieved January 21, 2016.

5. Ard, K.L. and Makadon, H.J. Addressing intimate partner violence in lesbian, gay, bisexual, and transgender patients. *J Gen Intern Med.* 2011, **26**(8):930–3.

Chapter

42

Alcohol Misuse

Monica Mendiola

Why Screen?

Alcohol misuse is a risk factor for a wide range of medical issues, psychosocial problems, and accident-related deaths. Short-term health risks include motor vehicle accidents, intimate partner violence, and unintended pregnancy; long-term risks include liver disease, cancer, and depression [1]. An estimated $250 billion per year is spent on the consequences of excess drinking [2]. Risks are compounded for reproductive-aged women who may face adverse effects on fertility and fetal development. The National Institute of Alcohol Abuse and Alcoholism (NIAAA) defines at-risk drinking for women as more than three drinks per occasion (binge drinking) and more than one drink per day (moderate drinking). The Centers for Disease Control and Prevention (CDC) estimates that in 2009, 25 percent of all individuals aged 18–24 engaged in binge drinking [3]. Among youth aged 12–20, 14 percent reported binge drinking [4]. Between 2011 and 2013, the prevalence of alcohol use among pregnant women was 10.2 percent and the prevalence of binge drinking was 3.1 percent [5]. An estimated 2–5 percent of first-grade students in the United States have fetal alcohol syndrome or disorder, which includes physical, behavioral, or learning impairments [6].

Rationale for Screening

Several studies have shown that brief interventions in at-risk patients produce a long-lasting overall reduction in alcohol consumption. Screening is important as it can be difficult for patients to differentiate normal from excessive alcohol consumption, and patients seldom bring concerns about personal alcohol use to the attention of their physicians. Screening patients at the well-woman exam provides an opportunity to encourage healthy behaviors, identify those at risk, and provide early intervention to mitigate poor outcomes.

Factors That Affect Screening

Age: Alcohol misuse may occur during all phases of life; however, there are vulnerable periods where the lifelong risk may be increased. Youth who start drinking before age 15 years are six times more likely to develop alcohol dependence than those who begin drinking after age 21 years [4].

Care-seeking behavior: Women suffering from alcohol misuse are less likely to attend well-woman visits [a]. Therefore, screening should be performed at any visit if it has not been done in the past 12 months.

Pregnancy: Since alcohol is a known teratogen, women who are pregnant or considering becoming pregnant should have additional screening in their first trimester, even if they have attended a well-woman visit within the past year.

Recommended Guidelines and How to Find Them

All major medical societies, including the American College of Obstetrics and Gynecology (ACOG) and the US Preventive Services Task Force (USPSTF), agree that annual evaluation and counseling is indicated for all adult patients [a, b]. The Well-Woman Task Force (WWTF) recommends annual screening for all patients by using a validated questionnaire and/or taking a history, but not laboratory data. In addition, the WWTF and the American Academy of Pediatrics (AAP) favor screening adolescents annually, although acknowledge that counseling has not been proven to be effective in this population.

How to Screen

The most readily available tools to identify alcohol misuse are screening questionnaires and not laboratory data. The mnemonic CAGE (Cut down, Annoyed,

Guilt, Eye-opener) is widely known; however, it lacks sensitivity and specificity and does not work well for women and minorities [7]. The screening tool T-ACE (Tolerance, Annoyed, Cut down, Eye-opener) has less gender bias, and a sensitivity of 69–88 percent, and specificity of 71–89 percent in the prenatal population [8]. T-ACE is recommended because it is widely known, highly reliable among several populations, and relatively short, which makes for ease of use in an ambulatory setting [a].

T-ACE: A total score of 2 or more indicates a positive screen for at-risk drinking.

- T – Tolerance: How many drinks does it take to make you feel high? (More than 2 drinks = 2 points)
- A – Annoyed: Have people annoyed you by criticizing your drinking? (Yes = 1 point)
- C – Cut down: Have you ever felt you ought to cut down on your drinking? (Yes = 1 point)
- E – Eye-opener: Have you ever had a drink first thing in the morning to steady your nerves or get rid of a hangover? (Yes = 1 point)

When a positive screen is encountered, a brief risk-reducing intervention should follow. There are many interventional strategies using the basic framework outlined below. Listed below are guidelines for motivational interviewing [c].

- Ask about alcohol use: Does the patient identify her at-risk drinking?
- Express concern by personalizing her alcohol consumption to her health and outcomes.
- Help her identify potential behavior changes. Allow her to set her own goals and then provide resources.
- Arrange a follow-up visit within a short timeframe to assess progress.

ACOG has a list of resources including various questionnaires, pocket guides for physicians, and intervention options at www.acog.org/About-ACOG/ACOG-Departments/Tobacco–Alcohol–and–Substance-Abuse/Alcohol. Additional counseling recommendations can be found in the chapter on *Promoting lifestyle modification and behavior change*.

New Developments Likely to Affect Future Guidelines

The WWTF recommendation to screen adolescents currently has mixed support due to inconclusive evidence that counseling is effective in this age group. Additional studies clarifying this issue may create more alignment between the various guidelines for adolescents. Studies are also underway to determine which screening tools perform the best in women and minorities.

Billing

Many health plans will pay for alcohol and substance use screening with a brief intervention when the visit includes a validated instrument such as T-ACE and documented counseling by a physician or mid-level health care professional lasting at least 15 minutes.

CPT codes are as follows:

- 99408: Alcohol and/or substance (other than tobacco) abuse structured screening and brief intervention services; 15–30 minutes
- 99409: Alcohol and/or substance (other than tobacco) abuse structured screening and brief intervention services; greater than 30 minutes

Medicare G codes are as follows:

- G0396: Alcohol and/or substance (other than tobacco) abuse structured assessment and brief intervention; 15–30 minutes
- G0397: Alcohol and/or substance (other than tobacco) abuse structured assessment and intervention; greater than 30 minutes

Medicaid H codes are as follows:

- H0049: Alcohol and/or drug screening
- H0050: Alcohol and/or drug services, brief intervention; per 15 minutes

Illustrative Cases

A healthy 20-year-old G0 presents for a well-woman visit. She is a freshman in college who is sexually active in a monogamous relationship and uses condoms for contraception.

All women should be screened even if they are younger than the legal drinking age. A study by the CDC noted that among nonpregnant women who reported binge drinking, those aged 18–20 reported the highest frequency (3.9 episodes) and intensity (7.1 drinks) [5]. As binge drinking in college is normalized, she may not be aware of her at-risk behavior. If she screens positive, motivational interviewing may help this patient set a goal to decrease her total alcohol intake and potentially avoid adverse outcomes.

Screen now? Yes

Laboratory testing now? No

Next screening: Annually

A healthy 40-year-old G3P3 presents for her well-woman visit. She has been seeing her health care provider for over 5 years and has a trusting relationship.

The recommendation is to screen all women annually, even patients who are well known to their physicians. Candid response to screening questions may become easier for patients over time as they establish more trust with their physicians.

Screen now? Yes

Laboratory testing now? No

Next screen: Annually

A 37-year-old G3P2A1 presents to reestablish care and reports symptoms of acute vaginitis. She does not have a primary care physician and has not been seen for a well-woman visit in over 3 years.

Women who drink at moderate levels are less likely to seek preventive care or attend annual visits. Consequently, women presenting for a problem-focused visit who have not attended annual well-woman visits should be screened for alcohol misuse. It takes less than 5 minutes to complete a screening questionnaire and provide a brief intervention to jumpstart a reduction in drinking.

Screen now? Yes

Laboratory testing now? No

Next screen: Annually

A 35-year-old G1 who is 8 weeks pregnant reports for her first prenatal care visit. Screening at her well-woman visit 6 months ago was negative.

Alcohol is a known teratogen and its use in pregnancy should be discouraged. Pregnancy provides a strong incentive for change, and in conjunction with motivational interviewing, it has been shown to modify behavior even in heavy drinkers. Of note, a recent study showed that the highest prevalence of late pregnancy alcohol use was in women who were least likely to be screened, specifically white college graduates aged 35 or older [9].

Screen now? Yes

Laboratory testing now? No

Next screen: Annually

Guidelines

a. American College of Obstetricians and Gynecologists. At-risk drinking and alcohol dependence: Obstetric and gynecologic implications. Committee Opinion No. 496. *Obstet Gynecol.* 2011, **118**:383–8.

b. US Preventive Services Task Force. *Final Recommendation Statement: Alcohol Misuse: Screening and Behavioral Counseling Interventions in Primary Care.* May 2013. Available at: www.uspreventiveservicestaskforce.org/Page/Document/RecommendationStatementFinal/alcohol-misuse-screening-and-behavioral-counseling-interventions-in-primary-care.

c. American College of Obstetricians and Gynecologists. Motivational interviewing: A tool for behavior change. ACOG Committee Opinion No. 423. *Obstet Gynecol.* 2009, **113**:243–6.

References

1. Available at: www.cdc.gov/alcohol/fact-sheets/alcohol-use.htm.

2. Sacks, J.J., Gonzales, K.R., Bouchery, E.E., Tomedi, L.E., and Brewer, R.D. 2010 National and state costs of excessive alcohol consumption. *Am J Prev Med.* 2015, **49**(5):e73–9.

3. Kanny, D., Liu, Y., and Brewer, R.D. Binge drinking – United States, 2009. Centers for Disease Control and Prevention (CDC). *MMWR Surveill Summ.* 2011, **60**(Suppl):101–4.

4. Substance Abuse and Mental Health Services Administration. *Results from the 2013 National Survey on Drug Use and Health: Summary of National Findings.* NSDUH Series H-48, HHS Publication No. (SMA) 14-4863. Rockville, MD: Substance Abuse and Mental Health Services Administration, 2014.

5. Tan, C., Denny, C., and Cheal, N., Alcohol use and binge drinking among women of childbearing age – United States, 2011–2013. Centers for Disease Control and Prevention (CDC). *MMWR Wkly.*

6. May, P.A., Baete, A., Russo, J. et al. Prevalence and characteristics of fetal alcohol spectrum disorders. *Pediatrics.* 2014, **134**:855–66.

7. Volk, R.J., Cantor, S.B., Steinbauer, J.R., and Cass, A.R. Item bias in the CAGE screening test for alcohol use disorders. *J Gen Intern Med.* 1997, **12**:763–9.

8. Burns, E., Gray, R., and Smith, L.A. Brief screening questionnaires to identify problem drinking during pregnancy: A systematic review. *Addiction.* 2010, **105**:601–14.

9. Cheng, D., Kettinger, L., Uduhiri, K., and Hurt, L. Alcohol consumption during pregnancy: Prevalence and provider assessment. *Obstet Gynecol.* 2011, **117**:212–7.

Screening for Tobacco or Nicotine Use

Sharon T. Phelan

Why Screen?

Despite public awareness that smoking is dangerous, the rates of tobacco or nicotine use are unacceptably high. Approximately 17 percent of reproductive-aged women smoke or vape with half continuing these habits into pregnancy [a]. Although this represents a decrease from over 43 percent in 1965, the rates among teens under 18 have not kept pace with this declining trend. In 2012, it was estimated that each day almost 4,000 children under the age of 18 in the United States try their first cigarette with over 2,000 per day quickly becoming addicted [1]. With the emergence of flavored E-cigarettes as an alternative source of nicotine for teens, there has been a ten-fold increase in their use among high school students who see them as a "safer" option [2].

Smoking contributes to the development of lung and cervical cancers, chronic pulmonary disease, heart disease, and pregnancy complications [3]. In the United States, over 1,000 individuals die each day due to smoking-related illness. Electronic cigarettes and similar devices allow users to decrease smoke-related risks but do not reduce nicotine-related risks. Vaporized nicotine causes cardiovascular disease, pregnancy complications, addiction, and nicotine poisoning [4]. Hence, although novel nicotine delivery systems may be less harmful in certain ways, they are not safe and should be included in tobacco screening and prevention efforts for women and their family members, regardless of age. Second-hand smoke, although not as dangerous as smoking, is associated with the same list of health consequences and exposes individuals who may not be in a position to consent, such as children.

Rationale for Screening

Combustible tobacco exposure (smoking) or nicotine exposure (vaping or using Electronic Nicotine Delivery Systems [ENDS]) are among the most

modifiable risks for women. Effective interventions are available for individuals who want to quit smoking. Due to the highly addictive nature of nicotine, multiple quit attempts are common before a person is truly smoke/nicotine free. Success rates for a single quit attempt range from 4 to 7 percent *without* the use of medication or other assistance. However, *with* medication about 25 percent who quit are smoke free at 6 months. There are medications that work on the central nervous system, decreasing the urge to smoke. Numerous studies indicate that these are effective in helping individuals quit. Most heavy and/or long-term smokers will typically require combinations of such aids to be successful. Since the damage done is reversible to some degree, cessation of tobacco/nicotine use at any age can provide benefits.

Recommended Guidelines and How to Find Them

The American College of Obstetricians and Gynecologists (ACOG) [a, b] US Preventive Services Task Force (USPSTF) [c, d], US Department of Health and Human Services [e], Center for Disease Control and Prevention (CDC) [f], and National Cancer Institute (NCI) [g] have all published guidelines for smoking screening and treatment. In forming its recommendations, the Well-Woman Task Force (WWTF) reviewed guidelines from the USPSTF, ACOG, American Academy of Family Physicians (AAFP), and American Academy of Pediatrics (AAP). Screening recommendations for all ages include the use of systematic and consistent inquiries to identify users followed by counseling interventions and assistance/referral to facilitate successful cessation. For adolescents and young adults who are non-smokers, the WWTF also encourages counseling to prevent initiation of tobacco use. In mature women

[h], there is an additional recommendation to NOT screen for lung cancer in smokers.

The established guidelines focus on traditional use of tobacco by smoking. Studies involving snuff or chew are limited but seem to show very similar consequences when used, so that current guidelines are relevant to the use of any tobacco product. The use of nicotine in ENDS is not as well studied. For this reason, it is assumed, but not proven that the screening and initial interventions for patients vaping/using ENDS should be similar.

Factors That Affect Screening

Age: In the past, if individuals made it to the age of 18 without taking up the habit of smoking, it was very rare that they would ever smoke. Today, successful marketing of new delivery systems has attracted initiation of tobacco/nicotine use well into the 20s and 30s [5]. This provides a sound rationale to extend anti-initiation counseling from adolescence into early adulthood. Women who use combined oral contraception (OCPs) must either discontinue tobacco products or OCPs after age 35 due to the increased risk of severe cardiovascular and thromboembolic complications.

Preconception: Given the complications of tobacco/nicotine use in pregnancy, it is important to identify women who are nicotine dependent prior to pregnancy and help them become smoke free before conception [4]. Nicotine replacement aids can be used in pregnancy or by women who may become pregnant. However, due to fetal concerns, they tend to be used in a more limited fashion [a].

Surgical planning: A Cochrane review of interventions for preoperative smoking cessation found a decrease in all postoperative complications, and in particular wound complications, if a comprehensive approach of counseling and medications was initiated at least 4 weeks prior to the surgery and continued through the postoperative care [6].

How to Screen, Counsel, and Intervene

Simply asking a patient if she smokes is an easy question. Unfortunately, it allows many patients to misrepresent their smoking status with a simple answer of NO. Given the societal pressures against tobacco use when pregnant or around children, many women want to depict themselves as nonsmokers even if they only "quit" that morning. More accurate screening results are achievable through a survey using standardized questions such as those in Box 43.1 [7]. The phrases added to include vaping make the questions more inclusive but have not been studied for their impact on the performance of this screening tool.

If a patient identifies with statements 1 or 2, the provider should offer praise and continue to screen at least yearly. Patients selecting statements 3 or 4 should receive praise and be informed that the provider is available to help with a relapse during the ongoing

---

BOX 43.1 Common Screening Questions for Tobacco or Nicotine Use*

1. I have never smoked or vaped
2. I currently do not smoke or vape but have used <100 cigarettes in my lifetime
3. I currently do not smoke or vape but have over a year ago
4. I currently do not smoke or vape but have in the past year
5. I currently smoke or vape but have recently cut down on the amount
6. I currently smoke or vape and have not changed the amount

*Screening questions are modified from the original wording; they include vaping so they are applicable to patients who use electronic nicotine delivery systems
Source: American College of Obstetricians and Gynecologists. *Smoking Cessation during Pregnancy: A Clinician's Guide to Helping Pregnant Women Quit Smoking*. Washington, DC: American College of Obstetricians and Gynecologists, 2011. Available at: www.acog.org/-/media/Departments/Tobacco-Alcohol-and-Substance-Abuse/SCDP.pdf?dmc=1&ts=20160927T0816274891. Retrieved September 27, 2016.

BOX 43.2 Counseling Steps for Tobacco/Nicotine Cessation

5 A's*: for all patients
1. Ask – whether the patient smokes. This is a key component of screening.
2. Advise – to quit. "Quitting is the most important thing you can do for your health."
3. Assess – willingness to quit. "Are you willing to quit within the next 30 days?"
4. Assist – in developing a quit strategy including counseling and medication as needed.
5. Arrange – follow-up in 30 days to see how the patient is doing.
   5 R's: for patients who are not ready to modify their smoking
1. Relevance – why personally relevant.
2. Risks – list the negative consequences.
3. Rewards – list the benefits of cessation.
4. Roadblocks – identify barriers to quitting.
5. Repetition – review these every visit.

*After the first three A's, the patient may be referred to a local smoking cessation resource or the national 1–800-QUITNOW line
Source: American College of Obstetricians and Gynecologists. *Smoking Cessation during Pregnancy: A Clinician's Guide to Helping Pregnant Women Quit Smoking.* Washington, DC: American College of Obstetricians and Gynecologists, 2011. Available at: www.acog.org/-/media/Departments/Tobacco-Alcohol-and-Substance-Abuse/SCDP.pdf?dmc=1&ts=20160927T0816274891. Retrieved September 27, 2016.

---

quit effort. Patients selecting statements 5 or 6 should be provided education and assessment using the steps listed in Box 43.2 [8]. This process is commonly called the 5 A's. Patients who are willing to quit in the next 30 days can be referred to local resources or the national quit line. A CDC-supported virtual clinic program can provide an interactive method for practicing the 5 A's [9]. Smokers not interesting in changing are counseled using the 5 R's, a brief intervention designed to increase motivation to quit [10]. Additional counseling recommendations can be found in the chapters on *Promoting Lifestyle Modification and Behavior Change* [11].

New Developments Likely to Affect Future Guidelines

Clarifying the harms associated with the new ENDS will provide clearer guidelines for patient education and counseling. Since the ENDS products do not create smoke, they do minimize smoke-related risks. ENDS vaporize "juice" which includes nicotine, flavorings, and propellant. The risks of these vaporized chemicals are not known. Nicotine by itself has a lengthy list of health concerns and risks. ENDS are not necessarily safer for the children, since the nicotine in the juice can be either ingested (it often smells like candy) or absorbed transdermally if spilled, resulting in nicotine poisonings. Studies are

underway to determine if ENDS can be a successful cessation tool. Early studies do not support this approach [12].

Billing

Coding is divided into tobacco use screening (Z13.89), tobacco use without nicotine dependence (Z72.0), or tobacco use with nicotine dependence (F17.2- -). The first spacer is used for the type of product used (0 – unspecified, 1 – cigarettes, 2 – chewing tobacco, and 9 – other products). The second spacer is used for the complexity of the dependence (0 – uncomplicated, 1 – in remission, 3 – in withdrawal, 8 – with other nicotine-induced disorders, and 9 – unspecified nicotine disorders). When screening in the context of an annual well-woman visit, the procedural code should be an evaluation and management (E/M) Preventive Medicine code stratified by age group and new or established patient.

Under the Affordable Care Act (ACA), all state Medicaid programs are required to provide benefits as defined by the USPHS to enrolled pregnant women. For nonpregnant individuals, coverage for cessation services are encouraged but not required resulting in coverage variation from state to state. Medicare and Federal Employee insurance covers individual cessation counseling and prescriptions for a maximum of two quit attempts per year. Reimbursement is based on the time spent on the patient counseling.

Illustrative Cases

A 33-year-old G3P3 currently using oral contraceptive pills (OCPs) presents for an annual well-woman visit. She has three children between 1 and 5 years old. During her last pregnancy, she became smoke-free. Her 5-year-old son has asthma. Upon screening, she admits to having resumed smoking partially due to depression and to help lose pregnancy weight. She is currently smoking ½ pack per day. She reports that she only smokes outside and never in the car.

It is important to screen everyone, since she may not have volunteered her relapse. It is now important to address her concerns and advise her to become smoke free again. Points to make might include the following:

- Smoking cessation will improve her son's asthma symptoms.
- Although she smokes outside, she still has third-hand smoke on her clothes and skin.
- There are medications that are less expensive, less dangerous, and more effective for her depression.
- The harms from smoking exceed the help with weight loss she is expecting.
- In 2 years, the OCPs she is happy using for contraception will not be an option.

Screen, counsel, and intervene now? Yes

Next screening: N/A – Because she is currently smoking, follow-up visits will be arranged to track her progress, reinforce education and counseling points, and adjust interventions/treatment.

A 44-year-old G2P2 patient presents for her annual examination. She recently moved to town and is seeking an Obstetrician-Gynecologist (Ob–Gyn) for well-woman care but also for potential hysterectomy for leiomyomas. Routine screening discovers that she smokes 1 pack per day for 28 years. On examination, her uterus is 22-week size and is creating increasing pain and discomfort.

Smoking is a significant risk factor for perioperative complications. Screening allows the provider to know that this patient should stop smoking at least 4 weeks prior to a major abdominal surgery. The patient should be advised about the need to quit to minimize operative complications and optimize postoperative recovery [5]. This patient might be referred to a hospital-based smoking cessation program for individuals being scheduled for surgery.

She then asks if it would be as important for her to quit if she was not to get surgery. Can't you just screen for lung cancer?

The patient needs to be told it is never too late to quit. Quitting now will benefit her health and may reduce the risks of developing cancer and COPD. She should be informed that screening asymptomatic patients for lung cancer is not effective. Chest x-rays do not detect cancer at an early enough stage to be useful so they are not recommended as screening.

Screen, counsel, and intervene now? Yes

Next screening: N/A – Because she is currently smoking, follow-up visits will be arranged to track her progress, reinforce education and counseling points, and adjust interventions/treatment.

A 27-year-old G0 presents for her annual examination. She asks when she should have her intrauterine device (IUD) removed since she plans to get pregnant in 6 months. Her screening reveals she smokes 2 packs per day for the past 6 years.

At 2 packs per day, this patient is nicotine dependent. She will have a difficult if not unsuccessful quit attempt without medications. Since the effectiveness and safety of some of these medications during pregnancy are unclear, it would be best to quit prior to conception. She should be advised of the risks of smoking in pregnancy. Then, she should be either offered treatment or referred for therapy.

Screen, counsel, and intervene now? Yes

Next screening: N/A – Because she is currently smoking, follow-up visits will be arranged to track her progress, reinforce education and counseling points, and adjust interventions/treatment.

A 16-year-old G0 presents for her human papillomavirus (HPV) vaccination. During her health screen, she reports that although she has not tried smoking or vaping, many of her friends are encouraging her. She is feeling pressure that to be cool she needs to at least try cigarettes.

The patient should be provided with information about the risks of smoking and the marketing strategies being used to get teens to try cigarettes. As the number of adults who smoke decrease through death or smoking cessation, companies need to recruit new users. Teens are targeted because they are more vulnerable to peer and media influences, and their brains are more susceptible to nicotine addiction. The patient can improve her chances of remaining nicotine free by participating in activities where smoking is rare and not seen as cool. The provider should help her identify role models (parents, coaches, teachers, celebrities, etc.) who do not smoke cigarettes and who have made healthy life choices.

Screen, counsel, and intervene now? Yes

Next screening: At least annually. In addition, follow-up visits will be arranged to track her status and reinforce counseling points, to prevent initiation of smoking.

Guidelines

a. American College of Obstetricians and Gynecologist. Smoking cessation during pregnancy. Committee Opinion No. 417. *Obstet Gynecol.* 2010, 116:1241–44.

b. American College of Obstetricians and Gynecologist. Tobacco use and women's health. Committee Opinion No. 503. *Obstet Gynecol.* 2011, 118:746–50.

c. Moyer, V.A. Primary care interventions to prevent tobacco use in children and adolescents: USPSTF recommendation statement. *Ann Intern Med.* 2013, 159:552–7.

d. US Preventive Services Task Force. Tobacco Smoking Cessation in Adults, Including Pregnant Women: Behavioral and Pharmacotherapy Interventions. September 2015. Available at: www .uspreventiveservicestaskforce.org/Page/Document/Up dateSummaryFinal/tobacco-use-in-adults-and-preg nant-women-counseling-and-interventions1. Retrieved December 26, 2016.

e. Fiore, M.C., Jaen, C.R., Baker, T.B. et al. *Treating Tobacco Use and Dependence: 2008 Update: Clinical Practice Guidelines.* Rockville, MD: US Department of Health and Human Services. Public Health Service, 2008.

f. Center for Disease Control and Prevention. Smoking and Tobacco Use. December 8, 2016. Available at: www .cdc.gov/tobacco/index.htm. Retrieved December 26, 2016.

g. National Cancer Institute (NIH). Cigarette Smoking: Health Risks and How to Quit: Health Professional Version. November 2016. Available at: www.cancer.gov/about-cancer/causes-prevention/ris k/tobacco/quit-smoking-hp-pdq. Retrieved December 26, 2016.

h. Conry, J.A. and Brown, H. Well-woman task force: Components of the well-woman visit. *Obstet Gynecol.* 2015, 126:697–701.

References

1. US Department of Health and Human Services. *Preventing Tobacco Use Among Youth and Young Adults: A Report of the Surgeon General.* Atlanta, GA: US Department of Health and Human Services, Centers for Disease Control and Prevention, National Center for Chronic Disease Prevention and Health Promotion, Office on Smoking and Health, 2012. Retrieved March 21, 2016.

2. Ambrose, B.B.K., Day, H.R., Rostron, B. et al. Flavored tobacco product use among US youth aged 12–17 years, 2013–2014. *JAMA.* 2015, **314**:1871–3.

3. Carte, B.D., Abnet, C.C., Feskanich, D. et al. Smoking and mortality – Beyond established causes. *N Engl J Med.* 2015, 371:631–40.

4. England, L.J., Bunnell, R.E., Pechacek, T.F. et al. Nicotine and the developing human: a neglected element in the electronic cigarette debate. *Am J Prev Med.* 2015, **49**:286–93.

5. Leventhal, A.M., Strong, D.R., Kirkpatrick, M.G. et al. Association of electronic cigarette use with initiation of combustible tobacco product smoking in early adolescence. *JAMA.* 2015, **314**:700–7.

6. Thomsen, T. Villebro, N., and Moller, A.M. Interventions for preoperative smoking cessation. *Cochrane Database Syst Rev.* 2014:CD00294. DOI:10.1002/14651858.CD00294.pub4. Available at: http://onlinelibrary.wiley.com/doi/10.1002/14651858 .CD002294.pub4/full. Retrieved December 17, 2016.

7. Jamal, A., Dube, S.R., Malarcher, A.M. et al. Tobacco use screening and counseling during physician office visits among adults – National Ambulatory Medical Care Survey and National Health Interview Survey, United States, 2005–2009. *MMWR.* 2012, 61(2):38–45.

8. Center for Disease Control and Prevention. *Protocol for Identifying and Treating Patients Who Use Tobacco: Action Steps for Clinicians.* Atlanta, GA: Centers for Disease Control and Prevention, US Dept of Health and Human Services, 2016. Available at: https://million hearts.hhs.gov/files/Tobacco-Cessation-Action-Guide .pdf. Retrieved December 27, 2016.

9. Smoking Cessation for Pregnancy and Beyond: A Virtual Clinic. Joint Project of CDC, ACOG and Dartmouth Interactive Media Laboratory. World Two Systems, LLC, Grantham NH, 2016. Available at: www .smokingcessationandpregnancy.org.

10. The 5 R's for Those Not Ready to Quit. Part of the ACOG Tobacco and Nicotine Cessation Toolkit. 2016. Available at: www.acog.org/About-ACOG/ACOG-Dep artments/Toolkits-for-Health-Care-Providers/Tobacco- and-Nicotine-Cessation-Toolkit/Treatment-and-Cessat ion/Pocket-Card-Counseling-Steps-for-Tobacco-and- Nicotine-Cessation. Retrieved December 27, 2016.

11. Zimmerman, G.L., Olsen, C.G., and Bosworth, M.F. A "Stages of Charge" approach to helping patients change behavior. *Am Fam Physician.* 2000, March 1, **61**(5):1409–16.

12. Joint statement from AAP, ACOG, AACP, AMA. Electronic Nicotine Delivery Systems. American College Ob-Gyn, 2016. Available at: www.acog.org/-/media/Departments/Toolkits-for-Health-Care-Providers/Smoking-Cessation-Toolkit/Smoking-Cessation-Toolkit-Electronic-Nicotine-Delivery-Systems.pdf?dmc=1&ts=20161226T1744112105 Retrieved December 27, 2016.

13. Lavinghouze, S.R., Malarcher, A., Jama, A. et al. Trends in quit attempts among adult cigarette smokers – United States, 2001–2013. *MMWR.* Morb Mortal Wkly Rep. 2015, **64**(40):1129–35. Available at: www.cdc.gov/mmwr/preview/mmwrhtml/mm6440a1.htm. Retrieved December 27, 2016.

Chapter

44

Drug Use

Michelle M. Isley

Why Screen?

Addiction to both prescription and nonprescription drugs is a major public health problem in the United States. Substance abuse leads to $193 billion annual costs related to crime, lost work productivity, and health care [1]. Drug abuse crosses all age, socioeconomic, cultural, and ethnic lines. The percentage of individuals aged 12 or older reporting illicit drug use has increased from 8.3 percent in 2002 to 10.2 percent in 2014 [1]. In 2013, 8.0 percent of females aged 12 and older reported current illicit drug use, a decrease from 9.5 percent in 2012 [2]. One in five individuals aged 18–25 reports using illicit drugs in the past month [1]. Excluding tobacco and alcohol use, misuse of prescription drugs now falls just after illicit use of marijuana as the nation's most common drug problem. Addiction leads to impaired health and harmful behaviors. Accidental deaths from narcotic overdose outnumber deaths caused by motor vehicle accidents or suicide. Drug use at the onset and throughout pregnancy can cause fetal harm [3]. Drug use screening and intervention is a key component of well-woman care.

Rationale for Screening

Screening is important, since despite the prevalence and scope of the problem, only a fraction of people who need treatment for drug abuse actually receive it. Routine screening can identify affected individuals and intervention can impact their usage of drugs.

Screening and intervention in general medical settings have been shown to make a difference in drug use behaviors [4]. This difference has been well established in the reduction of alcohol and tobacco use. Evidence also supports the same benefits for illicit or nonmedical prescription drug use [5].

While screening and intervention for drug abuse may be effective, few primary care physicians report that they screen patients. Physician reluctance to

screen and counsel may reflect inadequate formal education and training of health care providers [6]. Even if screening is performed, the physician may not be aware of appropriate treatment options or available community resources.

Patients may also be reluctant to discuss substance abuse issues with their health care provider. Fear of consequences including possible criminal punishment, rejection from partners, jeopardized child custody, and care of family may prohibit patients from seeking treatment. Pregnant women may be even more reluctant due to fear of repercussions, including prosecution, loss of custody, or termination of parental rights in the event of fetal harm [7].

The well-woman visit provides a unique opportunity for screening in a nonthreatening atmosphere in which women already share private and sensitive information with their health care provider. Through routine screening and identification, important intervention and referral can be accomplished.

Factors That Affect Screening

Age: Teens are an especially vulnerable population. Drug abuse often begins during adolescence and young adulthood. Developmentally, adolescents are programmed to be impulsive, seek new experiences, and be easily swayed by peers, making risk-taking behavior appealing. By their senior year, 64 percent of high school students have tried alcohol, 49 percent have taken an illegal drug, 31.1 percent have smoked cigarettes, and 18.3 percent have used a prescription drug for nonmedical reasons [8]. There is an urgency to identify and intervene early in the adolescent population because drug use at an early age is an important predictor of a substance abuse disorder later on, with the likelihood of developing a substance disorder greatest for those who begin use in their early teens. Adolescent substance abuse can affect key developmental and social milestones and can affect normal brain maturation, underscoring the importance of identifying and addressing adolescent drug use.

Sexual activity: Sexually active women of reproductive age are another group of women in which drug abuse screening is especially important. Drug abuse can result in higher-risk sexual behaviors, exposing women to infectious diseases and sexually transmitted infections (STIs), and pregnancy risk. If women are identified as at risk, screening should also be provided for hepatitis B, hepatitis C, HIV, and other sexually transmitted diseases (STDs). Pregnancy testing should also be provided. Effective contraception should be recommended, if not drug free.

Pregnancy: In the United States, despite well-known risks, it is estimated that between 2.8 and 7 percent of pregnant women will continue to use illicit drugs during pregnancy [9]. If an obstetric patient is identified as using drugs, special care will need to be taken. If available, the patient may need to be referred or comanaged with a specialist, and due to the higher fetal risks, additional antepartum surveillance may be indicated. Communication with the pediatrician will also be important to ensure that all infant issues are addressed. Neonatal abstinence syndrome occurs in 50–95 percent of infants who have been prenatally exposed to illicit substances [10].

Recommended Guidelines and How to Find Them

The Well-Woman Task Force recommends at least annual screening for substance abuse by history (not lab testing) in women of all ages. Counseling or referral of patients is also strongly recommended. This recommendation is informed by guidelines from several organizations, including the American College of Obstetrics and Gynecology (ACOG) [a, b, c] and the American Academy of Pediatrics (AAP) [d]. The National Adolescent and Young Adult Health Information Center [e] as well as the AAP Bright Futures [d] have guidelines

specific for adolescent women available on their websites. The Centers of Disease Control and Prevention (CDC) action plan for preconception health and health care recommends that all health care providers taking care of reproductive-aged women take a careful history to identify the use of illegal substances as a part of preconception risk assessment [f]. Resources for health care providers are available on the Preconception Health and Health Care Resource Center website (www.cdc.gov/preconception/index.html). Neither the US Preventive Services Task Force (USPSTF) [g] nor the American Academy of Family Physicians (AAFP) [h] have guidelines for drug use screening, stating insufficient evidence to assess the balance of benefits and harms to screening adolescents, adults, and pregnant women.

How to Screen

Adolescents and women of all ages should be screened at least annually for drug abuse. In addition to routine drug screening, health care providers should advise adolescents against the use of alcohol, tobacco, and other illicit drugs. All pregnant women should be screened for drug abuse at their initial pregnancy visit due to the risk of fetal harm and adverse outcomes.

Screening for drug abuse is a sensitive issue. Maintaining a caring, nonthreatening, and nonjudgmental atmosphere will make patients more comfortable and more likely to disclose information on substance use. All types of drug misuse should be explored including illicit drugs, prescription drugs, over-the-counter-drugs, tobacco, and alcohol use. Screening often starts with a general statement, such as: "Substance use is so common in our society that I now ask all of my patients what, if any, substances they are using." The standard practice of screening all patients should be explained including ramifications in pregnancy for the fetus. All patients should be reassured that the information will be kept confidential.

Routine screening should rely on validated screening tools, as this improves accuracy of detecting substance abuse or dependence. There are a number of evidence-based screening tools available to the practitioner. These tools are easy to use and available at no cost (Table 44.1). For adults, the National Institute on Drug Abuse (NIDA) online tool guides clinicians through a series of questions to identify high-risk

Table 44.1 Guide to Evidence-Based Screening Tools for Adults and Adolescents

Screening Tool	Substance Type: Drugs	Validated for Adults	Validated for Adolescents	Tool Is Self-Administered	Tool Is Clinician Administered
NIDA Drug Use Screening Tool	X	X			X
CRAFFT	X		X	X	X
Opioid Risk Tool	X	X		X	
Drug Abuse Screen Test (DAST-10)	X	X		X	X
DAST-20: Adolescent version	X		X	X	X

Source: Adapted from the National Institute on Drug Abuse (NIDA). Available at: www.drugabuse.gov/nidamed-medical-health -professionals/tool-resources-your-practice/screening-assessment-drug-testing-resources/chart-evidence-based-screening-tools-adults. Retrieved May 19, 2015.

BOX 44.1 Center for Adolescent Abuse Research, Children's Hospital Boston. The CRAFFT Screening Interview

CRAFFT – Substance Abuse Screen for Adolescents and Young Adults

C	Have you ever ridden in a CAR driven by someone (including yourself) who was high or had been using alcohol or drugs?
R	Do you ever use alcohol or drugs to RELAX, feel better about yourself, or fit it?
A	Do you ever use alcohol or drugs while you are by yourself or ALONE?
F	Do you ever FORGET things you did while using alcohol or drugs?
F	Do your FAMILY or friends ever tell you that you should cut down on your drinking or drug use?
T	Have you ever gotten in TROUBLE while you were using alcohol or drugs?

Scoring: Two or more positive items indicate the need for further assessment.

---

substance use in their adult patients. It provides resources that assist clinicians in providing patient feedback and referral for specialty care [11]. For adolescents, the CRAFFT screening interview is an easy-to-use tool (Box 44.1) [12].

Routine screening should be limited to history. Urine drug testing may be indicated in some situations as an adjunct to screening. Urine drug testing should only be performed with the patient's consent and in compliance with state laws. Pregnant women need to be informed of potential consequences of positive test results, including mandatory reporting requirements.

Providers may be able to identify at-risk patients through observation, especially in their pregnant patients. Some signs or symptoms that may suggest illicit drug use include late prenatal care, poor attendance to appointments, poor weight gain, somnolence, intoxication, and erratic behavior. On physical examination, patients may demonstrate skin changes including track marks, lesions from intradermal injections, abscesses, or cellulitis.

The ability to provide comprehensive addiction care and follow-up is often out of the scope of primary health care providers. Routine screening will identify patients who are at risk for substance abuse or dependence. The clinician can identify the patient, provide initial counseling, then recommend and facilitate appropriate referral for further evaluation and treatment.

New Developments Likely to Affect Future Screening

Recommendations for drug abuse screening are unlikely to change dramatically in the future. However, clinicians will need to be aware of new trends in drug use and abuse. The website for the National Institute on Drug Abuse for Medical and Health Professionals (NIDAMED) is an excellent resource.

Billing

When screening for drug abuse reveals that a patient needs additional counseling or referral, physicians may code for a higher-level office visit. To do so, the amount of face-to-face time must be documented and there must be documentation that over 50 percent of the visit time was spent in counseling related to medical risks, benefits of therapy, coping strategies, and other aspects of comprehensive care.

Illustrative Cases

A healthy 17-year-old presents for a well-adolescent visit. She reports that she has tried alcohol a couple of times with her friends. She has been sexually active since age 15.

Recommendations from ACOG and AAP are to screen this patient for drug abuse by history at least annually. The conversation should be initiated with a statement that you talk to all of your patients about substance use. Use an evidence-based screening tool specifically validated in adolescents, such as the CRAFFT screening interview (Box 44.1). Determine if further assessment is needed and refer as appropriate. As a part of the discussion, strongly advise against the use of alcohol, tobacco, and other illicit drugs. Since she is sexually active and drug use may lead to higher-risk behaviors, discuss the importance of condom use for STD protection, and recommend and provide reliable and safe contraceptive options.

Screen now? Yes

Next screening: At least annually, although short-term follow-up may be indicated for adolescents at risk

A 30-year-old woman presents for a problem visit. On review of records, you find that she has been in the emergency room three times over the last 3 months for pelvic pain. Each time she has received a prescription for pain medication, but has run out.

She asks for another prescription for oxycodone for the pain.

Unplanned problem visits are another opportunity to screen for drug abuse. In this situation, the provider must maintain a caring and nonjudgmental approach. A full substance use history should be obtained. An online screening tool, such as the NIDA Drug Use Screening Tool, may be helpful. If a problem is identified, the patient should be referred for additional evaluation and treatment. Since she is of reproductive age, contraception and STI testing should be offered.

Screen now? Yes.

Next screen: At least annually or short-interval follow-up as needed

A 25-year-old G1P0 woman presents for her first prenatal care visit. Estimated gestational age is 8 weeks by last menstrual period.

All pregnant women should be routinely asked about their use of alcohol and drugs, including prescription opioids, at the initial prenatal care visit. Pregnant women may be especially hesitant to disclose this information due to fear of retaliation or loss of parental rights, so it is essential that patients know that the information disclosed will be kept confidential. They should be informed of the potential adverse consequences to the fetus.

Screen now? Yes

Next screen: As needed during pregnancy

A 36-year-old G4P3003 woman presents for her first prenatal care visit at 20 weeks. On examination, she is underweight and has multiple healing skin lesions on her arms.

All pregnant women should be routinely asked about their use of alcohol and drugs at the first prenatal care visit. This patient is presenting later than usual for prenatal care. She also has signs on physical examination of possible drug use. She should be informed that questions about substance use are asked of all pregnant women and that all information is kept confidential. Emphasize that the information will be used to ensure proper care for her and her fetus. Educate the patient about the adverse outcomes associated with drug use during pregnancy and encourage cessation. The patient should be screened for STIs and other infectious diseases. Referral for drug counseling and multispecialty care should be initiated. Additional antepartum surveillance may be indicated. Pediatrics should be notified at the time of delivery. Close postpartum follow-up is important.

Screen now? Yes

Next screen: As needed during pregnancy

A 60-year-old woman presents for annual well-woman visit. She has no complaints.

It is recommended to screen women for drug use at least annually, regardless of age. Initiate the conversation by stating that you talk to all of your patients about substance use. Use an evidence-based screening tool, such as the online NIDA Drug Use Screening Tool. Determine if further assessment is needed and refer as appropriate. Screening for STIs and other infectious disease should be done as appropriate based on history.

Screen now? Yes

Next screen: At least annually

Guidelines

a. American College of Obstetricians and Gynecologists. *Well-Woman Recommendations.* Washington, DC: American College of Obstetricians and Gynecologists, 2015. Available at: www.acog.org/About-ACOG/ACOG-Departments/Annual-Womens-Health-Care/Well-Woman-Recommendations. Retrieved May 18, 2016.

b. American College of Obstetricians and Gynecologists. Opioid abuse, dependence, and addiction during pregnancy. Committee Opinion No. 524. *Obstet Gynecol.* 2013, **119**:1070–6.

c. American College of Obstetricians and Gynecologists. *Guidelines for Adolescent Health Care [CD-ROM]*, 2nd edition. Washington, DC: American College of Obstetricians and Gynecologists, 2011.

d. Tanski, S., Garfunkel, L.C., Duncan, P.M., and Weitzman, M., editors. *Performing Preventative Services: A Bright Futures Handbook.* Elk Grove Village, IL: American Academy of Pediatrics, 2010. Available at http://brightfutures.aap.org/continuing_education.html. Retrieved May 18, 2016.

e. National Adolescent and Young Adult Health Information Center. *Summary of Recommended Guidelines for Clinical Preventive Services for Young Adults Ages 18–26.* San Francisco, CA: National Adolescent and Young Adult Health, 2015.

f. Jack, B.W., Atrash, H., Coonrod, D.V. et al. The clinical content of preconception care: An overview and preparation of this supplement. *AJOG.* 2008, **199**:S266–79.

g. US Preventive Services Task Force. *Final Recommendation Statement: Drug Use, Illicit: Screening.* Rockville, MD: USPSTF, 2008. Available at: www.uspreventiveservicestaskforce.org/Page/Document/RecommendationStatementFinal/drug-use-illicit-screening. Retrieved May 18, 2016.

h. American Academy of Family Physicians. *Illicit Drug Use: Clinical Preventive Service Recommendations.* Leawood, KS: AAFP, 2015. Available at: www.aafp.org/patient-care/clinical-recommendations/all/illicit-drug-use.html. Retrieved May 18, 2016.

References

1. Substance Abuse and Mental Health Services Administration. *Behavioral Health Barometer: United States, 2014.* HHS Publication No. SMA-15-4895. Rockville, MD: Substance Abuse and Mental Health Services Administration, 2015.

2. Substance Abuse and Mental Health Services Administration, *Results from the 2013 National Survey on Drug Use and Health: Summary of National Findings,* NSDUH Series H-48, HHS Publication No. (SMA) 14-4863. Rockville, MD: Substance Abuse and Mental Health Services Administration, 2014. Available at: www.samhsa.gov/data/sites/default/files/NSDUHresultsPDFWHTML2013/Web/NSDUHresults2013.htm#2.5..

3. Wendell, A.D. Overview and epidemiology of substance abuse in pregnancy. *Clin Obstet Gynecol.* 2013, **56**:91–6.

4. Babor, T.F., McKee, B.G., Kassebaum, P.A. et al. Screening, brief intervention, and referral to treatment (SBIRT): Toward a public health approach to the management of substance abuse. *Substance Abuse.* 2007, **28**:7–30.

5. Bernstein, E., Edwards, E., Dorman, D. et al. Screening and brief intervention to reduce marijuana use among youth and young adults in a pediatric emergency department. *Acad Emerg Med.* 2009, **16**:1174–85.

6. Missed Opportunity: National Survey of Primary Care Physicians and Patients on Substance Abuse. The National Center on Addiction and Substance Abuse at Columbia University. April 2000. Available at: www.centeronaddiction.org/addiction-research/reports/national-survey-primary-care-physicians-patients-substance-abuse. Retrieved May 18, 2016.

7. Flavin, J. and Paltrow, L.M. Punishing pregnancy drug-using women: Defying law, medicine, and common sense. *J Addict Dis.* 2010, **29**:231–44.

8. Johnston, L.D., O'Malley, P.M., Miech, R.A., Bachman, J.G., and Schulenberg, J.E. *Monitoring the Future National Survey Results on Drug Use, 1975–2015: Overview, Key Findings on Adolescent Drug Use.*

Ann Arbor, MI: Institute for Social Research, The University of Michigan, 2016, 98 pp. Available at: www.monitoringthefuture.org/data/15data/15drtbl1 .pdf. Retrieved May 18, 2016.

9. Greenfield, S., Manwani, S., and Nargiso, J. Epidemiology of substance use disorders in women. *Obstet Gynecol Clin North Am.* 2003, **30**:412–46.

10. Kelly, J.J., Davis, P.G., and Henschke, P.N. The drug epidemic: Effects on newborn infants and health resource consumption at a tertiary perinatal center. *J Paediatr Child Health.* 2000, **36**:262–4.

11. National Institute on Drug Abuse Screening Tool. *Clinician Screening Tool for Drug Use in General Medical Settings.* Available at: www.drugabuse.gov/n massist. Retrieved May 19, 2016.

12. Center for Adolescent Substance Abuse Research, Children's Hospital Boston. *The CRAFFT Screening Interview.* Boston, MA: CeASAR, 2009. Available at: www.ceasar-boston.org/CRAFFT/screen CRAFFT.php. Retrieved May 19, 2016.

Sleep Disorders

Lee A. Learman and David Chelmow

Why Screen?

Inadequate sleep has become increasingly common in the United States over the past 30 years. Between 1997 and 2009, the prevalence of short (<5 hours) or very short sleep (5–6 hours) increased from 21.4 to 29.1 percent [1]. Longitudinal studies controlling for other explanatory factors show positive associations between inadequate sleep and obesity, diabetes, hypertension, and cardiovascular disease, as well as lost workplace productivity, performance, and safety [1–3].

Sleep disorders are more prevalent across the life span in women than men and are common in the peripartum period [4], when they may be associated with a concurrent or future mood disorder [5]. Insomnia and sleepiness during the menopause transition may be from vasomotor symptoms or psychosocial issues warranting counseling or treatment. Persistent symptoms are more likely to reflect medical conditions, mood disorders, or obstructive sleep apnea (OSA) [6], a disorder characterized by repetitive upper airway obstruction during sleep, diminished sleep quality, and daytime sleepiness [7]. Patients with OSA have an increased risk of motor vehicle accidents [8], although evidence is inconclusive to establish OSA as a cause of mortality, stroke, hypertension, and cardiovascular disease.

Rationale for Screening

Patients may not disclose sleep problems without being asked and may not appreciate their underlying significance, particularly women who are pregnant, postpartum, or in the menopause transition. Screening women for disordered sleep can lead to identification of morbid conditions that can be successfully treated, including depression, anxiety, thyroid disease, obesity, OSA, and gastroesophageal reflux disease (GERD).

Factors That Affect Screening

Age: The increasing prevalence of mood disorders, psychosocial issues, chronic medical conditions, and OSA with age warrants a lower threshold for screening older women than younger women.

Weight: The strong association of obesity, metabolic disorders, and OSA warrants a lower threshold for screening overweight and obese women than normal weight women.

Recommended Guidelines and How to Find Them

At the time of the Well-Woman Task Force (WWTF) report, there were no major society guidelines available. The WWTF drew their single recommendation from the American College of Obstetrics and Gynecology (ACOG) Well-Woman Recommendations [a] which was a qualified recommendation that assessment for sleep disorders is recommended as part of depression screening or evaluation of other psychosocial issues in women aged 65 and older.

Since the Task Force convened, the American College of Physicians (ACP) has developed guidelines for the diagnosis of OSA in adults [b]. They recommend:

1. A sleep study for patients with unexplained daytime sleepiness (Grade: weak recommendation, low-quality evidence).
2. Polysomnography for diagnostic testing in patients suspected of OSA. ACP recommends portable sleep monitors in patients without serious comorbidities as an alternative to polysomnography when polysomnography is not available for diagnostic testing (Grade: weak recommendation, moderate-quality evidence).

How to Screen

The standard review of systems should include screening questions related to fatigue, insomnia, and sleep disorders. The ACP guidelines provide [b] useful additional guidance. Patients with suggestive symptoms on initial review of symptoms should be asked about common presenting symptoms for OSA, which include the following:

- Unintentional sleeping during wakefulness
- Daytime sleepiness
- Unrefreshing sleep
- Fatigue
- Insomnia
- Snoring

The most common risk factor is obesity. Particularly in women aged 65 and older, depression and other psychosocial issues should be considered, and if suspected, additional screening is performed as described in Chapter 40. Other causes such as thyroid symptoms, GERD, and other respiratory causes should also be considered.

If, after initial assessment, OSA is still being considered, current ACP guidelines recommend the patient should be referred to a sleep center for diagnostic testing with polysomnography. Their recommendations prefer polysomnography as first line for testing, but allow testing with portable sleep monitors in patients without serious comorbidities if polysomnography is not available.

New Developments Likely to Affect Future Guidelines

The US Preventive Services Task Force (USPSTF) finalized a draft research plan [7] for screening for OSA in adults in November 2015. Given the weight applied to the USPSTF guidelines, their recommendations will inform practice. Currently, major unanswered questions include refining whom to screen, whether there are screening tools that can narrow the number of women sent for diagnostic testing, and the effectiveness of methods other than polysomnography for diagnosis. Given that current screening recommendations are weak recommendations from a single professional organization based on low-quality evidence, it is anticipated that the recommendations will evolve over time. Given the accepted OSA-related morbidity, there will likely be a series of changing recommendations in the near future.

Billing

Initial screening for sleep disorders through review of system would be covered as part of the preventive visit codes. There are many sleep-related diagnosis codes. A number appear particularly relevant when evaluation of past initial screening questions is indicated:

Z72.820 – Sleep deprivation: Lack of sleep, insomnia

Z72.821 – Inadequate sleep hygiene

G47.39 – Other sleep apnea

F51.12 – Insufficient sleep syndrome

G47.9 – Sleep disorder, unspecified

G47.33 – Obstructive sleep apnea

Illustrative Cases

A 34-year-old woman presents for a well-woman visit. She delivered her third child 3 months ago. The pregnancy was complicated by nausea and vomiting, which resolved by the second trimester. The patient reports she is doing well, other than daytime sleepiness improved with napping. The baby awakens for a feed one to two times each night, and the patient's partner does not participate in the nighttime feeds. Her fatigue is similar to what she experienced after her first two pregnancies.

Screen now? No. Her daytime sleepiness is explained by the nighttime feedings and has not occurred at other times.

Next screen: As needed, for example, if the sleepiness does not improve after her baby sleeps through the night consistently, or if sleep-disordered breathing is suspected.

A 46-year-old woman presents for a well-woman visit. She reports general fatigue and worsening of her baseline depression. She naps daily. She has difficulty waking in the morning, and reports her husband has begun sleeping on the couch because of her snoring. Her body mass index is 27.

Screen now: Yes. While her sleep symptoms may be a sign of worsening depression, the patient's loud snoring is suggestive of OSA. She should be referred for polysomnography.

Next screen: As needed. OSA screening is prompted by symptoms, with no requirement for periodic testing.

Guidelines

a. American College of Obstetricians and Gynecologists. *Well-Woman Recommendations.* Washington, DC: American College of Obstetricians and Gynecologists, 2015. Available at: www.acog.org/About-ACOG/AC OG-Departments/Annual-Womens-Health-Care/ Well-Woman-Recommendations. Retrieved April 23, 2016.

b. Qaseem, A., Dallas, P., Owens, D.K. et al.; Clinical Guidelines Committee of the American College of Physicians. Diagnosis of obstructive sleep apnea in adults: A clinical practice guideline from the American College of Physicians. *Ann Intern Med.* 2014, **161**(3): 210–20.

References

1. Jean-Louis, G., Williams, N.J., Sarpong, D. et al. Associations between inadequate sleep and obesity in the US adult population: Analysis of the national health interview survey (1977–2009). *BMC Public Health.* 2014, **14**:290.

2. Buxton, O.M. and Marcelli, E. Short and long sleep are positively associated with obesity, diabetes, hypertension, and cardiovascular disease among adults in the United States. *Soc Sci Med.* 2010, **71**:1027–36.

3. Rosekind, M.R., Gregory, K.B., Mallis, M.M. et al. The cost of poor sleep: Workplace productivity loss and associated costs. *J Occup Environ Med.* 2010, **52**:91–8.

4. Abbott, S.M., Attarian, H., and Zee, P.C. Sleep disorders in perinatal women. *Best Pract Res Clin Obstet Gynaecol.* 2014, **28**(1):159–68.

5. Bei, B., Coo, S., and Trinder, J. Sleep and mood during pregnancy and the postpartum period. *Sleep Med Clin.* 2015, **10**(1):25–33.

6. Bruyneel, M. Sleep disturbances in menopausal women: Aetiology and practical aspects. *Maturitas.* 2015, **81**(3): 406–9.

7. US Preventive Services Task Force. Draft Research Plan for Obstructive Sleep Apnea in Adults: Screening (New Topic). November 2015. Available at: www .uspreventiveservicestaskforce.org/Page/Document/ draft-research-plan167/obstructive-sleep-apnea-in-adults-screening. Retrieved April 23, 2015.

8. Terán-Santos, J., Jiménez-Gómez, A., and Cordero-Guevara, J. The association between sleep apnea and the risk of traffic accidents. Cooperative Group Burgos-Santander. *N Engl J Med.* 1999, **340**:847–51.

Mental Health and Psychosocial Issues
Suicide and Behavioral Assessment

Jonathan Schaffir

Why Screen?

When thinking of a well-woman exam, many practitioners concentrate on the physical and corporeal elements of health. However, psychosocial and behavioral issues may have a profound impact on various aspects of health and deserve equal attention. According to the World Health Organization (WHO), mental health is more than the absence of mental illness. They define it as a "state of well-being in which every individual realizes his or her own potential, can cope with the normal stresses of life, can work productively and fruitfully, and is able to make a contribution to her or his community" [1]. In order to assess whether their patients are meeting these goals, health care providers must inquire about the lifestyle and behavioral issues that constitute mental health screening.

Taking a careful psychosocial history may uncover problems such as chronic stress, social isolation, relationship problems, and unproductive thought patterns. Such difficulties may indirectly have an adverse impact on physical health by impairing a woman's ability to assess her health needs, her propensity to seek out medical attention, and her capacity to follow medical recommendations. They may also have direct effects by leading to destructive thoughts and behaviors including substance abuse, violence or victimization, and at worst, suicide. This overview on screening for mental health issues will discuss screening for psychosocial factors in general. Screening for depression, injury prevention, and substance abuse, as well as domestic and intimate partner violence are addressed in separate chapters.

Rationale for Screening

Ensuring wellness involves making sure that a woman can navigate normal developmental stages and challenges, and providing counseling during periods of emotional adjustment and difficulty. Building identity and self-esteem, forming meaningful relationships, and achieving goals in school and work are stages associated with adolescence and adulthood. Challenges include the experience of loss (whether of a job, a physical or mental ability, or a loved one) and traumatic situations such as victimization or abuse. By exploring such issues, a health care provider can anticipate difficulties with achieving healthy milestones and with overcoming challenges that put health at risk.

Many disorders that involve destructive or harmful behaviors, such as substance abuse, eating disorders, self-mutilation, and suicidality, share similar risk factors. Social isolation, an inability to cope with stress, diminished self-esteem, and feelings of loss may all contribute to these behaviors. Women who are subjected to traumatic experiences such as abuse, rape, or domestic violence may be particularly vulnerable to such feelings [2].

A woman's capacity to process challenges and maintain a healthy outlook may change across her life span. Adolescence is a time of particular vulnerability when self-identity and self-esteem are forged, and when some girls feel ill-equipped to deal with social pressure from school and peers. Adolescents may experience unique circumstances that increase their risk of attempting suicide, including serious adverse childhood events, family history of suicide, and a history of being bullied (often associated with discrimination due to sexual orientation or sexual identity) [3].

Older age is another phase when women may be presented with unique psychosocial challenges. With advancing age and increasing physical challenges, a woman may be more concerned about her needs when she is incapacitated; consideration of advance directives becomes appropriate. Deficits in cognition may present a challenge, and age-related changes may be difficult for patients to discern from more serious conditions. Mild cognitive impairment (MCI), which is defined as impairment that is not severe enough to interfere with daily living, is identified variably in 3–42 percent of adults over age 65 [4]. This change may be predictive of greater deficits in function, or dementia, over time.

Factors That Affect Screening

Age: Psychosocial concerns and stressors vary considerably with age; issues of concern for adolescents will be different from those of elderly adults. Adolescents may be concerned about interpersonal and family relationships, school experience, aspects of sexual orientation and gender identity, personal goal development, peer relationships, and bullying. Aspects of social life for older adolescents and young adults may also include acquaintance rape prevention, work satisfaction, lifestyle and stress, and sleep disorders. Older women may have entirely different concerns including advance directives and end-of-life plans, neglect and abuse, and cognitive functioning.

History of mental health disorders: Suicide screening is not recommended in the general population of women aged 19 and older. However, women of any age with a history of depression are at elevated risk and should be screened for recurrent depression and suicide.

Sexual orientation and gender identity: Being in a sexual minority (lesbian, gay, bisexual, transgender, or questioning) is a risk factor for suicide, and the American College of Obstetricians and Gynecologists (ACOG) recommends that adolescents who fall into this category deserve special concern.

Recommended Guidelines

Most authorities agree on the value of exploring psychosocial issues at the time of a routine annual visit. ACOG recommends that assessment of various aspects of psychosocial health should be incorporated into the well-woman visit [a]. Evaluation and counseling should include interpersonal and family relationships, intimate partner violence, work satisfaction, lifestyle and stress, and sleep disorders. Screening for depression and neglect/abuse should also be included [b]. The American Academy of Pediatrics (AAP) also recommends that psychosocial and behavioral assessment should be a part of annual preventive

pediatric health care through age 21 [c]. In keeping with ACOG's recommendations, the Well-Woman Task Force (WWTF) recommends that girls and women under the age of 40 should be counseled about acquaintance rape prevention, and women aged 40 and older should be counseled about formulating advance directives.

The WWTF encountered noteworthy differences in other aspects of mental health and psychosocial screening. Both ACOG and AAP advise that screening for self-injurious thoughts or suicidal ideation should be carried out annually in adolescents, and ACOG continues to include suicide screening in its list of topics to evaluate in the well-woman assessment for all ages. Both the American Academy of Family Physicians (AAFP) and the US Preventive Services Task Force (USPSTF) maintain that there is insufficient evidence to screen for suicide risk in the general population including adolescents [d, e].

Recommendations are also not uniform for screening for cognitive impairment. Both AAFP and USPSTF agree that there is insufficient evidence to recommend screening older adults for cognitive impairment [f, g]. However, the National Institute for Health and Care Excellence (NICE) in the United Kingdom suggests that all primary health care staff should consider screening for MCI as a possible precursor for dementia, although they agree that screening for dementia is not indicated [h].

The final WWTF recommendations were developed primarily around areas of common agreement. Due to the particular vulnerability perceived in adolescents, annual screening is recommended for mental health disorders and suicide in women under age 19. Women aged 65 and older should be screened for MCI and screen-positive women should be referred for additional memory assessment. Routine screening of asymptomatic older adults for dementia, however, is not recommended.

How to Screen

The WWTF recommends that evaluation of psychosocial aspects of health should be conducted at each routine health assessment. Screening for psychosocial issues begins with a thorough social history. Many of the topics that are recommended for evaluation (including interpersonal and family relationships, school and work satisfaction, lifestyle and stress, and sexual orientation and gender identity) are elements of a social history as taught in introductory medicine classes [5], and may be part of routine discussions that a practitioner has with her patients to get the full picture of their life stories. Such conversations do not only help to elicit problems and difficulties that the patient may face. By demonstrating caring in a holistic way, they strengthen the clinician–patient relationship, which is a key element of the annual well-woman visit.

For adolescents below the age of 19, specific annual assessment is recommended for mental health disorders and for emotions and behaviors that may increase the risk of suicidality. While there is no screening instrument that is universally accepted for this purpose, the AAP provides a list of suggested questions and strategies for anticipatory guidance in their Bright Futures guidelines for pediatric care [c]. For clinicians who prefer to use a standardized questionnaire, they suggest using the Pediatric Symptom Checklist [6], a 35-item tool that has been validated for use in children up to the age of 16. Similarly, there is no standard method for assessing the risk of an adolescent killing or harming herself. Validated options include the Suicide Risk Screen, a 20-item screening instrument geared toward high school–age individuals, or simply asking about thoughts of suicidality within the past month. A more complete description of screening instruments and tools for suicide prevention can be obtained through the Suicide Prevention Resource Center (SPRC) at www.sprc.org/webform/primary-care-toolkit.

For women over the age of 64, screening for MCI is recommended. Although there have been several tools described to assess for dementia in the elderly adults, there is no agreement about a threshold that would provide a diagnosis of mild impairment. Since the definition of MCI is cognitive decline not severe enough to interfere with daily functioning, it may be up to the discretion of the clinician whether additional exploration is necessary based on the details of a frank conversation about daily activities. If using a standardized questionnaire, the best tool to determine whether such exploration is indicated is the Dementia Screening Indicator recommended by the National Institute for Aging. This seven-item yes/no questionnaire (available at http://bit.ly/1pxk5rl) provides a numerical score that suggests whether additional screening for cognitive impairment is indicated [7].

Specific screening instruments for depression, interpersonal violence, sexual health, injury prevention, and substance abuse will be discussed in separate chapters.

New Developments Likely to Affect Future Recommendations

The WWTF recommendations against screening for suicide and dementia in asymptomatic general populations are based on USPSTF guidelines, which note that there is insufficient medical evidence to recommend routine screening. In both cases, recommendations may change as new research clarifies the gaps in the existing medical information.

In the case of suicide screening, there is currently insufficient evidence to justify screening asymptomatic women older than 18 in the general population. Further research is needed to demonstrate whether screening instruments can reliably detect those who are likely to carry out a suicide attempt and whether any interventions are beneficial for screen-positive individuals.

For cognitive impairment screening, the deficit in evidence is primarily in predicting which individuals with MCI will progress to functional impairment, and which interventions can slow progression. Evidence that progression can be delayed or prevented would support the value of routine screening in older patients.

Billing

Taking a social history that includes screening for psychosocial issues would be an included and expected part of any periodic assessment, which could be billed with the ICD-10 code for gynecological examination (general, routine) without abnormal findings (Z01.419) or periodic health assessment, general screening (Z00.00). When screening specifically for depression or mental health issues, one may use the code Z13.89. Screening for cognitive impairment or dementia may be billed under the code Z13.4.

Although such screening may be done as part of the well-woman visit, Medicare Preventive Services will also cover a separate annual depression screening up to 15 minutes, coded with the special HCPCS code G0444.

For women with Medicare, two CPT codes have been added that specifically cover discussions on advance directives: 99497 is to be used for the first

30 minutes of face-to-face discussion, and 99498 may be used for each additional 30 minutes. When this service is documented concurrently with an annual wellness visit on the same date, these codes are payable in full with the use of modifier -33.

Illustrative Cases

A 17-year-old student presents for her first gynecological visit. She has not yet been sexually active and is not interested in an examination. She would like to establish care in case of future needs.

As this is her first visit, establishing trust and rapport will be particularly important. A careful social history should be obtained to explore family and school interactions, mood and behavioral issues, sexual orientation and gender identity, and history of physical or sexual abuse. Counseling at the visit should include information about acquaintance rape prevention. Because she is less than 19 years old, screening for emotions and behaviors that indicate recurrent or severe depression and thoughts of killing or harming herself is also recommended. If questioning about sexual orientation and identity suggests that she is a member of a sexual minority, she may be at risk of discrimination, bullying, and social isolation, which are risk factors for suicide independent of a depression diagnosis. This patient should be screened specifically for suicidality, either with directed questions or with a standardized screener.

Screen now? Yes

Next screen? Annually and/or with future clinical encounters

A 32-year-old woman returns for a routine gynecological visit. She was last seen 2½ years ago. She apologizes for being so late in returning and mentions that it has been hard to keep track of time due to so much stress with her children and her job.

As with all women at a routine checkup, her psychosocial history should be explored, particularly interpersonal and family relationships, work satisfaction, sleep disorders, acquaintance rape prevention, and lifestyle/stress. Screening for depression and intimate partner violence is also appropriate. Keep in mind that psychosocial issues may be a factor in noncompliance with medical care and may be at the root of her lapse in visits.

Screen now? Yes

Next screen? Annually

A 72-year-old woman presents for an annual checkup. When questioned about her medications, she off-handedly mentions that sometimes she forgets to take them.

Forgetfulness in an elderly woman should be examined more closely. Screening for MCI should include questioning to determine whether her level of cognition is interfering with her activities of daily living or her ability to care for herself. If the patient or her family expresses concerns about how she is affected by loss of memory or confusion, referral should be made for additional dementia screening.

In addition to the other psychosocial issues that are routinely discussed at the well-woman visit, advance directives should also be brought up with this woman. According to the ACOG recommendations [b], a discussion about values and wishes regarding future care is best held while the patient is healthy at a routine visit. The patient should be encouraged to describe her future wishes in writing (a "living will") and designate a proxy who can make medical decisions if she is unable to do so.

Screen now? Yes

Next screen? Annually and/or with future clinical encounters

Guidelines

a. American College of Obstetrician and Gynecologists. *Well-Woman Recommendations*. Washington, DC: American College of Obstetricians and Gynecologists, 2015. Available at: www.acog.org/About-ACOG/ACOG-Departments/Annual-Womens-Health-Care/Well-Woman-Recommendations. Retrieved December 29, 2016.

b. American College of Obstetricians and Gynecologists. End-of-life decision making. Committee Opinion No. 617. *Obstet Gynecol.* 2015, 125:261–7.

c. American Academy of Pediatrics. *Bright Futures: Guidelines for Health Supervision of Infants, Children, and Adolescents*, 3rd edition. Elk Grove, IL: American Academy of Pediatrics, 2014. Available at: https://brightfutures.aap.org/materials-and-tools/guidelines-and-pocket-guide/Pages/default.aspx. Retrieved December 29, 2016.

d. American Academy of Family Physicians. Clinical Preventive Service Recommendation: Suicide. 2014. Available at: www.aafp.org/patient-care/clinical-recommendations/all/suicide.html. Retrieved December 29, 2016.

e. LeFevre, M.L. Screening for suicide risk in adolescents, adults, and older adults in primary care: US Preventive Services Task Force recommendation statement. *Annals Internal Med.* 2014, **160**:719–26. Available at: www .uspreventiveservicestaskforce.org/Page/Document/Upd ateSummaryFinal/suicide-risk-in-adolescents-adults-and -older-adults-screening.

f. American Academy of Family Physicians. Clinical Preventive Service Recommendation: Dementia. 2014. Available at: www.aafp.org/patient-care/clinical-recommendations/all/dementia.html. Retrieved December 29, 2016.

g. Moyer, V.A. Screening for cognitive impairment in older adults: US Preventive Services Task Force recommendation statement. *Ann Intern Med.* 2014, **160**:791–7. Available at: www .uspreventiveservicestaskforce.org/Page/Document/ UpdateSummaryFinal/cognitive-impairment-in-older-adults-screening.

h. NICE Guidelines: Dementia: Supporting people with dementia and their carers in health and social care. National Institute for Health and Care Excellence, 2006. Available at: http://nice.org.uk/guidance/cg42/chapter/ 1-recommendations. Retrieved December 29, 2016.

References

1. World Health Organization. *Mental Health: Strengthening Our Response.* Fact Sheet #220. Geneva: World Health Organization, 2014. Available at: www.who.int/mediacentre/factsheets/fs220/en/. Retrieved December 29, 2016.

2. Cowley, D. and Lentz, G.M. Emotional aspects of gynecology. In: Lentz, G.M., Lobo, R.A., Gershenson, D.M., and Katz, V.L., editors. *Comprehensive Gynecology*, 6th edition. Philadelphia, PA: Mosby, 2012. pp. 137–71.

3. LeFevre, M.L. Screening for suicide risk in adolescents, adults, and older adults in primary care: US Preventive Services Task Force recommendation statement. *Ann Intern Med.* 2014, **160**:719–26.

4. Lin, J.S., O'Connor, E., Rossom, R.C., Perdue, L.A., and Eckstrom, E. Screening for cognitive impairment in older adults: A systemic review for the US Preventive Services Task Force. *Ann Intern Med.* 2013, **159**:601–12.

5. Bickley, L.S. and Szilagyi, P.G. Interviewing and the health history. In: Bickley, L.S., editor. *Bates' Guide to Physical Examination and History Taking*, 10th edition. Philadelphia, PA: Lippincott Williams & Wilkins, 2009. pp. 55–98.

6. Jellinek, M.S., Murphy, J.M., Robinson, J. et al. Pediatric symptom checklist: Screening school-age children for psychosocial dysfunction. *J Pediatrics.* 1988, **112**:201–9. Available at: http://brightfutures.org/mentalhealth/pdf/ professionals/ped_sympton_chklst.pdf. Retrieved December 29, 2016.

7. National Institute on Aging. *Assessing Cognitive Impairment in Older Patients: A Quick Guide for Primary Care Physicians.* Bethesda, MD: National Institute on Aging, 2014. Available at: www.nia.nih .gov/alzheimers/publication/assessing-cognitive-impairment-older-adults. Retrieved December 29, 2016.

Chapter

47

Breastfeeding

Andrea B. Joyner

Why Counsel?

Oftentimes, women have already made a decision about infant feeding by the time they reach the first trimester of pregnancy [1]. The factors that play into that decision can vary greatly based on each patient's personal knowledge about breastfeeding. Patients may form opinions about infant feeding based on their own experiences, familial and societal influences, and information they can glean from available media. Negative views may be based on misinformation and it is the provider's responsibility to ensure that women are given the opportunity to make an evidence-based informed decision about how to feed their children.

Health care providers can influence a woman's decision to breastfeed and her ability and desire to continue breastfeeding [2]. Because breastfeeding has significant individual and public health benefits, the American College of Obstetricians and Gynecologists (ACOG) calls on women's health care providers to support their patients in choosing to breastfeed [3]. Likewise, the US surgeon general released *The Surgeon General's Call to Action to Support Breastfeeding* in 2011 to encourage better support from health care workers [2]. Since 2014, the Joint Commission has been collecting hospital breastfeeding data as a part of their perinatal core measures. As breastfeeding rates are now considered a reflection of quality of care, physicians themselves may eventually be held individually responsible for the breastfeeding rates in their own practices.

Rationale for Counseling

Multiple research studies and systematic reviews support breastfeeding and human milk being the normative standards for infant feeding and nutrition. Breastfeeding protects infants against respiratory tract infections, otitis media, gastrointestinal tract infections, necrotizing enterocolitis, sudden infant death syndrome, infant mortality, allergic disease, celiac disease, inflammatory bowel disease, obesity, diabetes, childhood leukemia, and childhood lymphoma. There also appear to be significant positive effects on neurodevelopment [4].

Both short- and long-term benefits are seen by mothers who breastfeed, as well. In the immediate postpartum period, breastfeeding decreases postpartum blood loss and causes more rapid involution of the uterus. Additionally, decreases in the incidence of postpartum depression and increased child spacing from lactational amenorrhea have been shown to benefit mothers who breastfeed. Long-term maternal benefits such as postpartum weight loss, protection against type 2 diabetes, and decreased risks of rheumatoid arthritis, cardiovascular disease, hypertension, hyperlipidemia, breast cancer, and ovarian cancer have been associated with breastfeeding [4].

The Agency for Healthcare Research and Quality (AHRQ) estimated a saving of $13 billion each year if 90 percent of US mothers would comply with recommendations related to exclusive breastfeeding. This estimate included healthcare savings through decreased incidence of childhood illnesses, but did not include additional savings related to reduction in parental absenteeism from work and reduction in adult-onset diseases that are prevented by breastfeeding [4].

Studies show that the optimal duration of exclusive breastfeeding is about 6 months, followed by continued breastfeeding as complementary foods are introduced [5]. It should then be continued for 1 year or longer, as mutually desired by the breastfeeding dyad [4]. Nevertheless, many women who have a general understanding of breastfeeding still experience difficulty fulfilling these recommendations because they may not have access to information about how to breastfeed or may receive incorrect information [2].

Fortunately, a number of interventions have been shown to be successful in helping women meet the recommended breastfeeding goals. Multiple counseling methods have been evaluated by both Cochrane reviews and the US Preventive Services Task Force (USPSTF). These studies offer strong evidence that formal education and printed materials alone do not affect breastfeeding rates [2]. Instead, these resources should be used as a part of a multifaceted, personalized intervention to be effective [6].

Factors That Affect Counseling

Maternal infections: Human T-cell lymphotrophic virus type I or II, untreated brucellosis, and HIV are all maternal infections in which breastfeeding is contraindicated. In addition, mothers with herpes simplex lesions on the breasts, active varicella, H1N1 influenza, and active untreated tuberculosis may provide expressed breast milk to their infants but should not breastfeed until their infections have cleared.

Street drugs: Use of street drugs such as PCP, cocaine, and cannabis are contraindicated in breastfeeding.

Maternal medications: Maternal amphetamine, chemotherapy, ergotamine, or statin use is not compatible with breastfeeding.

Infant medical conditions: Infants born with galactosemia should not be breastfed [4].

Psychological aversion: Some women have a psychological aversion to breastfeeding, perhaps due to a history of sexual trauma [7]. They should be counseled that they can feed expressed breast milk by bottle to achieve the same infant health benefits.

Additional factors: A history and breast examination will detect additional medical conditions that can be associated with breastfeeding difficulty (Box 47.1). It is important that providers set expectations appropriately so that patients can be better prepared to navigate breastfeeding challenges specific to their medical conditions.

Recommended Guidelines and How to Find Them

ACOG's Well-Woman Task Force (WWTF) adopted the USPSTF and Institute of Medicine's recommendations that providers should promote breastfeeding

---

BOX 47.1 Maternal Conditions Associated with Breastfeeding Difficulty [7]

- Primiparity
- Cesarean delivery
- Long second stage of labor
- Maternal fluid loads in labor*
- Type 1 diabetes mellitus
- Labor analgesia†
- Obesity
- Lupus
- Inverted nipples
- Polycystic ovarian syndrome
- Theca lutein cysts
- Retained placenta
- Sheehan's syndrome
- Stress
- Hypothyroidism
- Breast surgery‡
- Hypoplastic breasts

* Total amounts and flow rate of IV fluids in labor may play a role in edema-related breastfeeding difficulties

† IV or IM opiates given in labor can decrease infants' ability to suckle effectively during breastfeeding initiation. The effect of epidural analgesia on breastfeeding is still controversial

‡ A history of breast surgery is associated with a three-fold higher risk of lactation insufficiency. This is especially true in the case of reduction mammoplasty

---

for all women of reproductive capacity during pregnancy and after birth to ensure successful initiation and duration. Comprehensive lactation support and counseling should include information about obtaining breastfeeding equipment, such as breast pumps [8,9].

There are many easily accessible resources to aid women's health care providers in counseling. For basic education about the benefits of breastfeeding and why breast milk is superior to infant formula, providers can easily access a free copy of the American Academy of Pediatrics (AAP) *Breastfeeding and the Use of Human Milk* paper via internet search [4]. ACOG has published a number of helpful physician and patient resources available at www.acog.org/breastfeeding [a]. There are several resources for the safety of specific medications with breastfeeding, including Hale's "Medications & Mothers' Milk" [b]. LactMed is an online drugs and lactation database that has a corresponding app for quick reference [c]. The Academy of Breastfeeding Medicine (ABM) has free clinical practice protocols available for reference on their website under the "Protocols & Statements" tab [d]. The AAP and ACOG coauthored a comprehensive reference text for physicians called *Breastfeeding Handbook for Physicians, 2nd Edition* [e]. An online comprehensive resource can be found in the breastfeeding section of the Centers for Disease Control and Prevention (CDC) website [f] including *The CDC Guide to Strategies to Support Breastfeeding Mothers and Babies* as well as links to other useful resources such as La Leche League International and the US Breastfeeding Committee [g, h].

How to Counsel

Periodic Well-Woman Visits

There are many opportunities outside of maternity care to advocate for breastfeeding to all reproductive-aged women. A history and physical performed during a well-woman visit might reveal potential barriers to breastfeeding that could be addressed in someone preparing for pregnancy, such as obesity or history of breast surgery (Box 47.1). Additionally, displaying breastfeeding educational materials in the office setting invites questions about breastfeeding among patients of all ages, which in turn can improve knowledge and support.

Prenatal Visits

Patients rely heavily on the advice and support of their providers when deciding whether to breastfeed. Starting with the first prenatal visit, providers should encourage or reinforce the decision to breastfeed by emphasizing the advantages of breastfeeding compared with formula feeding. The benefits of exclusive breastfeeding should be emphasized because mothers who intend to breastfeed and formula feed are less likely to meet their breastfeeding goals. Breastfeeding education groups can increase duration of breastfeeding and should be offered to patients as part of their prenatal care [1]. During the history and physical that is performed when a patient establishes prenatal care, careful screening should be performed to identify risk factors for delayed lacto genesis and problems of breastfeeding. If risk factors are recognized, the patient should be offered additional prenatal lactation support and counseled regularly so that they are better prepared for additional challenges they may face in the immediate postpartum period (Box 47.1) [7].

Intrapartum Care

When making pain management decisions in labor, patients should be aware that breastfeeding initiation is negatively affected by some medications such as narcotics. Skin-to-skin contact and early breastfeeding should be encouraged within the first hour of birth. Efforts should be made to avoid separating newborns from their mothers for procedures that can be performed on the maternal chest or delayed until after the first feed [1].

Postpartum Care

Immediately after delivery, patients should be instructed on breastfeeding basics and skin-to-skin contact should be continued. They should be counseled that rooming-in with their newborns decreases infant crying, increases maternal and infant sleeping, helps infants learn to breastfeed, and increases milk production. Whenever possible, newborn procedures should be performed without taking infants out of their mothers' rooms. Prior to leaving the hospital, mothers should feel comfortable feeding at the breast on demand and expressing breast milk manually. Mothers should be counseled that an initial 5–7 percent weight loss is common in breastfeeding newborns. They should also be aware that all breastfed infants need close pediatric follow-up after hospital discharge to ensure weight gain resumes. Patients should be provided with information on outpatient lactation services and should know who to call if they have questions when they get home [1]. At the postpartum visit, providers should continue to encourage breastfeeding mothers and specifically inquire about any new breastfeeding concerns.

New Developments Likely to Affect Future Recommendations

The body of evidence proving that human breast milk is superior to infant formula continues to grow and efforts to reestablish breastfeeding as a norm in the American culture will likely become more robust. In order to help providers better support breastfeeding patients, health care provider education on breastfeeding is becoming more formalized across all levels of training. Physician-specific curricula developed by both ABM and AAP are being incorporated with increasing frequency in medical school, residency, and specialist training programs.

Now that breastfeeding is considered a form of preventive health care because of its protective effects on maternal and infant well-being, obstetrician-gynecologists will be responsible for ensuring that their patients are educated appropriately. In the same way, a growing number of hospitals are taking responsibility for increasing breastfeeding rates by following the practices outlined in the World Health Organization's *Ten Steps to Successful Breastfeeding* and seeking accreditation by Baby-Friendly USA to enforce these policies.

Billing

The Affordable Care Act requires new health plans to fully cover the cost of prenatal and postpartum breastfeeding counseling and supplies [2]. When performed by licensed professionals, counseling can be billed as preventive care counseling in addition to routine maternity care billing. If performed during a routine prenatal visit, the global charge for maternity care (or correlate evaluation and management [E/M] visit charge if unbundled) can be billed along with a preventive procedure codes (99401–99404) using the modifier -25 and the ICD-10 code Z39.1 (Care and Examination of Lactating Mother). If the patient is seen for a routine maternity care visit and a breastfeeding problem is addressed, the appropriate ICD-10 problem diagnosis code should be used and a co-pay may apply. Again, modifier -25 should accompany a separate E/M code in order to bill for the additional care. Lactation classes attended in addition to routine maternity visits can be separately billed using the S9443 procedure code and the Z39.1 diagnosis code [10].

Illustrative Cases

A 25-year-old G1P0 presents for new prenatal visit at 8 weeks' gestation. She told your nurse that she plans to breastfeed and formula feed because she has to go back to work after 6 weeks and the baby will need formula eventually anyway.

The patient should be asked first about what she has heard about breastfeeding and the workplace to assess her fund of knowledge. The benefits of breastfeeding should be reviewed with her. After acknowledging her concerns, she should be reassured that she can continue to exclusively breastfeed after returning to work by expressing and storing milk while she is separated from her infant [7]. It is important for her to

understand that the Affordable Care Act mandates that breastfeeding supplies such as pumps be covered by her insurance carrier [2]. She should be advised to speak to her employer about accommodations that can be made for her since there are laws that protect the rights of breastfeeding mothers who work outside of the home [7]. Online resources can be given.

Counsel now? Yes

Next counseling? This topic should be revisited throughout prenatal care until both the provider and patient are confident that an informed decision has been made about infant feeding.

A 34-year-old G2P1001 presents for routine prenatal visit at 16 weeks' gestation. She states that she tried to breastfeed for about a week with the first child but was unable to make enough milk. To avoid struggling again, she plans to give her second baby formula.

A mother's perception that she has insufficient milk is the most commonly cited breastfeeding problem worldwide. The diagnosis of true insufficient milk supply only occurs when there is insufficient breast milk production to sustain normal infant weight gain, despite appropriate feeding routines, maternal motivation to continue breastfeeding, and skilled assistance with breastfeeding problems [7]. If the patient indicates that she is motivated to breastfeed and her history reveals that she probably had the more common diagnosis of perceived insufficient milk supply, she should be reassured that successful breastfeeding can be achieved with her second child with better support. The patient should be offered outpatient prenatal lactation consultation, if available. Alternatively, if it appears that the patient has made an informed decision to feed with formula after counseling and support are offered, she should be supported in her decision.

Counsel now? Yes

Next counseling? If the patient wants to try to breastfeed again after this discussion, counseling and support should continue at each subsequent prenatal and postpartum visit. If the patient has made an informed decision to feed with formula, additional breastfeeding counseling is not indicated.

A 40-year-old G4P1203 presents for routine prenatal visit at 32 weeks' gestation. She recently attended a hospital tour and is upset because she did not know that your hospital became "Baby Friendly." She states she has been educated numerous times about the benefits of breastfeeding but that she will not change her mind. Furthermore, she is not interested in any practices that would disrupt her rest and recovery after the delivery.

The first step in addressing this patient's concerns starts with gaining an understanding about her knowledge base by asking open-ended, nonjudgmental questions. For example, she could be asked, "What have you heard about breastfeeding and the Baby-Friendly Hospital Initiative (BFHI)?" If her answers indicate that she is adequately educated about benefits of breastfeeding and she chooses to feed with formula, she should be supported in her decision. She should be informed that the BFHI does not aim to force patients to breastfeed, but rather aims to decrease barriers to mothers who have chosen to do so. She can expect to benefit from new hospital practices such as rooming-in because studies indicate that mothers and babies actually sleep better when they share a room [7]. She should be reassured that there will be plenty of support for her if she becomes overtired after her delivery. Any other new hospital procedures that may have changed since becoming Baby Friendly should be reviewed with her so that expectations are set appropriately.

Counsel now? Yes

Next counseling? To adequately address this patient's concerns and set appropriate expectations about her inpatient stay, it is important to continue this conversation at subsequent prenatal visits until she indicates that she is well-informed about the new hospital procedures.

A 28-year-old G1P0 presents for routine prenatal visit at 36 weeks' gestation. Her history is significant for polycystic ovarian syndrome, obesity, and well-controlled hypothyroidism. She became pregnant with dichorionic-diamnionic twins as the result of in vitro fertilization. The babies are in breech/breech presentation and she is scheduled for a planned cesarean delivery. She is very excited about breastfeeding her twins and wants to know if she will be able to make enough milk for both babies.

This patient should be reassured that many mothers of multiples are able to supply most if not all the milk necessary to feed twins. She should be advised that her personal medical history and planned cesarean for twin gestation put her at risk for delayed lactogenesis [7]. Setting her expectations appropriately will help her feel empowered to overcome challenges she may expect to encounter after the babies are born. It is not uncommon for twin mothers to supplement breastfeeding with expressed milk until

the feeding relationship is better established. Expressing milk for her babies within 2 hours of giving birth will help her to be more successful in meeting her breastfeeding goals [7]. She should be given information about inpatient and outpatient lactation support prior to delivery and be instructed on how to obtain a breast pump.

Counsel now? Yes

Next counseling? The patient should be offered continued counseling at each prenatal visit until she delivers since she is quickly approaching her delivery date. She will need enhanced lactation support given her risk factors for difficulties. It will help her to have a coordinated care plan arranged prior to delivery.

A 21-year-old G1P1001 who is postpartum day #1 after a normal spontaneous vaginal delivery tells you that her baby is losing weight and she needs to give him formula. She is frustrated that her milk has not come in yet. You note that the baby is sleeping soundly in the bassinet and has a pacifier.

This patient's concern is very common among new breastfeeding mothers and is a reason for early cessation of breastfeeding. The patient should be reassured that weight loss is expected in breastfed newborns and that breast milk intake is reflected in the number of wet or soiled diapers. In order to facilitate the production of mature milk, she should feed the baby on demand [9]. Feeding cues can be missed with a pacifier in place and therefore pacifier use is best reserved for after the maternal milk supply has been well established. Inpatient lactation support should be arranged for one-on-one teaching.

Counsel now? Yes

Next counseling? The patient's concerns should be again addressed during rounds the following day. Prior to discharge home, the patient should have appointments arranged with her pediatrician and, if available, with an outpatient lactation consultant to ensure continued support. Counseling should be continued at her postpartum visit and she should be encouraged to follow up sooner if any additional concerns arise.

Guidelines

a. American Congress of Obstetricians and Gynecologists. ACOG Departments & Activities – Breastfeeding. Available at: www.acog.org/breastfeeding. Retrieved January 17, 2016.

b. Hale, T.W. and Rowe, H.E. *Medications & Mother's Milk*, 2nd edition. Plano, TX: Hale Publishing, 2014.

c. US National Library of Medicine. Toxnet Toxicology Data Network Databases – Breastfeeding & Drugs: LactMed. Available at: http://toxnet.nlm.nih.gov/new toxnet/lactmed.htm. Retrieved January 17, 2016.

d. Academy of Breastfeeding Medicine. Protocols & Statements. Available at: www.bfmed.org/Resources/Pr otocols.aspx. Retrieved January 17, 2016.

e. American College of Obstetricians and Gynecologists and American Academy of Pediatrics. *Breastfeeding Handbook for Physicians*, 2nd edition. Elk Grove Village, IL, Washington, DC: American Academy of Pediatrics and American College of Obstetricians and Gynecologists, 2014.

f. Centers for Disease Control and Prevention. Division of Nutrition, Physical Activity, and Obesity – Breastfeeding. Available at: www.cdc.gov/breastfeeding. Retrieved January 17, 2016.

g. La Leche League International. Available at: www .lalecheleague.org. Retrieved January 17, 2016.

h. United States Breastfeeding Committee. Available at: www.usbreastfeeding.org. Retrieved January 17, 2016.

References

1. American College of Obstetricians and Gynecologists. ACOG clinical review. Special report from ACOG: Breastfeeding: Maternal and infant aspects. *Obstet Gynecol.* 2007, **12**(suppl):1S–16S.

2. Centers for Disease Control and Prevention. *Strategies to Prevent Obesity and Other Chronic Diseases: The CDC Guide to Strategies to Support Breastfeeding Mothers and Babies.* Atlanta, GA: US Department of Health and Human Services, 2013.

3. American College of Obstetricians and Gynecologists. Breastfeeding: Maternal and infant aspects. ACOG Committee Opinion No. 361. *Obstet Gynecol.* 2007, **109** (2 pt 1):479–80.

4. Eidelman, A.I. and Schanler, R.J. Breastfeeding and the use of human milk. *Pediatrics.* 2012, **129** (3):827–41. Available at: http://pediatrics.aappublications.org/con tent/129/3/e827. Retrieved January 17, 2016.

5. Kramer, M.S. and Kakuma, R. Optimal duration of exclusive breastfeeding (review). *Cochrane Database Syst Rev.* 2012:1–131.

6. Renfrew, M.J., McCormick, F.M., Wade, A., Quinn, B., and Dowsell, T. Support for healthy breastfeeding mothers with healthy term babies. *Cochrane Database Syst Rev.* 2012:1–121.

7. Wambach, K. and Riordan, J. *Breastfeeding and Human Lactation*, 5th edition. Burlington, MA: Jones & Bartlett Learning, 2016.

8. U.S. Preventive Services Task Force. Primary care interventions to promote breastfeeding: US Preventive Services Task Force recommendation statement. *Ann Intern Med.* 2008, **149**:560–4.

9. Committee on Preventive Services for Women, editor. *Clinical Preventive Services for Women: Closing the Gaps.* Washington, DC: Institute of Medicine, 2011. Available at: http://www .nap.edu/download.php?record_id=13181. Retrieved February 21, 2016.

10. American Academy of Pediatrics. *Supporting Breastfeeding and Lactation: The Primary Care Pediatrician's Guide to Getting Paid.* Available at: http://www2.aap.org/breastfeeding/files/ pdf/coding.pdf. Retrieved January 17, 2016.

11. Dyson, L., McCormick, F., and Renfrew, M.J. Interventions for promoting the initiation of breastfeeding. *Cochrane Database Syst Rev.* 2005:1–40.

Neural Tube Defect Prevention

Jody Stonehocker

Why Prevent?

Neural tube defects (NTDs) are abnormalities in the formation of the fetal central nervous system, which result from failure of the neural tube to close properly during embryogenesis. They are the second most common congenital birth defect, following congenital heart disease, affecting approximately 4,000 pregnancies and 2,660 live births in the United States each year [1]. The two most common types of NTDs are anencephaly and spina bifida. Anencephaly (Figures 48.1 and 48.2) occurs when the top of the neural tube fails to close and the majority of the brain, skull, and scalp fail to form. Anencephaly is uniformly fatal. Live-born affected infants generally survive only hours. Spina bifida (Figure 48.3) occurs when the lower portion of the neural tube fails to close, causing a defect in the formation of the spinal cord and surrounding spine. Often a sac, or myelomeningocele, protrudes through the back and contains a portion of the spinal cord. The severity of disease depends on the level the spinal defect occurs, but often includes paralysis of the lower extremities, loss of bowel and bladder control, hydrocephalus, and learning disabilities. Most infants born with spina bifida survive. Folic acid supplementation has been shown to be an effective primary prevention for NTDs, reducing incidence by 30 percent and preventing 1,300 affected infants in the United States each year [2].

Rationale for Prevention

As an embryo develops, the neural plates, the precursor to the neural tube, appear in week 3 after conception. These develop into the neural folds that

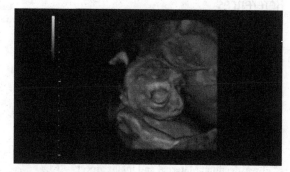

Figure 48.2 3D Image of Fetus Affected by Anencephaly. Courtesy of Rebecca Hall, University of New Mexico.

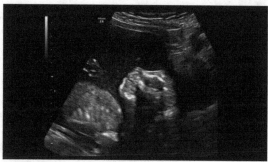

Figure 48.1 Fetus Affected by Anencephaly in Profile. Courtesy of Rebecca Hall, University of New Mexico.

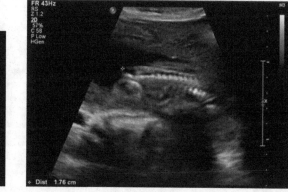

Figure 48.3 Spina Bifida Affecting the Lower Spine. Courtesy of Luis Izquierdo, University of New Mexico.

then fuse in the midline to form the completed neural tube. The entire process is complete by day 30 after conception. This means that most NTDs occur between 4 and 6 weeks after a woman's missed menses, before many women are even aware they are pregnant.

Researchers in the United Kingdom noted the association of NTDs and lower socioeconomic status and discovered women who had affected fetuses had lower plasma concentrations of folate. This finding, coupled with reports that aminopterin, a folic acid antagonist used for a short time to induce therapeutic abortion, resulted in anencephalic fetuses, spurred them to perform the first randomized controlled trial of folic acid supplementation for the prevention of recurrent NTDs. The trial enrolled only 111 women, but showed a reduction in disease [3]. In 1991, the Medical Research Council Vitamin Study Research Group confirmed the protective effect of folic acid supplementation to prevent recurrent NTDs. Their prospective, double-blinded study enrolled 1,817 women with a previously affected pregnancy from 33 centers in 7 countries. These women were then randomized to receive folic acid, other vitamins, both, or neither. Women assigned to take 4 mg of folic acid per day before pregnancy and through week 12 of gestation experienced a 72 percent reduction in their recurrence risk (odds ratio (OR) 0.28; 95 percent confidence intervals (CI) 0.15–0.53) [4]. In 1992, the role of folic acid for primary prevention of NTDs was confirmed with a double-blind, placebo-controlled, randomized trial [5]. That same year, the Centers for Disease Control and Prevention (CDC) made the first US recommendation that all women of reproductive potential (aged 15–44 years) should take 0.4 mg of folic acid daily. In 1996, the US Preventive Services Task Force (USPSTF) made their first recommendation that all women planning pregnancy take a daily multivitamin containing folic acid at a dose of 0.4–0.8 mg beginning at least 1 month before conception and continuing through the first trimester to reduce the risk of NTDs. In the United States, folic acid fortification of all grain products was introduced in 1996 and compliance was required by 1998 from all food manufacturers. The USPSTF recommendation was reconfirmed in 2009 [a] based on a growing body of confirmatory evidence, including population data showing a decline in NTDs after the implementation of nationwide grain fortification.

Examination of the National Health and Nutrition Examination Study (NHANES) data [6] shows a slight decrease in overall US population serum folate concentrations recently, likely related to the popularity of low-carbohydrate and gluten-free diets. The World Health Organization (WHO) has established recommended serum levels of folate for entire populations to guide public health interventions internationally [7]. When compared to the WHO serum folate guidelines, data from the 2007 to 2012 NHANES found that 22.8 percent of reproductive-aged women in the United States have folate concentrations considered deficient, putting them at risk for NTDs when they conceive.

The exact mechanism explaining how folic acid prevents NTDs is unknown. The most important metabolic reaction that requires folate is the conversion of homocysteine to methionine. Methionine is important because it provides the methyl group necessary for gene regulation and many metabolic reactions essential for tissue growth and development, especially in the rapidly developing early embryo. Interruption of this conversion pathway appears important in the genesis of NTDs. It is possible that folic acid supplementation helps to ensure adequate production of methionine from homocysteine.

Hypothesized harms of routine folic acid supplementation have included masking symptoms of vitamin B12 deficiency allowing neurologic complications to progress untreated, drug interactions, allergic reactions, carcinogenic effects, and effects on the rate of twinning. The current USPSTF review [a] found no evidence to support these concerns 10 years after recommending routine, daily supplementation and implementation of nationwide grain fortification.

Factors That Affect Prevention

Planned pregnancy: In the United States, half of all pregnancies are unplanned. NTDs occur early in gestation, prior to many women being aware they are pregnant. In each of the randomized controlled trials that established the efficacy of folic acid supplementation to prevent NTDs, supplements were given prior to conception and continued through the first trimester of pregnancy. Starting supplementation prior to conception ensures adequate serum folate levels at the time of neural tube formation. Unfortunately, this approach only reaches half of the at-risk population leading to recommendations for all women planning or capable of pregnancy (aged 15–44 years) to routinely take a daily folic acid supplement [a–g].

History of NTDs: While 95 percent of NTDs occur in couples with no personal or family history, a personal history of having an NTD, family history of affected children, and personal history of a previously affected pregnancy all increase the risk of recurrence. Recurrence risk for couples is 1 in 33 with 1 previously affected pregnancy, and 1 in 10 for couples with 2 previously affected pregnancies. Sisters of women with an affected child have a 1 in 100 risk and sisters of a man with an affected child have a 1 in 300 risk of having an affected child. Initial research on folic acid supplementation to prevent NTDs was conducted in these high-risk populations, used the increased dose of 4 mg daily, and showed significant reductions in disease. Although lower doses of folic acid supplementation may be efficacious in preventing disease in this population, the daily dose of 4 mg of folic acid per day is consistently recommended in this high-risk group [c–g].

Anticonvulsant medication: Congenital malformations in general are increased in infants exposed to anticonvulsant medications in utero, yet there is a specific, significant association between valproate and carbamazepine use and development of spina bifida. The prevalence of spina bifida with valproate exposure is approximately 1–2 percent and with carbamazepine 0.5 percent. There is insufficient data to support the benefit of increased folic acid supplementation to prevent NTDs in women taking anticonvulsant medications during pregnancy, but these studies are problematic with small sample sizes and recall bias from retrospective study design [8]. All invested expert bodies recommend using a daily increased dose of 4 mg of folic acid daily in this high-risk group [c–g].

Diabetes: Women with insulin-dependent diabetes have an increased risk of congenital malformations, which increases with worsening glycemic control (Hgb A1C) in the first trimester.

They have a 7.9-fold increased rate of NTDs in their offspring. A smaller increase has been noted in women with gestational diabetes requiring insulin in the third trimester, likely because of intermediate glucose abnormalities in the first trimester. No increased risk was seen for gestational diabetes not requiring insulin [9]. Despite the increased risk in diabetics, there are currently no special recommendations for increased folic acid supplementation in pregnancy.

Obesity: Obesity increases the risk for NTDs. In a review of a birth defect surveillance system, the women weighing 50–59 kg were considered to have baseline risk of NTDs. Women weighing 80–89 kg had an OR of 1.9 (95 percent CI 1.2–2.9) and women weighing 110 kg or more had an OR of 4.0 (95 percent CI 1.6–9.9). Intake of 0.4 mg of folic acid or more reduced risk of NTDs by 40 percent among women weighing less than 70 kg, but no risk reduction was observed among heavier women [10]. Despite the increased risk in this population, there are currently no special recommendations for increased folic acid supplementation.

Elevated maternal temperature: Maternal fever in the first trimester elevates NTD risk (OR 2.9; 95 percent CI 1.5–5.7). Women who took fever-reducing medications showed a lower risk (OR 2.4; 95 percent CI 1.0–5.6) than those who did not (OR 3.8; 95 percent CI 1.4–10.9). First-trimester maternal exposure to heat devices such as hot tubs, saunas, or electric blankets were associated with an OR of 3.6 (95 percent CI 1.1–15.9) [11].

Ethnicity: Hispanic women have a higher prevalence of NTDs than non-Hispanic white women, who have slightly higher prevalence than Black or Asian women in the United States. In the NHANES through 2010, Hispanic women reported lower folic acid intake and had serum folate levels lower than non-Hispanic white women. This trend was more significant in less acculturated Hispanic women [6]. Polymorphisms in the methylenetetrahydrofolate reductase (MTHFR) genes are also more common in the Hispanic population and are associated with reduced folate absorption. These mutations, coupled with lower overall folic acid intake, may explain the increased risk of NTDs in the US Hispanic population.

Folic acid source: While folate and folic acid are often used interchangeably to refer to the same B-vitamin, there are distinctions. Folate is found naturally in food sources – especially legumes, leafy green vegetables, citrus fruits, and liver. Folic acid is the synthetic form of folate and is found in supplements and used in grain fortification. It has a simpler structure and is better absorbed than natural folate.

Recommended Guidelines and How to Find Them

The USPSTF [a] and CDC [b] recommend that all women planning or capable of pregnancy take 0.4–0.8 mg of folic acid daily. Both guideline documents are publicly available at their respective websites. The American Academy of Pediatrics [c], American Academy of Family Physicians [d], American College of Obstetricians and Gynecologists [e], Healthy Mothers and Healthy Babies [f], and March of Dimes [g] have uniformly adopted this recommendation and also recommend increased folic acid (4 mg daily) in women who have previously delivered a baby with NTDs, have a personal or family history of NTDs, or are taking anticonvulsant medications. The Well-Woman Task Force (WWTF) adopted the USPSTF guidelines for low-risk women as well as the guidelines of the other organizations for high-risk women.

How to Prevent

All women planning or capable of pregnancy should be counseled to take a daily supplement containing 0.4–0.8 mg (400–800 µg) of folic acid. The recommended dose should be increased to 4 mg per day in those taking anticonvulsant medications or who have a personal or family history of NTDs or who have delivered a baby affected by NTDs in an earlier pregnancy. The increased dose should be started 1 month prior to attempting conception and continued until the end of the first trimester.

There are a number of potential sources for folic acid. The USPSTF and WWTF specifically recommend a daily supplement. This supplement can be folic acid alone, or as part of a multivitamin.

While the most recent USPSTF update [b] did not examine the evidence related to food fortification or dietary counseling, concerns exist regarding reliance on dietary folate intake for the prevention of NTDs. Appropriately counseled patients who refuse supplementation can be counseled about dietary alternatives. The CDC recommendations include the alternatives of daily consumption of a fortified breakfast cereal containing 100 percent of the recommended daily folic acid dose, or increased consumption of folate rich foods. Women in high-risk populations should be counseled to take daily folic acid supplementation, as diet alone may not be sufficient to meet their increased needs. These women typically take a prenatal vitamin with 1 mg of folic acid and three 1 mg folic acid supplements.

While not specifically in any guidelines, given the recognized association between first-trimester fever and NTD, it seems prudent to counsel women who are seeking pregnancy or who are pregnant to avoid heat producing sources and to manage any fever in the first trimester with fever-reducing medications.

New Developments Likely to Affect Future Guidelines

Questions remain about the best dose and route of folic acid supplementation. Doses ranging from 0.36 to 6 mg a day have proven effective in preventing both occurrence and recurrence of NTDs [12]. These studies have been performed worldwide. The large dose variation and response to supplementation may be influenced by the baseline blood folate concentrations in the different populations studied. High-risk populations other than patients with prior NTDs have not been studied to determine appropriate dosing. Some public health researchers have proposed weekly instead of daily supplementation. The use of 5-methyltetrahydrofolate (5-MTHF) has been proposed as an alternative to folic acid supplementation. Most dietary folate and folic acid are metabolized to 5-MTHF during their passage across the intestinal mucosa. The 5-MTHF may be a better supplement for those with the MTHFR gene mutation, less likely to mask symptoms of vitamin B12 deficiency, and interact less with antifolate medications (methotrexate, antimalarials, etc.). Preliminary studies suggest equal efficacy with folic acid in the prevention of NTDs. Further research to clarify optimal dosing and route of administration may lead to future refinements in the guidelines.

Billing

Counseling reproductive-aged women on the need to use supplemental folic acid for the prevention of NTD can be billed under the diagnosis of preconception counseling or preconception management, medication discussion. Both of these diagnoses are billed with the ICD-10 code Z31.69.

Illustrative Cases

A healthy 16-year-old presents for a well-adolescent visit. She has been sexually active since age 15. She is using oral contraceptive pills for the prevention of pregnancy.

Prevent now? The WWTF recommends counseling the patient to take a daily supplement of 0.4–0.8 mg of folic acid. She is not seeking pregnancy, but has the potential to become pregnant.

When to stop prevention? She should continue supplementation until no longer capable of pregnancy.

A healthy 25-year-old G1P0010 presents for a well-woman visit. Her previous pregnancy was complicated by anencephaly and ended in an 18-week intrauterine fetal demise. She would like to seek pregnancy once again, but is worried she will have the same outcome.

Prevent now? Her risk of recurrent NTD is increased (1:33) given the previous affected pregnancy. She should begin 4 mg of folic acid supplementation daily 1 month prior to conception and continue through the completion of the first trimester in pregnancy to decrease the risk of a recurrent NTD.

When to stop prevention? After the first trimester she should reduce supplementation to 0.4–0.8 mg, typically as a prenatal vitamin. She should continue supplementation until no longer capable of pregnancy.

A 35-year-old G2P2 with epilepsy well controlled on levetiracetam (Keppra) presents for a well-woman visit. Her previous pregnancies have been uncomplicated, but she was diagnosed with epilepsy after her last delivery. She has no history of NTDs personally, in her family, or in her offspring. She is considering another pregnancy.

Prevent now? Women taking anticonvulsants in pregnancy have an increased risk of congenital malformations, including NTDs. While valproate and carbamazepime are the anticonvulsants most associated with spina bifida, and levetiracetam has no known specific association, she will still have increased general risk. She should take 4 mg of folic acid daily starting 1 month prior to conception and continuing through the completion of the first trimester of pregnancy for prevention of NTDs.

When to stop prevention? After the first trimester she should reduce supplementation to 0.4–0.8 mg, typically as a prenatal vitamin. She should continue supplementation until no longer capable of pregnancy.

A 39-year-old Hispanic G4P4 presents for a well-woman visit. She has recently become involved with a new partner who has no children and they would like to conceive. Her past medical history is significant for insulin-dependent diabetes mellitus, with her most recent HbgA1c measuring 8.3. Her body mass index (BMI) is 40. She has stopped her contraceptive method.

Prevent now? This patient has multiple risk factors for the development of a NTD in the desired pregnancy. There is no recommendation for universal screening of Hispanic women for the MTHFR gene mutation. Weight loss and improved glycemic control prior to conception should be recommended to this patient and she should take 0.4–0.8 mg of folic acid daily.

When to stop prevention? She should continue folic acid supplementation until no longer capable of pregnancy.

Guidelines

a. U.S. Preventive Services Task Force. Folic acid for the prevention of neural tube defects: US Preventive Services Task Force recommendation statement. *Ann Intern Med.* 2009, **150**:626–31.

b. Centers for Disease Control and Prevention. *Preventing Neural Tube Birth Defects: A Prevention Model and Resource Guide.* Atlanta, GA: Centers for Disease Control and Prevention, 2009. Available at: www.cdc.gov.ncbdd/orders/pdfs/09_202063-a_nash_neural-tube-bd-guide-final508.pdf. Retrieved January 27, 2016.

c. Folic acid for the prevention of neural tube defects. American Academy of Pediatrics. Committee on Genetics. *Pediatrics.* 1999, **104**:325–7.

d. American Academy of Family Physicians. *Neural Tube Defects: Clinical Preventive Service Recommendation.* Leawood, KS: American

Academy of Family Physicians, 2015. Available at: www
.aafp.org/patient-care/clinical-recommendations/all/neu
ral-tube-defects.html. Retrieved January 27, 2016.

e. Cheschier, N.; ACOG Committee on Practice
Bulletins-Obstetrics. ACOG practice bulletin. Neural
tube defects. Number 44, July 2003 (Replaces Committee
Opinion Number 252, March 2001). *Int J Gynaecol
Obstet.* 2003, **83**(1):123–33.

f. National Healthy Mothers, Healthy Babies Coalition.
*National Healthy Mothers, Healthy Babies Mother's Day
Call to Action* [press release]. Alexandria, VA: National
Healthy Mothers, Healthy Babies Coalition, 2012.
Available at: www.hmhb.org/press_release/mothers-day
-call-to-action/. Retrieved January 27, 2016.

g. March of Dimes. *Birth Defects.* White Plains, NY: March
of Dimes, 2012. Available at: www.marchofdimes.org/b
aby/neural-tube-defects.aspx. Retrieved January 27,
2016.

References

1. Parker, S.E., Mai, C.T., Canfield, M.A. et al. Updated
national birth prevalence estimates for selected birth
defects in the United States, 2004–2006. *Birth Defects
Res A Clin Mol Teratol.* 2010, **88**(12):1008–16.

2. Williams, J., Mai, C.T., Mulinare, J. et al. Updated
estimates of neural tube defects prevented by mandatory
folic acid fortification – United States, 1995–2011.
MMWR Morb Mortal Wkly Rep. 2015, **64**(1):1–5.

3. Laurence, K.M., James, N., Miller, M.H., Tennant, G.B.,
and Campbell, H. Double-blind randomised controlled
trial of folate treatment before conception to prevent
recurrence of neural-tube defects. *Br Med J (Clin Res
Ed).* 1981, **282**(6275):1509–11.

4. Prevention of neural tube defects: Results of the
Medical Research Council Vitamin Study. MRC
Vitamin Study Research Group. *Lancet.* 1991, **338**
(8760):131–7.

5. Czeizel, A.E. and Dudás, I. Prevention of the first
occurrence of neural-tube defects by periconceptional
vitamin supplementation. *N Engl J Med.* 1992, **327**(26):
1832–5.

6. Marchetta, C.M. and Hamner, H.C. Blood folate
concentrations among women of childbearing age by
race/ethnicity and acculturation, NHANES 2001–2010.
Matern Child Nutr. 2014, June 17. DOI: 10.1111/
mcn.12134. [Epub ahead of print]

7. World Health Organization. *Guideline: Optimal Serum
and Red Blood Cell Folate Concentrations in Women of
Reproductive Age for Prevention of Neural Tube Defects.*
Geneva: World Health Organization, 2015. Available
at: http://apps.who.int/iris/bitstream/10665/161988/1/
9789241549042_eng.pdf.

8. American Academy of Neurology. Practice parameter:
Management issues for women with epilepsy
(summary statement). Report of the quality standards
subcommittee of the American Academy of
Neurology. *Epilepsia.* 1998, **39**:1226–31.

9. Becerra, J.E., Khoury, M.J., Cordero, J.F., and
Erickson, J.D. Diabetes mellitus during pregnancy and
the risks for specific birth defects: A population-based
case–control study. *Pediatrics.* 1990, **85**(1):1–9.

10. Werler, M.M., Louik, C., Shapiro, S., and
Mitchell, A.A. Prepregnant weight in relation to
risk of neural tube defects. *JAMA.* 1996,
275(14):1089–92.

11. Suarez, L., Felkner, M., and Hendricks, K. The effect of
fever, febrile illnesses, and heat exposures on the risk of
neural tube defects in a Texas-Mexico border
population. *Birth Defects Res A Clin Mol Teratol.* 2004,
70(10):815–9.

12. De-Regil, L.M., Peña-Rosas, J.P., Fernández-Gaxiola,
A.C., and Rayco-Solon, P. Effects and safety of
periconceptional oral folate supplementation for
preventing birth defects. *Cochrane Database Syst Rev.*
2015, (**12**):CD007950.

Diabetes Postpartum

Shari M. Lawson

Why Screen?

Gestational diabetes mellitus (GDM) is one of the most common medical complications of pregnancy. In the United States, the prevalence ranges from 2.5 percent in non-Hispanic whites to over 10 percent in African Americans and Asians. The prevalence of GDM in the United States has been increasing due to increased rates of obesity and sedentary lifestyle, as well as population growth of ethnic groups disproportionately affected by diabetes, which include Hispanic, African American, Asian, Native American, and Pacific Islander women [1]. Women with GDM are at increased risk of adverse perinatal outcomes including developing hypertensive disorders of pregnancy or requiring cesarean delivery. These women are at risk of having impaired fasting glucose, impaired glucose tolerance, or undiagnosed type 2 diabetes. Up to 50 percent of women with GDM will develop DM in the future, so the postpartum and well-woman visits present important opportunities to screen, intervene, and appropriately refer these at-risk women.

Rationale for Screening

The rationale for the early diagnosis and treatment of diabetes in general is discussed in detail in the chapter on Diabetes. Postpartum screening of women with GDM presents a unique opportunity to identify women with preexisting diabetes. Up to 3 percent of women diagnosed with GDM may have overt diabetes. In a population-based study of women with GDM, 3.7 percent were diagnosed with diabetes by 9 months postdelivery [2]. After 9 years, 18.9 percent of women with GDM developed diabetes compared to 1.95 percent among women with no previous diagnosis of GDM. Once a patient with DM has been identified, her glucose can be controlled prior to a subsequent pregnancy to reduce the risk of spontaneous abortion and the development of hyperglycemia-related fetal

anomalies such as cardiovascular, neurologic, and musculoskeletal defects. Identification and management of preexisting diabetes also allows initiation of treatment to improve long-term outcomes as noted in the chapter on Diabetes. Screening in the postpartum period also provides an opportunity to intervene with lifestyle modification or medical therapy to delay or prevent onset of diabetes in women diagnosed with prediabetes.

Factors That Affect Screening

Physiologic changes related to pregnancy and delivery: Glycosylated hemoglobin levels may be lower during pregnancy and during the 12 weeks postpartum due to increased red blood cell turnover related to different types of anemia, which may affect optimal timing of performing screening with Hgb A1C testing.

Glycemic control in the third trimester: Hgb A1C levels during the 6–12 weeks postpartum may also be artificially low due to tight glycemic control achieved through diet or medication use in the third trimester, which may affect optimal timing of performing screening with Hgb A1C testing.

Compliance: There are a number of potential screening methods for diabetes, some of which require fasting, multiple blood draws, or a glucose load. While more complex tests may increase diagnostic accuracy, testing may need to be individualized. Patients who are unlikely to return fasting or comply with a glucose load test may benefit from a test like Hgb A1c performed after 12 weeks postpartum, which can be done with a single blood draw.

Recommended Guidelines and How to Find Them

Guidelines for diabetes screening after a diagnosis of GDM have been established by the American

College of Obstetricians and Gynecologists (ACOG) [a] and the American Diabetes Association (ADA) [b]. Each organization endorses screening at 6–12 weeks postpartum. The ADA recommends that women with GDM undergo the 75 g 2-hour oral glucose tolerance test (OGTT) at 6–12 weeks postpartum using nonpregnant criteria for diagnosis. ACOG recommends that women be screened at 6–12 weeks postpartum with either the 75 g OGTT or fasting plasma glucose (FPG). The Well-Woman Task Force recommends laboratory screening 6–12 weeks postpartum with follow-up screening at least every 3 years in women who screen negative for DM.

How to Screen

Women diagnosed with GDM should be screened 6–12 weeks postpartum with either the 75 g OGTT or FPG. While more inconvenient, the 75 g OGTT has the additional advantage over FPG of detecting impaired glucose tolerance, one type of prediabetes. Both OGTT and FPG can diagnose overt diabetes and impaired fasting glucose, the second type of prediabetes.

In preparation for the 75 g OGTT, the patient should fast for 8 hours. After the first blood draw, she should drink the glucose solution and have the second sample drawn 2 hours later.

If the patient misses the postpartum visit, she should be screened for diabetes at the next encounter. If the screening takes place after the 6–12-week postpartum period, screening can be conducted with FPG, 2-hour OGTT, or Hgb A1C. The FPG levels <100 mg/dL are normal, 100–125 mg/dL indicate impaired fasting glucose, and ≥126 mg/dL indicate diabetes. With the 2-hour OGTT, <140 mg/dL is normal, 140–199 mg/dL indicates impaired glucose tolerance, and ≥200 mg/dL indicates diabetes. Hgb A1C <5.7 percent is normal, 5.7–6.4 percent indicates impaired glucose tolerance, and ≥6.5 percent indicates diabetes [3].

Women diagnosed with prediabetes should be referred for counseling and possible medical therapy and retested every 1–2 years. Women who test negatively should be rescreened every 1–3 years based on risk factors. All women with a previous history of GDM should also be screened for diabetes preconception and at initiation of prenatal care with subsequent pregnancies.

New Developments Likely to Affect Future Guidelines

Currently, there is a lack of consensus on the ideal screening test for diabetes 6–12 weeks postpartum in women who had GDM. The ADA has identified the OGTT as its preferred screening modality, while ACOG recognizes screening with either the FPG or 2-hour OGTT. Requiring the patient to fast or make a 2-hour commitment for the testing are significant barriers to screening for new mothers. An ideal test would be a single draw blood test like Hgb A1C that does not require fasting. New research is focusing on identifying parameters for using Hgb A1C during pregnancy and in the first 12 weeks postpartum as a screening tool for overt diabetes.

Intensive lifestyle modification (7 percent weight loss with 150 minutes moderate exercise per week) and metformin use twice daily have both been found to be superior to placebo in reducing the incidence of diabetes among those at highest risk for developing diabetes [4]. Identification of effective strategies for preventing or delaying diabetes may lead to a greater push for unifying recommendations for screening for prediabetes and overt diabetes.

Billing

Screening for DM is typically covered under the ICD-10 code Z13.1, encounter for screening for diabetes mellitus. Medicare will cover one screening per year for those never tested for diabetes or those previously tested but not diagnosed with prediabetes. It will cover two screening tests per year if an individual has been diagnosed with prediabetes.

Illustrative Cases

A 33-year-old presents for her well-woman exam 10 months after a vaginal delivery. She was diagnosed with GDM in her pregnancy. She was not able to attend her postpartum visit because she had already returned to work.

Recommendations are for screening at 6–12 weeks postpartum with the 2-hour 75 g OGTT or FPG. Although the patient has missed this window, she is still at risk for having DM and should be screened at the earliest opportunity.

Screen now? Yes. Patient may be screened with OGTT, FPG, or Hgb A1C.

Next screening: If negative, repeat in 3 years. If prediabetes (impaired FPG, impaired glucose tolerance, or both), repeat in 1–2 years.

A 31-year-old G1P1 presents for her 6-week postpartum visit. She was diagnosed with GDM during her pregnancy and successfully managed with glyburide. She had an uncomplicated vaginal delivery.

Due to this patient's history of GDM, she should be screened for diabetes with a 75 g OGTT or FPG between 6 and 12 weeks postpartum.

Screen now? Yes. She should be screened within the next 6 weeks.

Next screening: If negative, repeat in 3 years. If prediabetes (impaired FPG, impaired glucose tolerance, or both), repeat in 1–2 years. The patient should also be screened preconception.

A 25-year-old presents for an initial prenatal visit. She had gestational diabetes in her last pregnancy and a negative screen for diabetes at her postpartum visit 18 months ago. She is 7 weeks pregnant.

Euglycemia is important during organogenesis to reduce the risk of fetal anomalies or spontaneous abortion. Early pregnancy is an opportune time to intervene with lifestyle modification or medication if DM is diagnosed.

Screen now? Yes

Next screening: 24–28 weeks gestation, if this screen negative

A 37-year-old presents for problem visit for vaginal discharge. She is concerned that she may have another yeast infection. Her last pregnancy (6 months ago) was complicated by GDM, and at her 8-week postpartum visit, she was scheduled for a 2-hour OGTT. She did not complete the test because she does not like the taste of the glucose solution.

Although she is outside the window for postpartum screening, she still should be screened for diabetes given her history of GDM. The patient could also be counseled that frequent yeast infections may be a sign of hyperglycemia.

Screen now? Yes. Patient may be screened with OGTT, FPG, or Hgb A1C.

Next screening: If negative, repeat in 3 years. If prediabetes (impaired FPG, impaired glucose tolerance, or both), repeat in 1–2 years.

Guidelines

a. American College of Obstetricians and Gynecologists. Gestational diabetes mellitus. Practice Bulletin No. 137. *Obstet Gynecol.* 2013, **122**(2 pt 1):406–16. Available at: www.acog.org/Resources-And-Publications/Practice-Bulletins-List. Retrieved March 1, 2016.

b. American Diabetes Association. Management of diabetes in pregnancy. *Diabetes Care.* 2016, **39**(Suppl 1):S94–8. Available at: http://care.diabetesjournals.org/site/misc/2016-Standards-of-Care.pdf. Retrieved March 2, 2016.

References

1. Hunt, K.J. and Schuller, K.L. The increasing prevalence of diabetes in pregnancy. *Obstet Gynecol Clin North Am.* 2007, **34**(2):173–vii.

2. Feig, D.S., Zinman, B., Wang, X., and Hux, J.E. Risk of development of diabetes mellitus after diagnosis of gestational diabetes. *CMAJ: Can Med Assoc J.* 2008, **179**(3):229–34.

3. American Diabetes Association. Classification and diagnosis of diabetes. *Diabetes Care.* 2016, **39**(Suppl 1): S13–22. Available at: http://care.diabetesjournals.org/site/misc/2016-Standards-of-Care.pdf. Retrieved April 9, 2016.

4. Diabetes Prevention Program Research Group. Reduction in the incidence of type 2 diabetes with lifestyle intervention or metformin. *N Engl J Med.* 2002, **346**:393–403.

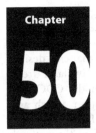
Preconception/Interconception Care

Dean V. Coonrod

Why Counsel?

Pregnancy complications are common, costly, and burdensome to women, families, and society. Gestational diabetes (2–5 percent of pregnancies), preterm birth (7–10 percent), and preeclampsia (5–7 percent) produce substantial morbidity and can recur in subsequent pregnancies [1]. Obesity, diabetes mellitus, and hypertensive disorders are now more common among nonpregnant women than in past decades. These conditions produce lifelong consequences for women's health as well as adverse perinatal outcomes. Approximately half of all pregnancies are unintended meaning that many women enter pregnancy without advanced planning [2]. Contraceptive failure explains 40 percent of unintended pregnancies [3].

Rationale for Counseling

The Institute of Medicine (IOM), in their review of women's services, included preconception care as an essential element [a]. Preconception care and interconception care, health care prior to or between pregnancies, improves pregnancy outcomes for mothers and infants, and is a critical aspect of health care for all women of reproductive capacity. In 2006, a Select Panel of the Centers for Disease Control and Prevention (CDC) published a report focusing national attention on the untapped potential of women's health care before and between pregnancies [4]. The Panel defined preconception care as, "interventions that aim to identify and modify biomedical, behavioral, and social risks to a woman's health or pregnancy outcome through prevention and management by emphasizing those factors that must be acted on before conception or early in pregnancy to have maximal impact. It includes care before a first pregnancy or between pregnancies (commonly known as 'interconception care')" [4]. At least 63 million reproductive-aged women in the United States may be impacted [5].

Unprecedented access to prenatal care in the 1990s did not improve pregnancy outcomes, leading some to conclude that prenatal care occurs too late to implement effective prevention [4]. Data supporting that prenatal care is too late comes from randomized trial data of interventions specifically done in the preconception period which have demonstrated benefit such as folic acid [b]. Teratogen exposure may occur before a woman learns she is pregnant and establishes prenatal care [4]. Improving disease status in women with obesity, diabetes, hypertension, and other chronic conditions may decrease the risk of associated pregnancy complications while improving women's health. Preventive care normally thought of as prenatal, such as updating Rubella immunity, is more appropriate to address prior to pregnancy. Interconception care provides lead time to plan interventions early in pregnancy such as progesterone to reduce recurrence of preterm birth, aspirin to reduce recurrence of severe, early-onset preeclampsia, and optimal glycemic control to reduce consequences of gestational diabetes [1]. Interconception care also facilitates counseling and prevention of chronic diseases associated with gestational diabetes, preeclampsia, tobacco use, as well as other diseases and health habits identified in pregnancy. A final compelling rationale for preconception care is that it represents good women's health care, making it an end in itself. When considering the rate of unintended pregnancy, each well-woman visit provides a critically important opportunity to make an important impact on preconception health.

Factors That Affect Counseling

Intent for future pregnancy: The most crucial aspect to preconception care is to know a women's intent for future pregnancy in the short and long term. Studies have shown women to be segmented into those who actively plan on becoming or not becoming pregnant (planners) and those who do not (nonplanners) [6]. Thus, a provider must ascertain a woman's intent or reproductive life plan, which sets the stage for preconception care (see "How to counsel"). Past, current, and intended use of contraception is important to address in planners as well as nonplanners.

Prior pregnancy complications: Understanding prior pregnancy complications and outcomes may alter the approach to preconception care and spur further evaluation prior to another pregnancy. Counseling regarding interpregnancy interval (birth-to-conception) is of importance, as intervals less than 18–24 months are associated with increased risk of infant mortality and other adverse outcomes [7,8].

Lifestyle behaviors and mental health issues identified in prior pregnancy: Medical, behavioral, and substance use issues, their detection and screening are other important factors to consider. As one example, screening and intervening for binge drinking has been shown in randomized trials to improvements by decreasing the incidence of fetal alcohol syndrome disorder [b].

Recommended Guidelines and How to Find Them

The Well-Woman Task Force includes general recommendations for preconception care; however, given that much of preconception care is synonymous with well-woman care, following the recommendations in other sections of this book is good preconception care. In developing its recommendations, the Task Force relied on evidence-based guidelines from the IOM and CDC [a, c]. An evidence-based approach of various interventions was published in a supplement to the *American Journal of Obstetrics and Gynecology* in 2008 [b]. All articles from this supplement are currently available at beforeandbeyond.org in the key articles section/supplements [9]. The recommendations have been updated on the CDC's website [c]. A more global perspective is provided by the World Health Organization [d].

How to Counsel

The most important element of preconception counseling is to know a woman's plans for childbearing. Tools for identifying a reproductive life plan group women into those desiring pregnancy, not wanting pregnancy, and uncertain. Others ask for the number of pregnancies desired and when. Examples of these are available freely online. One such example is from the CDC [10], and another is the One Key Question* which asks pregnancy intent in the next year [11].

The discussion is then tailored to the patient's plans with nuances in emphasis. For those not wanting pregnancy, the focus might be primarily on family planning and birth control methods and secondarily on health issues that may impact a pregnancy, with additional emphasis on health issues that affect the woman's health. Women desiring pregnancy would receive counseling focused on the timing of conception and the presence of any health issues that would increase maternal–fetal risk during pregnancy, as well as the woman's overall health. Postponing pregnancy may be a better course of action as in the case of transitioning to alternative hypertensive agents, optimizing glycemic control in diabetes, or achieving smoking cessation prior to conception. For those unsure of their desires for pregnancy, clarifying why a patient may be unsure, informing the patient of the risk associated with unintended pregnancy, and optimizing health prior to a pregnancy all deserve emphasis.

An itemization of potential actions based on a woman's reproductive life plan is available online at BeforeandBeyond.org in the toolkit [12]. It breaks down conditions including family planning, contraception, nutrition, infectious disease, immunizations, chronic disease, medication use, substance abuse, previous pregnancy outcomes, genetic history, mental health history, and intimate partner violence, with recommendations including information on the scope of the problem, preconception significance, risk identification and reduction strategies, and important talking points. As one example, for thyroid disorders it would recommend avoiding pregnancy within the 6 months after radioactive iodine treatment and assessing thyroid status prior to conception. For those not desiring pregnancy, emphasizing that there are no specific considerations of the type of contraceptive methods to use to avoid pregnancy and to be cautious of the increased fertility that may occur on initiating treatment for hypothyroidism due to ovulation.

The postpartum visit provides important opportunities to develop an interconception care plan. Women recently postpartum or in the interconception period should have their pregnancy reviewed for possible recurrence risks and development of a strategy for recurrence prevention. In addition, attention to conditions that are risk factors for later-onset chronic disease, such as gestational diabetes and preeclampsia, should be provided through periodic screening and preventive strategies. Similarly, continuity of care for lifestyle behaviors or mental health issues identified in pregnancy or postpartum should be assured.

Some patients with more complex medical issues may benefit from referral to maternal–fetal medicine or other specialists for more specific preconception or interconception care. In addition, anticipating future pregnancy may make for a more smooth transition to early prenatal care that is so often important for those with medical and behavioral health issues entering pregnancy.

New Developments Likely to Affect Future Guidelines

There are few high-quality studies demonstrating a specific benefit to preconception care [b]. It is possible that future randomized trials will provide evidence on the effectiveness of preconception care programs or specific components of care. A recent publication of the Clinical Workgroup of the National Preconception Health and Health Care Initiative proposes nine preconception wellness measures to assess the health care system's performance in this domain [13]. Campaigns to increase access to preconception and well-woman care in the United States may spur interest by some organizations to develop their own guidelines or endorse existing ones. Similar efforts in other countries may produce new and different guidance for preconception and interconception care.

Billing

It is regrettably uncommon to have a specific visit focused on preconception care and counseling. If this were the case, the specific ICD-10 code is Z31.69, with a short title of Encounter for Other General Counseling and Advice, Non Procreation. Some of the synonyms for this are preconception counseling, preconception management, and

medication counseling. Preconception and interconception care occurs most often during visits scheduled and billed for other primary purposes, including well-woman care, family planning counseling, or problem-oriented care for a chronic disease, health behavior, or mental health problem.

Illustrative Cases

A 16-year-old G0 is seen for an annual visit. She was treated recently for chlamydial infection following unprotected vaginal intercourse with her male partner. She became sexually active 3 months ago and uses no method of contraception.

In addition to the routine annual screening and counseling for a 16-year-old, additional counseling about prevention of sexually transmitted infection (STI) is also warranted, as well as screening for high-risk health behaviors. Barrier contraception would have preconception care benefit of avoiding repeat infection that could lead to tubal damage, risks in subsequent pregnancies of tubal pregnancy, and/or tubal infertility. Eliciting the patient's reproductive life plan could reveal that she is planning a pregnancy or could lead to a discussion about optimal contraception to allow for achievement of other goals, such as completion of school. Even if the patient plans to postpone pregnancy, it would be appropriate to offer folic acid supplementation in a multivitamin since she would remain at risk for pregnancy.

Counsel now? Yes

Next counseling: Next visit

A 24-year-old G2P0101 presents for a postpartum visit. This patient delivered at 28 weeks by a cesarean delivery following spontaneous preterm labor with a breech presentation. She seeks your advice on the timing of future pregnancies.

The postpartum visit presents an excellent time to review the patient's prior obstetric history and recent delivery. This visit may be considered the beginning of interconception care for a following pregnancy. In this case being a malpresentation, she may be at higher risk of a classical uterine scar. This could be reviewed in the operative note, and the patient counseled about the potential for vaginal birth after cesarean (VBAC). Counseling would include the use of contraception to achieve an interpregnancy interval of 18–24 months to reduce the risk of adverse pregnancy outcomes including uterine rupture. Other counseling points include the importance of early prenatal care in order to obtain accurate dating, the benefits of progesterone treatment in subsequent pregnancies, transvaginal cervical length surveillance, the value of a daily multivitamin including folic acid, and any other pregnancy complications, health habits, or chronic conditions that may put a future pregnancy at risk.

Counsel now? Yes

Next counseling: Next visit

A 42-year-old G6P4024 is seen for a well-woman visit. Her youngest child is 10 years old and her reproductive life plan is to have no more children. She does not believe she is at risk for pregnancy. She has not had a pregnancy for 5 years despite using no birth control and having regular vaginal intercourse with a monogamous partner. The patient is obese, reports irregular periods, and was diagnosed with diabetes 3 years ago. After being uninsured for several years, she now plans to get her diabetes and weight "under control."

It is possible that the patient, with improved control of her diabetes and weight loss, may have more regular ovulation, which may increase her risk of pregnancy. Risks of obesity and diabetes mellitus should be discussed with respect to her long-term health and to a future pregnancy should it occur, along with her age-related risk. Appropriate contraception would be recommended to help the patient achieve her life plan of no further pregnancy, and follow-up care for her chronic diseases would be arranged.

Counsel now? Yes

Next counseling: Next visit

A 27-year-old G0 presents for her annual exam. She indicates she is using no contraception at this time. She is monogamous with a same-sex partner, and at this time the couple is not planning on having children.

At this visit, it would be appropriate to acknowledge the couple's reproductive plan and invite a future preconception care visit if those plans change.

Counsel now? Yes

Next counseling: Next annual visit

A 32-year-old G3P1011 presents for a well-woman visit. Her blood pressure is 152/93. She is overweight and her prior pregnancy was complicated by gestational diabetes and preeclampsia at term. She notes that her blood pressure was treated with intravenous medication and her doctors and nurses were somewhat concerned about her liver. The patient had very limited care and did not attend her postpartum visit

6 months ago. She reports that today's office blood pressure reading is similar to blood pressures she has checked at her grocery store. She is considering another pregnancy.

In addition to routine screening and counseling, follow-up should be arranged to optimize the patient's blood pressure with medications compatible with pregnancy and to screen for adult-onset diabetes. Medical records from her last pregnancy should be requested to determine whether she a candidate for aspirin to prevent sequelae of preeclampsia in the subsequent pregnancy. The patient should be counseled to optimize her weight prior to pregnancy and to continue taking a folate-containing vitamin daily. A contraceptive method should be offered to help the patient postpone pregnancy while optimizing her health. The patient would be counseled that patients with pregnancy-related complications such as gestational diabetes and preeclampsia are at risk of developing chronic hypertension and diabetes later in life, and should be regularly screened.

Counsel now? Yes

Next counseling: Next visit

Guidelines

a. Institute of Medicine. Clinical Preventive Services for Women, 2011:1–4 Available at: www.nationalacademies.org/hmd/~/media/Files/Report%20Files/2011/Clinical-Preventive-Services-for-Women-Closing-the-Gaps/preventiveservicesforwomenreport brief_updated2.pdf. Retrieved January 9, 2017.

b. Jack, B.W., Atrash, H., Coonrod, D.V. et al. The clinical content of preconception care: An overview and preparation of this supplement. *Am J Obstet Gynecol.* 2008, 199.

c. Centers for Disease Control and Prevention. Preconception Health and Health Care: Content of Care for Women. 2016. Available at: www.cdc.gov/preconception/careforwomen/index.html. Retrieved January 9, 2017.

d. World Health Organisation. *Meeting to Develop a Global Consensus on Preconceptionternal and Childhood Mortality and Morbidity: World Health Organization Headquarters.* Geneva: World Health Organization, February 6–7, 2012.

References

1. Moore, L.E. Recurrent risk of adverse pregnancy outcomes. *Obstet Gynecol Clin North Am.* 2008, 35:459–71.

2. Finer, L.B. and Zolna, M.R. Unintended pregnancy in the United States: Incidence and disparities, 2006. *Contraception.* 2011, **84**:478–85.

3. Mosher, W.D., Jones, J., and Abma, J.C. Intended and unintended births in the United States: 1982–2010. *Natl Health Stat Rep.* 2012:1–28.

4. Atrash, H., Jack, B.W., Johnson, K. et al. Where is the "W"oman in MCH? *Am J Obstet Gynecol.* 2008, **199**:259–65.

5. Martin, J.A., Hamilton, B.E., Osterman, M.J., Curtin, S.C., and Matthews, T.J. Births: Final data for 2013. *Natl Vital Stat Rep.* 2015, **64**:1–65.

6. Squiers, L., Mitchell, E.W., Levis, D.M. et al. Consumers' perceptions of preconception health. *Am J Health Promot.* 2015, **27**:S10–9.

7. Bigelow, C.A. and Bryant, A.S. Short interpregnancy intervals: An evidence-based guide for clinicians. *Obstet Gynecol Surv.* 2015, **70**:458–64.

8. Hussaini, K.S., Ritenour, D., and Coonrod, D. V. Interpregnancy intervals and the risk for infant mortality: A case–control study of Arizona infants 2003–2007. *Matern Child Health J.* 2013, **17**:646–53.

9. The National Preconception Health and Health Care Initiative (PCHHC). The National Preconception Curriculum and Resources for Clinicians: Key Articles. Before, Between and Beyond Pregnancy, 2016. Available at: http://beforeandbeyond.org/key-articles/. Retrieved January 9, 2017.

10. Centers for Disease Control and Prevention. Preconception Health and Health Care: Reproductive Life Plan Tool for Health Professionals, 2016. Available at: www.cdc.gov/preconception/rlptool.html. Retrieved January 9, 2017.

11. One Key Question®. Would You Like to Become Pregnant in the Next Year? 2016. Available at: www.onekeyquestion.org/. Retrieved January 9, 2017.

12. Before, Between and Beyond Pregnancy. The National Preconception Curriculum and Resources for Clinicians: Tool Kit, 2016. Available at: http://beforeandbeyond.org/toolkit/.

13. Frayne, D.J., Verbiest, S., Chelmow, D., Clarke, H., Dunlop, A., Hosmer, J., Menard, M.K., Moos, M.K., Ramos, D., Stuebe, A., and Zephyrin, L. Health care system measures to advance preconception wellness: Consensus recommendations of the Clinical Workgroup of the National Preconception Health and Health Care Initiative. *Obstet Gynecol.* May 2016, **127**(5): 863–72. doi: 10.1097/AOG.0000000000001379.

Index

preventive health screenings for, 77
reproductive health care for, 76–8
resources for, 81
securing housing to improve health, 78
statistics regarding, 75
HPV. *See* Human papillomavirus (HPV)
HRSA. *See* Health Resources and Services Administration (HRSA)
Human immunodeficiency virus (HIV) screening. *See* HIV screening
Human papillomavirus (HPV). *See also* Cervical cancer screening
immunization for, 99, 100, 102
oral cavity examination, effect on, 110–11, 112
Hyperglycemia measurement in metabolic syndrome screening, 152
Hyperlipidemia, effect on kidney disease screening, 172
Hypertension screening, 132–5
for homeless women, 77
kidney disease screening, effect of hypertension on, 171
lifestyle modification and behavioral change, 48
metabolic syndrome screening and, 152
Hypothyroidism screening, 167–70
Hysterectomy
abdominal examinations, effect on, 122
cervical cancer screening, effect on, 209
pelvic examinations, effect on, 122

IDSA. *See* Infectious Diseases Society of America (IDSA)
Immunization, 99–103
for homeless women, 77
for LGBT persons, 66
Immunization Action Coalition, 100
Implementation of preventive care, practical considerations, 52
Incarcerated women
contraception for, 79
as disadvantaged, 78
Estelle v. Gamble (1976), 78
lack of standards regarding health care, 78
as medically underserved populations, 78–80
mental health of, 79
pregnancy and, 80
resources for, 81
sexually transmitted infection (STI) screening for, 79, 200
"sick call" basis of health care, 78–9

statistics regarding, 78
Incontinence screening, 177–80
Indian Health Service (IHS), 85
Individually purchased insurance, 84
Infectious diseases
adolescents (13–18 years), 95
Hepatitis screening (*See* Hepatitis screening)
HIV screening (*See* HIV screening)
mature women (46–64 years), 96
reproductive-aged women (19–45 years), 96
sexually transmitted infection (STI) screening (*See* Sexually transmitted infection (STI) screening)
women older than 64 years, 97
Infectious Diseases Society of America (IDSA)
on bacteriuria screening, 174–5, 176
on cervical cancer screening, 213
Inflammatory bowel disease, effect on colorectal cancer screening, 216
Injury prevention counseling, 115–17
Institute of Medicine (IOM)
"Closing the Gaps" recommendations, 86–8
on diet and nutrition screening and counseling, 137–8, 139, 140
on domestic and intimate partner violence screening, 247–8
on DSD, 68
guidelines, sources of, 5, 8, 32, 36
on patient-centered care, 42–3
on preconception/interconception counseling, 289, 290, 292
on preventive well woman care, 7
on transgendered individuals, 68
on women's preventive health care, 86–8
Women's Preventive Services section, 5
Insurance coverage
under Affordable Care Act, 58–9
commercial insurance, 84
evaluation and management (E/M) services, 59
individually purchased insurance, 84
LGBT persons and, 65
Medicaid (*See* Medicaid)
Medicare (*See* Medicare)
under Medicare, 59
practical considerations, 58–9
uninsured persons, 85
Integrated behavior model, 42
Interconception counseling, 289–92
tobacco use screening, effect on, 255
Internal Revenue Code, 89
International Agency for Research on Cancer, 205

International Diabetes Foundation (IDF), 150–1
Intimate partner violence screening, 247–9
for homeless women, 77
Task Force on, 8–9
Intrapartum care, breastfeeding counseling, 276
Intrauterine devices (IUDs)
Food and Drug Administration and, 181–2
homeless women and, 77
payment for well-women visits and, 90–1
IPV screening. *See* Domestic and intimate partner violence screening
Iron deficiency anemia screening, 155–6
IUDs. *See* Intrauterine devices (IUDs)

JNC 8. *See* Eighth Joint National Committee on Prevention, Detection, Evaluation and Treatment of High Blood Pressure (JNC 8)
JNC 7. *See* Seventh Joint National Committee on Prevention, Detection, Evaluation and Treatment of High Blood Pressure (JNC 7)
Joint Commission (JCAHO)
on breastfeeding counseling, 274
on DSD, 68
on transgendered individuals, 68

Kaiser Family Foundation, 83–4, 92
Keloid scarring, effect on piercing and tattooing counseling, 119
Kidney disease screening, 171–3

LactMed, 275
La Leche League, 276, 279
LARCs. *See* Long Acting Reversible Contraceptives (LARCs)
LGBT persons
adolescents and youth, 66
adults, 66
cancer risk in, 67
cisgender defined, 64
denial of health care services, 65
domestic and intimate partner violence screening for, 248, 249
DSD (*See* Disorders of sex development (DSD))
family planning for, 66–7
gender expression defined, 64
gender identity defined, 64
gender nonconforming defined, 64
historical background of medical treatment, 64–5

Printed in the United States
by Baker & Taylor Publisher Services